Ask for the accompanying software at
the circulation desk in this Library

DATE DUE

Mechanical
SHOULDER
Disorders

Perspectives in Functional Anatomy

Mechanical SHOULDER Disorders

Perspectives in Functional Anatomy

James A. Porterfield, PT, MA, ATC

Owner
Rehabilitation and Health Center, Inc.
Akron, Ohio

CEO
Venture Practice Services, Ltd.
Akron, Ohio

Carl DeRosa, PT, PhD

Professor and Chairman
Physical Therapy Program
Northern Arizona University
Flagstaff, Arizona

Co-founder and Owner
DeRosa Physical Therapy at Summit Center
Flagstaff, Arizona

Illustrator: Tina C. Cauller
Plano, Texas

SAUNDERS

An Imprint of Elsevier

SAUNDERS
An Imprint of Elsevier

11830 Westline Industrial Drive
St. Louis, Missouri 63146

Notice

Rehabilitation is an ever-changing field. Standard safety precautions must be followed, but as new research and clinical experience broaden our knowledge, changes in treatment and drug therapy may become necessary or appropriate. Readers are advised to check the most current product information provided by the manufacturer of each drug to be administered to verify the recommended dose, the method and duration of administration, and contraindications. It is the responsibility of the licensed prescriber, relying on experience and knowledge of the patient, to determine dosages and the best treatment for each individual patient. Neither the publisher nor the author assumes any liability for any injury and/or damage to persons or property arising from this publication.

International Standard Book Number 0-7216-9272-9

Acquisitions Editor: Marion Waldman
Developmental Editor: Sue Bredensteiner
Publishing Services Manager: John Rogers
Project Manager: Mary Turner
Design Manager: Bill Drone
Multimedia Manager: Bruce Robison
Cover Illustration: Hans Neuhart

Printed in the United States of America

Last digit is the print number: 9   8   7   6   5   4   3   2   1

PREFACE

Mechanical Shoulder Disorders: Perspectives in Functional Anatomy is the result of collaboration by two colleagues and friends whose professional passion has long been the study of clinical anatomy and exercise science. As in our previous *Perspectives in Functional Anatomy* texts, *Mechanical Low Back Pain* and *Mechanical Neck Pain*, the intent of this new multimedia package is to weave these two sciences into a clinically applicable model for the evaluation and treatment of the painful disorders of the shoulder. We also emphasize training considerations that will enhance performance for all aspects of living.

The DVD module that accompanies this textbook contains 2 hours of narrated cadaver dissection, which emphasizes the interdependence of physiologic structure and function. Commentary regarding clinical application is made throughout each dissection in order to allow both student and clinician to appreciate the musculofascial system as it works to direct forces into and through the skeleton.

The text module coordinates with the DVD. In Chapters 2, 3, and 4, the reader will find small circular icons marked "DVD" in the book's margins. These icons identify content that is enhanced by specific video clips on the DVD. The reader will increase learning benefit by inserting the DVD and playing the clips that are listed in the "Text Reference Section" while reading the book. This innovative method for learning presents a three-dimensional perspective of the glenohumeral and scapulothoracic regions. Additionally, more than 200 superb illustrations are positioned throughout the text to effectively satisfy the two primary methods of learning: multisensory (visual) and reading comprehension. Chapter 5 includes an effective assessment component with over 40 step-by-step photographs. Chapter 6 focuses on treatment options and includes an exercise section with 48 exercises and 160 photographs that clinicians, exercise physiologists, and patients will find useful.

Movement is anabolic, and sustaining strength and painless activities are important to the quality of life and a sense of well-being. A true appreciation of a healthy body can be clearly described only by someone who has lost the ability to move painlessly and then through hard work and effective guidance has regained it. Conversely, the process of aging is catabolic. The degenerative process, which is compounded by injury, is what ultimately must be managed. Understanding the close interrelationships between exercise (movement) and health maintenance, both physical and mental, has been our theme throughout our textbooks. We remain dedicated to the development of efficient patient care models that emphasize rehabilitation strategies and direct management of musculoskeletal problems. We are especially mindful of the need to quantify effective treatment outcomes and the importance of patient education in ensuring a return of body function within the medical, therapeutic, and economic realities of the current health care market. These themes, coupled with an understanding of the three-dimensional anatomy, continue in this new product.

James A. Porterfield
Carl DeRosa

ACKNOWLEDGMENTS

The process of developing and ultimately writing any scholarly publication provides many exceptional opportunities to interact with new people and work with lifelong friends. We have been fortunate to have had the opportunity to collaborate with numerous individuals during this unique project that integrates video and text. We would especially like to thank the following colleagues and friends for their insight and assistance: Brian Coote, PT, MBA; Debbie Benjamin, PTA; Kurt Lundquist, PT; Richard Monasterio (Monasterio Studios); Dick Fraser (Fraser Video Productions); Rob Bell, MD; Merrill Abeshaus, MD; our physical therapist colleagues at Rehabilitation and Health Center and DeRosa Physical Therapy at Summit Center, and the faculty at Northern Arizona University and the Cleveland State University Physical Therapy Program.

We also would like to extend a very special thanks to Tina Cauller and Sue Bredensteiner. The illustrations in this, and in all of our texts, have been drawn by Tina Cauller. Her patience and extraordinary talent significantly add to the quality of our work, and we thank her for her insight and persistence. Sue Bredensteiner, the developmental editor for this text, greatly assisted us in organizing and integrating the teaching materials. Her expertise and calm demeanor helped anchor the project.

"Teach Once, Learn Twice" supports the foundation of our growth, and we thank all of our students, past and present, for their interest and collaboration.

CONTENTS

CHAPTER 3

CHAPTER 4

CHAPTER 1

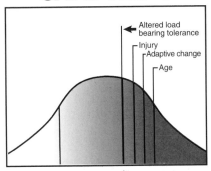

PRINCIPLES OF MECHANICAL SHOULDER DISORDERS

INTRODUCTION

Musculoskeletal disorders are a major health concern and remain one of the primary reasons for seeking health care. As we approach our 50s and 60s, disorders associated with bones, joints, and muscles are often the cause of worker disability, and there is little evidence to suggest that disability from musculoskeletal disorders is decreasing. While spinal disorders are the leading cause of musculoskeletal disability, they are followed by disorders of the extremities, especially disorders of the upper extremity.

Although low back, neck, and hand and wrist pain are commonly involved in work-related injuries, disorders of the shoulder are increasingly seen in the work environment, particularly when workers are required to do repetitive overhead lifting or under conditions where static shoulder postures need to be assumed. Work-related disorders associated with the shoulder are often referred to as "occupational cervicobrachial disorders" and are characterized by symptoms of diffuse pain in the paracervical, scapular, and glenohumeral regions.[4] As clinicians, we see that mechanical shoulder problems are not limited in their presentation to the shoulder girdle, but encompass a fairly extensive area of the upper quarter. The most common work-related disorders are associated with light industry, assembly line workstations, and office environments.

In this text we will endeavor to present the shoulder girdle complex in the context of its relationship to the surrounding body area including the neck and arm, as well as the trunk and lower extremities. As we continue to look for the best ways to treat shoulder disorders, it is valuable to integrate the typical local focus of the shoulder itself with a more global focus that includes its relationship with other areas of the appendicular and axial skeleton.

Many work environments are conducive to occupational injuries that result in cervicobrachial disorders. Required tasks often result in static postures of the upper trunk and shoulders and simultaneous rapid movements of the hands.[10,36,42] The disorders that result from occupations that require prolonged, static postures tend to be related to cumulative microtrauma to the musculoskeletal tissues, which can be compounded by reduced neuromuscular efficiency. On the opposite end of the injury spectrum, you find work environments that require heavy lifting and abrupt, rapid force generation. These occupations have a higher incidence of macrotraumatic injuries such as rotator cuff tears.

U.S. Bureau of Labor statistics from the past decade reveal an incidence of occupational cervicobrachial disorders that has increased and now ranks second to low back and neck pain in frequency.[46] Different occupations place such unique demands on the musculoskeletal system that the prevalence of occupational cervicobrachial disorders has a broad range, varying from 5% to 28%. In some occupations, such as musicians, it may be as high as 75%.[20,36]

1

The shoulder joint lacks inherent bony stability and therefore relies heavily on its associated muscles, joint capsules, and ligaments for stability. This places the soft tissues of the shoulder, particularly the connective tissue, at significant risk for injury.[29] The dependence on soft tissue for stability of the shoulder is best understood when you recognize that dislocations of the glenohumeral joint account for the largest percentage of dislocations when compared with all the other joints in the body.[27]

One of the most common clinical observations regards the differences seen between body regions of age-related changes of the specialized connective tissues. When considering the age-related changes of the spine, hips, and knees, for example, we are struck by the degenerative changes associated with the articular cartilage of those joints. In many shoulder disorders, however, the soft tissue of the region is the primary source of mechanical shoulder pain, for example, in the tendons and joint capsules, rather than articular cartilage. Certainly arthritis of the glenohumeral joint can be a major clinical problem, and advancing arthritic conditions of the glenohumeral joint are seen in the older adult population with approximately a 20% prevalence.[26,48] But we are often struck by the preponderance of soft tissue disorders related to the shoulder that we see in the clinic.

While industrial injuries have been a major impetus for analyzing the biomechanics of the anatomical regions that are associated with work-related injuries, it is really the sports sciences that have served as the stimulus for the study of shoulder biomechanics. Over the past several years, clinicians and scientists have begun to combine much of the emerging knowledge pertaining to the anatomy and biomechanics of the shoulder joints with the burgeoning understanding of tissue damage that results from industrial repetitive strain injuries. This has enabled us to gain a better understanding of the causes of shoulder injury, the response of the tissue of the shoulder complex to injury, the strategies that can be used to evaluate the shoulder, and, ultimately, the best ways to surgically and nonsurgically manage shoulder disorders.

The art and science involved in the evaluation and treatment of the shoulder depend largely on an understanding of the tissue's response to abnormal or excessive stress, as well as an application of this knowledge to the clinical anatomy of the region. This type of an approach leads to sound treatment and positive outcomes.

In this text we present a carefully illustrated and comprehensive description of shoulder anatomy in a manner designed to help direct the examination process. Understanding tissue injury and the healing process, coupled with the recognition of the role of the neuromuscular system of the trunk and shoulder complex, is essential to the successful treatment. We also emphasize the manner in which the strength of the trunk and shoulder girdle contributes to loading patterns that ultimately reach the connective tissues of the shoulder complex. In this chapter we examine the science of connective tissue as it relates to the shoulder since this tissue is so often compromised in syndromes of the shoulder complex. Additionally, we introduce several examples of common connective tissue disorders of the shoulder girdle in order to set the stage for more complete consideration of these and other mechanical disorders later in the book.

PURSUIT OF AN ACTIVE LIFESTYLE

As a result of many medical advances, the average life expectancy increases each decade. Consequently many of us are now pursuing sporting and recreational activities well into our eighth decade. Among the many stimuli for maintaining a healthy and active lifestyle are advances in the understanding of the causes of osteoporosis and the ways to minimize its onset, the beneficial effect of activity on the joints and muscles, the adverse effect of inactivity on the cardiopulmonary system, and the emotional and social benefits of exercise. These factors motivate all of us to engage in activities that are enjoyable and also have the potential to optimize our general health.

Some common activities include weight training, aerobic dancing, golf, swimming, racquet sports such as tennis and racquetball, and throwing sports. Even rock climbing is capturing the interest of many. Others make time to learn and play a musical instrument. All of these activities can place extraordinary demands on the muscle and connective tissue of the shoulder complex. Likewise, range-of-motion requirements and trunk and shoulder muscle recruitment are very specific and precise for each activity. As a result of the increased number of individuals of all ages engaging in such varied activities, shoulder injuries now appear with greater frequency.

Rotator cuff tendon lesions provide a good example of the magnitude of shoulder disorders in the general population. The variability of rotator cuff lesions makes it extremely difficult to assess the incidence of these tears precisely because age plays such a significant factor in the pathogenesis of this injury. As a result of the wide variation in signs and symptoms, and lack of understanding with regard to the differences between the normal aging process and degeneration, incidence rates have been placed as low as 5% and as high as 90%.[55] Especially in the older adult population, incidence rates for cuff tears may be as high as 90%.[14] As is the case with many other areas of the body, it is difficult to determine what is normal, expected aging and degeneration of tissues and what is a true pathological lesion.

Rotator cuff tears vary from being partial to full thickness (see Chapter 3). These injuries may present as painful entities or may not be painful at all; cuff disorders may result in significant functional deficit or leave no functional limitation.[38]

Thus, despite our continued advances in the study of sport science and repetitive strain injuries in the workplace, the simple fact remains that the primary cause of rotator cuff degeneration is age. Age results in a decrease in tendon elasticity and tensile strength, and these changes occur in active, as well as sedentary, individuals. And this emphasizes an important clinical concept: tendon lesions have a limited capacity to heal, though symptoms may decrease. Therefore symptom reduction is an unreliable way to determine tendon integrity.

Regardless of the presence or absence of symptoms and signs that might indicate cuff tears, loss of tendon integrity compromises the stability of the shoulder. Furthermore, such soft tissue injury associated with the shoulder joints results in altered joint kinematics, which may result in additional degenerative changes to surrounding tissues of the shoulder complex.

Key Role of Tissue Mobilization Versus Immobilization

The advances in understanding the response of connective tissue to injury, age, and adaptive change have occurred simultaneously with an enhanced understanding of the clinical anatomy of the shoulder complex and the contribution by the various components of the complex to its remarkable mobility. We know that immobilization is tolerated very poorly because motions of the shoulder girdle encompass several articulations and interfaces. In fact, immobi-

lization of the shoulder can lead to irreversible changes and a permanent loss of function.[33,45,47,50]

The deleterious effect of prolonged immobilization and the pronounced effect of disuse on the connective tissues result in structural changes to the tissues. For example, as a result of immobilization, the fibers of ligaments become increasingly disorganized and lose their parallel structure. Ligaments lose their structural rigidity, and as a result, less energy is needed to deform them.[1,15] Fibrous tissue with fatty inlays begin to invade the connective tissue and then adhere to the articular cartilage surface in the absence of joint motion.[2]

The properties of all the key connective tissue structures, such as synovial membranes, joint capsules, ligaments, tendons, insertional sites of tendons and ligaments, and the bones, are all adversely affected with immobilization and inactivity. The result is that these tissues can no longer attenuate compressive, tensile, or shear loads.[7]

Concurrent with changes in the connective tissues, the muscle tissue loses its volume and its normal function is also altered. In as little as 2 weeks, the mass of muscle begins to decrease because of a loss of myofibrils, and the oxidative enzymes needed for mitochondrial activity begin to diminish.[13] The strength (torque-generating ability of the muscle) and the oxidative capacity (necessary for muscle endurance) of the muscle therefore are decreased. The relative muscle atrophy seen so often in the sedentary individuals is a major concern. The loss of lean muscle mass coupled with skeletal changes that occur during aging render our bodies less able to deflect the barrage of forces that reach the articulations during daily activities of living, work, and sport.

In Chapter 3 we describe the anatomy and mechanics of the shoulder girdle muscles in detail. In addition to the role of these muscles in the movement of the various bony levers, we also point out the mechanical linkages each muscle has with connective tissue structures such as the joint capsules, ligaments, and fascial networks. In order to better understand how muscles contribute to the stability of an inherently unstable region like the shoulder girdle, it is necessary to broaden our view of the role muscles play over the articulations. The intimate relationship between muscles and specialized connective tissues is illustrated by the linkages seen between the rotator cuff muscles and joint capsule: the various muscles attached to and lying within the infraspinatus fascia, the convergence of numerous powerful muscles at the inferior border of the scapula, and the relationship of the abdominal fascia to the muscles of the anterior chest wall.

In these and other instances you can compare the muscle–connective tissue dynamics to the way in which a tent is stabilized. The central pole of the tent equates to the pushing effect the muscles, encased within the fascial envelopes, have as a result of the broadening effect of their contraction. External to this same fascial envelope are the pulls of various muscles, which act like the guy wires of a tent in securing and tightening the structure. Stability of the tent is achieved when the central post is pushing with appropriate force, and the guy wires are pulling in a manner that maintains tension within the tent walls. An excellent example, detailed in Chapter 3, involves the role of the infraspinatus fascia and the muscles encased within (the center pole of the tent) and attached to the external aspect (the guy wires pulling on the tent).

As a result of our understanding of the importance the musculature plays, current rehabilitation concepts associated with management of mechanical shoulder disorders feature earlier initiation of motion exercises for all of the key components of the shoulder complex and strength training of the glenohumeral, scapulothoracic, and trunk muscles (see Chapters 3 and 6). The intent of a more aggressive but specific approach to continued mobilization is to minimize the atrophy of the glenohumeral musculature. This is important because the glenohumeral joint is so highly dependent on neuromuscular control of the humeral head within the glenoid, and full shoulder motion requires the synchrony of scapula motion on the thorax. Earlier rehabilitation is now possible as a result of advances in surgical techniques and arthroscopic procedures that minimize the morbidity of the surrounding tissues.[39]

Influence of Body Type on Musculoskeletal Syndromes

Similar to most regions of the appendicular skeleton, the joints and soft tissues are subject to varying loads and diverse combinations of forces. The mechanical loads that reach the various tissues of the shoulder are compression, tension, and shear. These forces can reach different tissues of the shoulder in many different ways. An analysis of a posteriorly directed shear force at the glenohumeral joint is a good example (Figure 1-1). A posterior shear between the head of the humerus and the glenoid fossa can be imparted to the joint via the alignment of the two bones during a push-up. A posterior shear force also can occur as a result of contraction of the posterior cuff muscles. In a completely different scenario, a tight anterior glenohumeral joint capsule may generate a posterior shear of the humerus on the glenoid when the humerus is brought backward toward hyperextension. And in yet another example, an examiner may apply a posterior shear force through the humerus with a simple anterior-to-posterior force as long as this force is applied in the plane of the scapula. Note in each of these examples that the forces of compression and tension are simultaneously reaching different tissues, and it is essential that these forces be modified by the connective tissues as well.

The response of the tissues to forces of compression, tension, and shear is dependent on many factors, but one that needs to be considered in the evaluation of the patient is the body type. This is especially true in the examination of a patient with shoulder pain (see Chapter 5). Forces applied to the ectomorphic, highly inflexible individual result in a much different tissue response than forces applied to a mesomorphic, muscular individual or an endomorphic, highly flexible individual. Recognition of the body type often directs the clinician toward a different hierarchy of treatment. For example, it may be more appropriate to place additional emphasis on strengthening in an individual with a seemingly lax connective tissue matrix than to focus on stretching techniques, while an emphasis on motion and flexibility may be a better approach for the individual with a more rigid connective tissue matrix. Consideration of body type is therefore essential in the evaluation and treatment of most shoulder disorders.

When we analyze the broad spectrum of shoulder disorders seen in the clinic, the *end result* of many mechanical shoulder disorders can be distilled into specific biomechanical conditions: compression problems especially within the coracoacromial arch, tensile overload especially within the cuff tendons, and glenohumeral joint instability that results in excessive translation of the humeral head on the glenoid as a result of the inability to attenuate shear forces. Two examples of these biomechanical conditions are increased compression of the soft tissues residing in the suprahumeral space, which might occur with elevation of the humeral head, and humeral head subluxation, which might result from a redundant glenohumeral joint capsule. In these two very different clinical examples, a change in the connective tissues has resulted in two distinctly different clinical conditions.

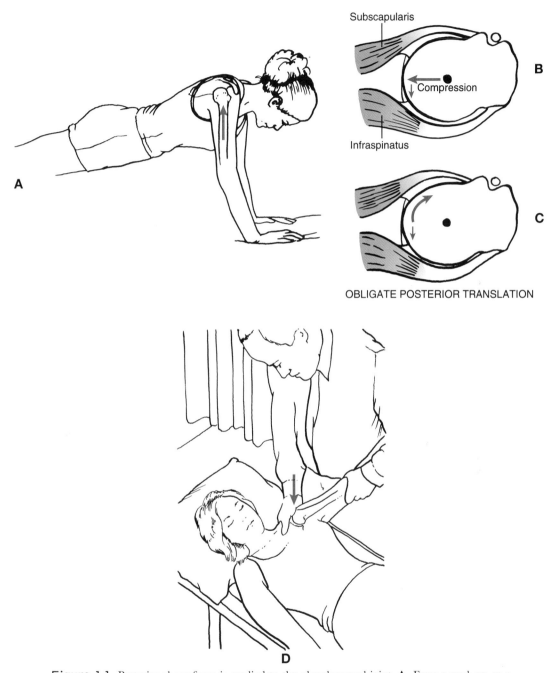

Figure 1-1. Posterior shear force is applied to the glenohumeral joint. **A,** From a push-up as a result of weight bearing. **B,** Through contraction of the posterior cuff muscles. **C,** As the result of a tight anterior glenohumeral joint capsule. **D,** As a result of the examiner applying posterior shear loads via the lever of the humerus. (**B** and **C** from Rockwood CA Jr, Matsen FA III, Wirth MA, et al: *The shoulder,* ed 2, Philadelphia, 1998, WB Saunders.)

The compression of the soft tissue that resides in the suprahumeral space might be due to the tightness of the posterior aspect of the glenohumeral joint capsule, which forces the head anteriorly during humeral elevation (see Chapter 4). Conversely, tightness of the anterior capsule pushes the humeral head posteriorly, and, more critically, tightness of the capsule in this anterior region does not allow the glenohumeral joint to reach full external rotation. Without full external rotation, the greater tuberosity cannot be cleared under the acromion during glenohumeral elevation.

Both syndromes result in increased compressive load to the subacromial tissues. Paradoxically, laxity of the glenohumeral joint capsule also may result in increased compressive loads to the subacromial tissues albeit for different reasons. The laxity of the glenohumeral joint capsule results in aberrational movement of the humeral head on the glenoid especially in the presence of a weak or fatigued rotator cuff. The subacromial tissues are again compromised via compression under the coracoacromial arch.

Again, body type is an important consideration because you may be able to estimate the magnitude of the abnormal or excessive loading patterns that reach the shoulder due to the activities in which an individual is engaged. For example, different swimming strokes have dissimilar requirements of the various shoulder tissues. Throwers have very specific biomechanical requirements for attenuating stresses. Again, the body type and the particular activity involved may influence the treatment priority hierarchy. A young female swimmer with a lax connective tissue matrix is a strong candidate for glenohumeral instability problems, which lead to secondary changes in the rotator cuff musculature. The glenohumeral joint of the baseball pitcher with a lax connective tissue matrix receives extraordinary shear loads between the humeral head and the glenoid during throwing, and the connective tissue framework may not reasonably contribute to stabilization of the joint.

On the other hand, the middle-age golfer who has a more rigid connective tissue matrix may have less glenohumeral and hip joint motion as a result of adaptive changes in the joint capsules. In order to carry out the golf swing, this golfer must compensate for lack of motion at these two proximal appendicular joints with excessive torsion of the lumbar spine.

Therefore it becomes important to closely examine the overall joint laxity of patients who present with mechanical shoulder problems. This is easily done by quickly screening the other joints of the body, such as the elbow or first metacarpal-phalangeal joint, for multiplanar mobility and the resistance imparted to the examiner's hands with endrange positions. Often the assessment of the turgor and elasticity of the skin can also provide the examiner with clues to the expected contributions of specialized connective tissues associated with the shoulder joints.

Can glenohumeral joint laxity be acquired through activity? Based on our knowledge of the response of connective tissue to different stresses (discussed later in this chapter), it is logical that excessive forces applied continuously and for extended periods of time may have the ability to alter the connective tissue matrix. You should always suspect instability of the glenohumeral joint in athletes or workers who engage in repetitive overhead activities that simulate the movements required in swimming, throwing, and racquet sports. Indeed, this possibility presents a dilemma: the joint capsule needs sufficient laxity in order to allow us to engage in the activity, yet the capsule must have enough stiffness to stabilize the joint. Perhaps no other joint in the body depends on such a fine line delineating the requirements for mobility versus the requirements for stability.

CONNECTIVE TISSUE WITH SPECIAL REFERENCE TO THE SHOULDER COMPLEX

There are a variety of different types of tissue in the human body, including epithelial, connective, blood, muscle, adipose, and nerve. All are considered tissues because they consist of cooperating cells that are formed into coherent associations, which are then surrounded by fibrous and amorphous intercellular substances. Each of the tissues of the body is represented in the shoulder complex, but this section will focus on connective tissue. The key components of the shoulder, including the rotator cuff tendons, biceps tendon, glenohumeral ligaments, glenohumeral joint capsules, bursal tissue, acromioclavicular capsule, and supporting ligaments, are prime examples of the connective tissues that are associated with mechanical disorders of the shoulder girdle.

Connective tissue is ubiquitous within the shoulder complex (Table 1-1). The whole family of connective tissue can be subdivided into connective tissue proper and the subclasses of specialized connective tissue (Figure 1-2). Even though there is a marked physical difference between connective tissue proper and specialized connective tissue, both tissues are considered

Table 1-1. Connective Tissues of the Shoulder Complex

Bone	Articular Cartilage	Ligaments	Joint Capsules	Joint Structures
Humerus	Humeral head	Glenohumeral	Glenohumeral	Glenoid labrum
Scapula	Glenoid fossa	Coracohumeral	Acromioclavicular	AC disc
Clavicle	Medial acromion	Coracoacromial	Sternoclavicular	SC disc
Sternum	Lateral clavicle	Transverse humeral	Cervical apophyseal	Bursae
Ribs	Medial clavicle	Coracoclavicular		Synovial lining
Cervical vertebrae	Sternum	Costoclavicular		Mechanoreceptors
	Cervical facets	Transverse scapular		

AC, Acromioclavicular; *SC,* sternoclavicular.

to reside within the same family because of the similarity among the building blocks, namely cells, intercellular matrix, and fibers.

Connective tissue proper can be subdivided into loose connective tissue and dense connective tissue. Loose connective tissue forms highly irregular matrices that help to protect and hold structures such as the vessels and nerves in place, or serve as tissue interfaces as seen in the case of bursal tissue. The axilla features an extensive array of loose connective tissue that also incorporates fat tissue into its weblike structure, providing additional support and cushion for the brachial plexus and the blood vessels in the axilla.

Dense connective tissue structures can be subdivided into regular and irregular tissue, with the clinically key subdivision being the dense regular type. Examples of dense regular tissue in the shoulder include the rotator cuff tendons, biceps tendons, the various ligaments of the glenohumeral joint, acromioclavicular joint, and sternoclavicular joint, and the joint capsules. Even though dense connective tissue has an abundant fiber framework, water still constitutes approximately 80% of its total makeup, followed by fibers (15% to 20%), and glycosaminoglycans (2%).[23] While we discuss the binding of water to these molecular elements later, in general, the greater the concentration of proteoglycans within the individual types of connective tissue, the greater the percentage of water.

Specialized connective tissue includes tissue with specific structures that allow for singular, individual-

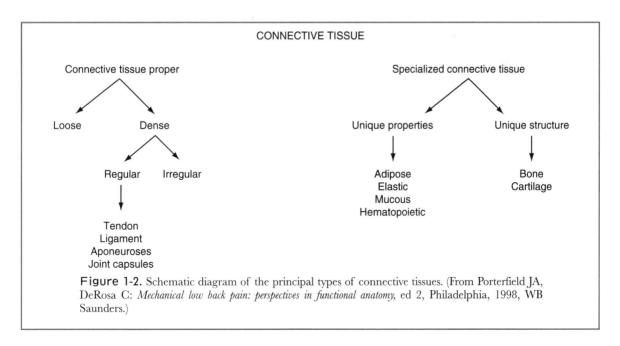

Figure 1-2. Schematic diagram of the principal types of connective tissues. (From Porterfield JA, DeRosa C: *Mechanical low back pain: perspectives in functional anatomy,* ed 2, Philadelphia, 1998, WB Saunders.)

ized physical properties. Two examples are bone and articular cartilage. The cellular and intercellular makeup of these two specialized connective tissues, as well as their physiology, are unique when compared with other forms of connective tissue. Despite such specialization, the general makeup remains similar to the general organizational scheme of tissues within the connective tissue proper, namely cells and an intercellular matrix composed of fibers and ground substance.

The distinguishing characteristics of the connective tissue are the result of distinct types of cells located within the specific tissues. These cells in turn synthesize the biochemical composition of the intercellular matrix. Although connective tissue cells are derived from the common mesenchyme precursor cell, that mesenchyme cell ultimately is differentiated into several cell types including the fibroblast, chondroblast, and osteoblast. These cells then become responsible for synthesizing the precursors of the fiber framework, as well as the molecules that form the matrix for the fibers and cells.

The capacity of connective tissue to resist different stresses such as compression, tension, and shear is due to the properties of its fibers and ground substance and the interaction between the two. For example, the resiliency and deformability of the articular cartilage of the humeral head and glenoid fossa, the structural rigidity of the scapula, clavicle, and humerus, and the ability of the glenohumeral ligaments and joint capsule to yield are all dependent on the specific types, proportions, and aggregations of glycosaminoglycans and proteins that form the ground substance of their specific connective tissue and the type, quantity, linkages, and orientation of intercellular fibers located within the matrix. In order to better understand the role of the matrix, we will look more closely at the key intercellular components: collagen fibers and glycosaminoglycans.

Intercellular Components of Connective Tissue

There are three basic types of fiber seen in the various connective tissues: collagen, which constitutes the majority of connective tissue fibers, elastic fiber, and reticulin fiber. Collagen, being the most abundant, is further classified into subtypes.[18] Tendons and ligaments—the tissues most often affected with shoulder disorders—are primarily composed of Type I collagen. Collagen typically makes up approximately 80% of the dry weight of connective tissue and is the only component of tendons, ligaments, or joint capsules resistant to tensile stresses. Such resistance to tensile stresses is an extremely important consideration for the shoulder since tensile stresses to the joint capsule and ligaments from repetitive motions or forced movement and eccentric loading of the rotator cuff tendons are among the more common etiologies for several of the mechanical disorders of the shoulder.[3]

The fundamental building block for collagen, which is synthesized by the fibroblast, is the tropocollagen molecule. A collagen precursor molecule is actually synthesized within the fibroblast cell and then secreted into the intercellular medium as tropocollagen. Tropocollagen consists of three polypeptide chains that are wound around one another in a helix and held together via cross-links through hydrogen bonding (Figure 1-3). As the building block of a tropocollagen molecule is added to other tropocollagen molecules end-to-end (in series) or side-by-side (in parallel), the collagen fiber begins to assume its shape (i.e., it begins to form the ligament, tendon, capsule, or other identifiable structure). Its orientation and bonding is directed, in part, by the stresses to which the cells and tissues are subjected. Tropocollagen molecules are held together in the formation of collagen fibers by strong covalent bonds. Because tropocollagen consists of polypeptide chains, collagen is essentially organized strands of protein molecules.

The second important class of chemicals that make up connective tissue is the glycosaminoglycans (GAGs), which also are produced by the fibroblasts. GAGs are chains of polysaccharides with repeating units: each unit is composed of a sugar molecule and a sugar with amine molecule (Figure 1-4). The number of repeating units (sugar amine and sugar) ultimately determines the length of the GAGs. Even though GAGs do not constitute as large a proportion of the dry weight of connective tissue as the collagen fiber, their importance lies in their affinity for water.

The final molecule to consider in a study of connective tissue is the proteoglycan. These large molecules consist of many GAGs linked to proteins. Several GAGs become linked to a core protein, which then forms a proteoglycan unit. In turn, a group of proteoglycan units can be linked together via hyaluronic acid to form a proteoglycan aggregate. The linkage of proteoglycan units through hyaluronic acid, for example,

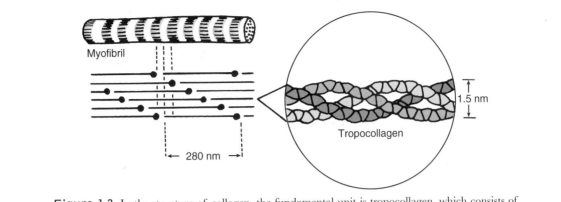

Figure 1-3. In the structure of collagen, the fundamental unit is tropocollagen, which consists of three separate polypeptide chains wound together in a helix.

provides the basis on which articular cartilage begins to assume its mechanical properties.

It is important to appreciate the physical structure of proteoglycan units and aggregates. The aggregates are twisted in various patterns resembling a fine mesh. The physical structure of the mesh, in combination with the electrical binding affinity of the proteoglycan to water, forms a structure that attracts and absorbs water and keeps it physically attached to the proteoglycan aggregates (Figure 1-5). This gives connective tissues with large concentrations of proteoglycan aggregates larger water content, such as occurs in articular cartilage, whereas a connective tissue with smaller proteoglycan content, such as a tendon, does not have the same quantity of water. Since different proteoglycans have different electrical charges, some are more adept at binding water than others. The loss of water from the various connective tissues as a result

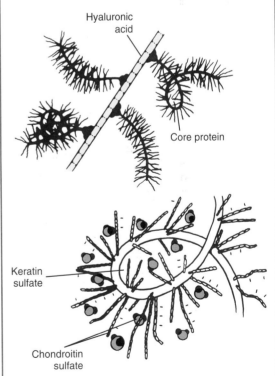

Figure 1-5. The convoluted shape of the proteoglycan aggregate, coupled with its affinity to water as a result of its electrical charge, makes it strongly attractive to the water molecule.

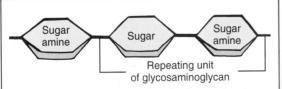

Figure 1-4. Repeating units of glycosaminoglycans appear as long chains of polysaccharides formed by a repeated sequence of a sugar molecule and a sugar with amine molecule.

of aging is due in part to two different factors associated with proteoglycans: a decrease in the absolute *number* of proteoglycans, as well as a changing *proportion* of the individual types of proteoglycans. As we age, different proteoglycans are no longer synthesized, which results in changes in number and proportion within the tissue.

While all of the features of the individual components of connective tissue contribute to its strength, one of the major factors is the ability of collagen and proteoglycan to bond together. This bonding gives connective tissue its ability to attenuate the various stresses it is subjected to, including compression, tension, and shear.

Basic Biomechanics of the Connective Tissues

The differences among the several types of connective tissue allow each to respond to stress in a different way. For example, the way in which bone responds to compressive loads is dissimilar to how tendons respond. Likewise, a tensile stress applied to ligaments will be modified in a different way than a tensile stress applied to articular cartilage.

The following discussion has significant clinical implications because there is often great attention to flexibility and range-of-motion exercises for many problems associated with the upper quarter. For example, a tight glenohumeral joint capsule that limits external rotation is going to have a significant impact on an individual's ability to raise his arm completely overhead. Quite simply, full elevation of the arm is dependent on achieving full external rotation of the glenohumeral joint. This is even more problematic in the glenohumeral joint because the rotator cuff tendons are intimately blended with the capsular tissue, so in essence the joint is a composite of ligamentous (glenohumeral ligaments), capsular (glenohumeral joint capsule), and tendinous (rotator cuff tendons) tissue (see Chapter 4). This begs the question, "Can a patient stretch a contracted, tight joint capsule in this instance?"

Much of the clinician's ability to actually modify connective tissue is dependent on several factors. These factors include the type of tissue, age of the tissue, thickness of the tissue, time since injury of the tissue, and inflammatory versus scarred condition of the tissue. You must recognize these factors because it is their various combinations that ultimately determine whether or not the connective tissue structures can, in fact, be stretched to a new resting position. Obviously, there are fundamental properties of connective tissues that ultimately influence and direct treatment approaches. Understanding the basic biomechanics involved will help you consider their implications in the evaluation and treatment process.

Stress and Strain on Connective Tissue

Clinical treatment protocols often include stretching maneuvers or techniques that are designed to elongate the nonosseous connective tissues. By definition, the force, which the clinician directs toward the tissue, is referred to as a *stress,* and the magnitude of the deformation that occurs as a result of the elongation force is known as the *strain.* Strain is thus measured as a length of change (in millimeters or inches) or as a percentage change from the initial length of the tissue. A tissue can deform if it is squeezed together (a compression strain) or if it is elongated (a tension strain).

The normal resting state of the collagen fiber is such that the individual collagen fibers have a wavy appearance (Figure 1-6). This characteristic of the collagen fiber is referred to as its *crimp.*[17] When a stress is applied to the collagen fiber in a direction parallel to the fiber orientation, the undulations are first taken out of the fiber (crimp is removed) and slight elonga-

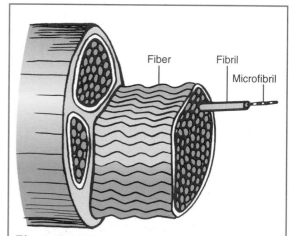

Figure 1-6. The wavy shape of the collagen fiber, the so-called "crimp" of the fiber, allows it to be slightly lengthened when an elongation force is applied.

tion occurs. Therefore the general "give" or elastic spring of the connective tissue that occurs as the joint is moved passively toward the endranges is responsible for this removal of crimp. Very little force is required by the examiner to remove the undulations from the collagen fiber because no chemical or electrical bonds have to be cleaved.

When the undulations of the resting collagen fiber are removed and the elongation force continues to be applied, the collagen fiber resists the force because of the bonding of the individual elements, specifically the linkage between the tropocollagen and the collagen fiber strands. As compared with the magnitude of force needed to remove crimp, the magnitude of force to induce strain in the collagen fiber without crimp is much greater because at this moment, the force is attempting to overcome the bonding of the connective tissue elements. Because the ligaments and joint capsules consist primarily of collagen fibers, the stress-strain curve for an individual collagen fiber is very similar to the stress-strain curve of the ligaments albeit with a few differences (Figure 1-7).[34,35]

As we just noted, the stress first removes the crimp from the collagen fiber and then greater energy is required to elongate the fiber because chemical and electrical bonds must be broken. When these bonds are broken, the fiber is less resistant to opposing the force and the stress results in a greater strain until the fiber fails completely. Capsules and ligaments are large, thick sheets of connective tissue, so in addition to the effect of the stress at the individual collagen fiber level, the stress will also cause the reorganization of the fibers as they attempt to align themselves in the direction of the stress. Once again, such reorganization would require that bonds be broken and thus energy is required.

You can also visualize that the reorganization of fibers that results from the elongation force squeezes the fibers together and water is expressed out from the molecule—again, a breaking of the chemical bonds that hold water (Figure 1-8). The breaking of chemical bonds that results in strain is a key point, because very often clinicians think of strain in terms of rupture

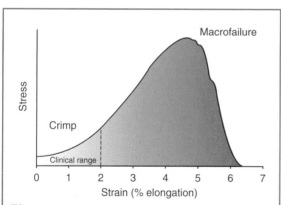

Figure 1-7. The stress-strain curve for ligaments is very similar to the stress-strain curve of collagen. First the stress removes the crimp from the collagen fiber, then increased energy is required to elongate the fiber because chemical and electrical bonds must be broken. When these bonds are broken, the fiber loses resistance and additional stress results in greater strain until the fiber fails completely. (From Porterfield JA, DeRosa C: *Mechanical low back pain: perspectives in functional anatomy,* ed 2, Philadelphia, 1998, WB Saunders.)

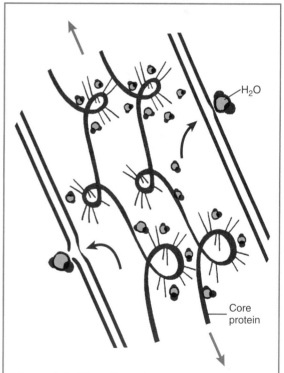

Figure 1-8. The collagen framework of large connective tissue structures such as joint capsules and ligaments is made up of closely approximated individual fibers. When elongation stresses are applied, the response is to squeeze out water.

of the collagen molecule itself, which is not quite accurate.[25]

One can see then that once the bonds between tropocollagen and the filaments of the collagen have been broken, it takes only minimal force (applied stress) to further disrupt the collagen matrix. This is part of the rationale for manipulation under anesthesia for the glenohumeral joint capsule that is rigorously adhered and tight. The manipulative thrust in this case is designed to break the chemical and electrical bonds in order to decrease the resistance to motion. Once those bonds are broken, the clinician must work with the tissue continuously and prudently in order to be sure that the healing process results in an elongated, more elastic scar that allows the maximal amount of glenohumeral motion to be achieved. This is achieved only if the tropocollagen framework begins to align itself along the natural lines of elongation stress.

In summary, an applied elongation stress has the potential to initiate a cascade of events. These include removal of crimp, breaking of bonds to separate tropocollagen molecules from collagen filaments, reorganization of the collagen fiber orientation, and the expression of water from the framework, nearly all as a result of breaking chemical and electrical bonds.

Within this cascade, approximately how much elongation can occur before bonds actually become broken? This is a difficult question because current research has been done with very specific but markedly different tissue such as ligament and tendon. Therefore determining a universal failing point is very difficult because such a failing point is dependent on factors including the rate at which the stress is applied and the cross-sectional area of the tissue. Generally stresses applied that result in a strain increasing tissue length by 1.5% to 3% are considered to be within the physiological limits of the tissue. Some mechanical failure is assumed to occur once the strain begins to surpass the 3% increase.[44,52]

Biomechanics of Connective Tissue Under Repetitive Loading

While a discussion focused on the application of a single stress that might exert strain above and beyond the physiological loading capacity of the connective tissue might be applicable to a one-time impact injury such as forced external rotation resulting in dislocation of the glenohumeral joint, it is also important to consider the effects of repetitive loading on connective

tissue. Many mechanical shoulder disorders are the result of such cumulative stresses. This was alluded to previously when we reviewed the increased rate of shoulder disorders resulting from workplace movement requirements. It is also obvious that the repetitive motions used by the swimmer, thrower, and musician are more akin to overload of the connective tissues via submaximal cumulative stresses than single-impact loading conditions.

The structural integrity and function of the shoulder complex depends largely on the ability of the musculoskeletal system to respond to repetitive loading. Because of the high degree of mobility found within nearly all components of the shoulder complex (e.g., the glenohumeral, acromioclavicular, and sternoclavicular joints and the scapulothoracic articulation) repetitive loading takes on great importance and can result in negative or positive consequences. It is not just the injury process that warrants the study of the influence of repetitive motion on injured tissue. *Controlled* loads can also *accelerate the repair* of damaged connective tissues, just as *uncontrolled* loading has the potential to *inhibit further healing.*[7]

In order to maintain optimal health of connective tissue, repetitive loading must be of a particular intensity, frequency, and range. If repetitive loading falls below or exceeds the optimal range, the various cells of the connective tissues begin to alter the intercellular framework.[19,49] Cells of the different connective tissues (fibroblast, chondroblast, osteoblast) interpret the signals related to the patterns of tissue loading and respond by redirecting the organization of the intercellular matrix. Unfortunately, the precise optimal physiological dose necessary to stimulate the various connective tissues is largely unknown and is difficult to predict because the dosage variability is influenced by multiple diverse factors such as age, endocrine factors, genetics, and environmental stress.

In previous texts we have used a bell curve model to illustrate the response of tissues to stress.[40,41] When the stress applied to tissues exceeds the physiological capacity of the tissues, tissue damage occurs. Likewise, when normal physiological loading of the tissue is decreased or absent, the tissue weakens. Several factors can influence this load bearing tolerance of the tissue, namely age, injury, and adaptive changes of the tissues themselves (Figure 1-9).

This concept of a bell curve can also be used to illustrate the principle of repetitive loading of the connective tissue of the shoulder, which must accommodate the many repetitive cycles inherent in sport and

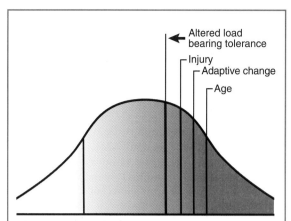

Figure 1-9. The optimal loading zone of tissues of the body can be changed as a result of age, injury, or adaptive change to the tissue.

work activity (Figure 1-10). When the loading cycles fall below the level necessary to stimulate the connective tissue cells, synthesis of intercellular matrix falls behind the process of tissue degradation and the tissue becomes substantially weakened. Conversely, increased rates of loading stimulate an adaptive cell response, which increases synthesis of intracellular

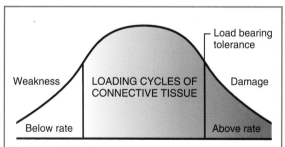

Figure 1-10. The concept of the optimal repetitive loading zone is important to the understanding of the potential for mechanical breakdown of the connective tissues. When the loading cycles fall below the rate necessary to maintain connective tissue integrity, synthesis of intercellular matrix falls behind the process of tissue degradation and the tissue becomes substantially weakened. Increased rates of loading first result in an adaptive cell response, which increases synthesis of intracellular matrix. If the loading intensity increases beyond the capacity of the cellular adaptive response, the tissue becomes damaged from the overload.

matrix. If the loading intensity increases beyond the capacity of the cellular adaptive response, however, the tissue becomes damaged from overload.

The rehabilitation process is framed around this concept of cellular response to stimulus. What is the optimal dose of exercise? What is the optimal dose of stretch? What is the optimal dose of rest? As simple as these questions may seem, they are the essence of rehabilitation program design. The intent of treatments to the shoulder is focused on optimization of the healing environment in order to restore anatomical relationships between the injured and noninjured tissues, maintain the normal function of the noninjured tissues, and prevent the patient from placing excessive stress and strain on the injured tissues while tissue strengthening treatment strategies are implemented (see Chapter 6). Training programs should be designed to progressively increase the frequency of exercise in order to take advantage of the cellular adaptive response. Changes can be expected to occur in ligament, bone, tendon, and cartilage as a result of the repetitive cyclic stress of exercise.[5,16] Repetitive loads that are applied to the tissues result in realignment of the intercellular matrix, and the repetitive stresses are transmitted to the cells of the tissue, resulting in further synthesis and alignment of the molecules comprising the matrix.[28,30] This is especially valuable to consider in cases of rotator cuff or glenohumeral joint capsule repair. Tensile loading of the repaired connective tissue results in the cells and collagen framework aligning parallel to the line of the applied tensile stresses, whereas the lack of applied tension leaves a more disorganized cellular and matrix environment.[5,6] Controlled loading of the repaired connective tissues also influences the rate of healing. Repaired tendons that are treated with controlled mobilization typically show significantly greater strength at nearly every point along the healing time frame than tendons that are left immobilized.[21,54]

Failure of Connective Tissue to Adapt to Repetitive Stress in the Rotator Cuff Tendon

The rotator cuff tendons provide a good example of the continuum of tissue damage, beginning with inflammation, progressing to degradation, and ending in fiber disruption. In many sports conditioning programs, the rotator cuff muscles must work at a high level both concentrically and eccentrically to control glenohumeral motion, as well as maintain the head of the humerus in the center of the glenoid fossa. Inappropriate training programs can potentiate the cascade of tissue injury events.[19] Training programs for many sports, such as swimming, throwing, tennis, and weightlifting, include so many repetitive loading cycles that the adaptive response of the fibroblasts within the cuff tendons may not meet the demands that are being imposed by the training program.

As might be expected, the initial changes that occur are usually at a microscopic level. The tissue may look macroscopically intact, but as discussed earlier, significant disruption and damage to the molecular framework of the cuff tendon matrix results in a markedly weakened tissue. This abnormal rearrangement of the molecular matrix results in a tendon that now can be more easily damaged by low-level loads. It is important to note that macromolecular reorientation can weaken the tissue. And this weakened tendon may rupture when subjected to an exceptionally high force, for example, a strong eccentric contraction when trying to throw at a maximum velocity, or attempting to lift a heavy object with a rapid, jerking motion.[11]

In contrast, decreased loading of the rotator cuff tendons is also damaging to the environment around the tendons. The rotator cuff tendons, just like other tendons, are subjected to tensile stresses through the concentric and eccentric contractions of the cuff muscles. When tissues that normally resist tensile stresses are not subject to this stimulus, the degradation of the intercellular matrix begins to exceed the synthesis of new matrix. Furthermore, as new matrix is synthesized, it is not oriented along lines of stress and is an inherently weaker tissue. The cellular changes that occur include a decrease in the amount and different proportions of GAGs, an obligatory loss of water as a result of GAG loss, and random orientation of the collagen fibrils.[9,56]

DISORDERS OF THE SHOULDER GIRDLE COMPLEX

In the preceding sections we attempted to provide a basic understanding of the mechanics of the specialized connective tissues at both the cellular and macroscopic levels. It is important to remember from the previous discussion that balance must be maintained between physiological stresses that enhance the tissue's health and physiological stresses that potentially break it down. Most of the mechanical disorders of the shoulder discussed in this text are largely the result of degenerative changes to or injury mechanisms in connective tissue structures. Additionally, nonsurgical management of such connective tissue injuries largely focuses on the education of the patient, emphasizing new biomechanical limits and exercise to enhance the neuromuscular elements that are now required for dynamic stabilization.

Because the shoulder complex encompasses several joints and a number of key structures, an in-depth discussion regarding the epidemiology of shoulder disorders is beyond the scope or intent of this book. Instead, in the final section of this chapter we provide an abridged review of several mechanical disorders of the shoulder commonly seen in the clinic, which are subsequently detailed in later chapters. The intent of this condensed discussion is to encourage you to think about both the impact that damage to these specialized connective tissues might have in regard to function and the objectives of treatment to restore function. The overview will include a brief discussion of the following topics:

- Injuries to the acromioclavicular joint
- Injuries to the sternoclavicular joint
- Fractures of the proximal humerus
- Instability of the glenohumeral joint
- Disorders of the rotator cuff
- Disorders of the biceps tendon
- Arthritis of the glenohumeral joint

Consider the functional anatomy presented in the following chapters in the context of these mechanical disorders. We hope you will gain an appreciation of the diversity of structures potentially responsible for mechanical shoulder pain while being able to visit and revisit the clinical anatomy through the text and the accompanying DVD. Together, the text and DVD present a comprehensive view of the alteration in function that might occur as a result of these disorders.

Injuries to the Acromioclavicular Joint

We present a detailed view of the anatomy and mechanics of this joint in Chapter 4. As this anatomy is reviewed, consider how trauma to the point of the shoulder could displace the scapula and tear the supporting ligaments. When such trauma occurs, the normal contour of the shoulder is lost as the upper extremity sags downward (Figure 1-11).

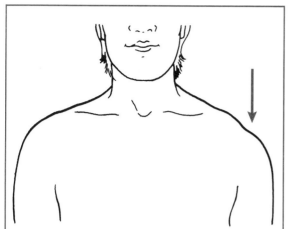

Figure 1-11. The normal contour of the shoulder can be changed as a result of downward force that displaces the scapula.

clavicular joint. When reviewing the anatomy, note also the relationship of the deltoid origins and trapezius insertions over the distal third of the clavicle and the potential for soft tissue to become wedged between the articulating surfaces of the joint.

Injuries to the Sternoclavicular Joint

We discuss the mobility and stability of the sternoclavicular joint, the articulation that literally suspends the upper extremity from the sternum, in Chapter 4. The most common causes of sternoclavicular joint injuries are motor vehicle accidents and sports injuries, suggesting that trauma is a primary mechanism of injury.[37] Posterior dislocations are of special concern because of the relationship of the medial end of the sternum to the major blood vessels and visceral structures such as the trachea and esophagus in the neck (Figure 1-12). Injuries include mild ligamentous sprains, subluxations, dislocations, and arthritic degeneration of the articulating partners of the joint.

Finally, the epiphysis on the medial end of the clavicle is the last epiphysis in the body to be seen on radiographs and it is the last to close. This epiphysis closes approximately between the ages of 23 and 26, and so as you review the anatomy of this region, you need to remember that subluxations or dislocations may

In some shoulder conditions, especially after acute injuries to the acromioclavicular joint region or as a result of repeated stress to the shoulder, the distal end of the clavicle can undergo demineralization and bony erosion.[32]

Finally, when you review the joint and understand its synovial joint characteristics, you can easily appreciate how degenerative joint disease may develop insidiously or as a sequelae to repair of the acromio-

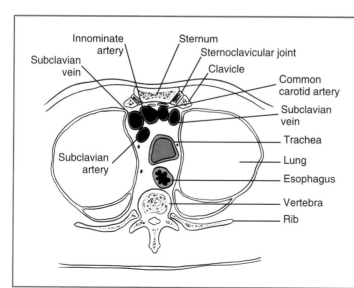

Figure 1-12. A cross section of the thorax shows the relationship of the medial end of the clavicle to the great vessels of the neck, trachea, and esophagus.

not in fact be sternoclavicular joint injuries, but rather epiphyseal plate injuries.[51]

Fractures of the Proximal Humerus

While studying the anatomy of the shoulder, it is important to keep in mind the different regions of proximal humerus, including its anatomical neck, epiphyseal line, and surgical neck (Figure 1-13). Note the attachments of the joint capsule and capsular ligaments (see Chapter 4), course of the peripheral nerves of the brachial plexus, especially the axillary nerve, in relation to this region (see Chapter 2), attachments of the rotator cuff and course of the long head of the biceps tendon (see Chapter 3), and course of the axillary artery (see Chapter 2). Injuries to the proximal humerus and these associated tissues have the potential to result in significant impairment with the consequence of disability.

Fractures of the proximal humerus are the most common fractures associated with the humerus.[43] In most cases these fractures occur as a result of falls and are a special concern in older adults since minimal trauma is needed to result in fracture in the presence of osteoporosis. Indeed, the incidence of proximal humeral fractures markedly increases in adults over 40 years of age. A careful review of the structures associated with this region provides us with a three-dimensional appreciation of its anatomy and the implications for evaluation of the extremity and post-fracture management.

Instability of the Glenohumeral Joint

While the unstable nature of the glenohumeral joint has long been discussed, it is only recently that the subtleties and complexities of that instability, especially those multidirectional in nature, have become understood (see Chapter 4). The functions of different portions of the capsule and the capsular ligaments acting as passive restraints have been coupled with a better understanding of the unique role of the rotator cuff (see Chapter 3) acting as an active restraint. These two features now are linked to our increased understanding of how afferent sensory input from the capsular and muscle tissues ultimately dictates motor output to the support muscles of the shoulder. Furthermore, we have a better understanding of the contribution of the scapulothoracic interface to maintenance of glenohumeral stability. Successful evaluation and treatment of glenohumeral joint instability relies on an integration of the neurologic, connective tissue, and exercise sciences.

You should especially consider the orientation of the connective tissue framework of the capsule and glenohumeral ligaments and the intimate blending of the cuff tendons and the capsule when reviewing shoulder

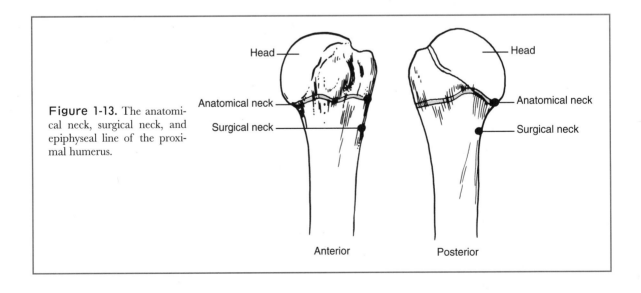

Figure 1-13. The anatomical neck, surgical neck, and epiphyseal line of the proximal humerus.

Head — Head
Anatomical neck — Anatomical neck
Surgical neck — Surgical neck
Anterior   Posterior

anatomy. As pointed out in this chapter, once the connective tissue matrix has been compromised (breakdown of the cellular bonding of the connective tissues), static restraints cannot check aberrational motions. Trivial forces may result in abnormal translations. It is at this point that exercise training of the neuromotor system becomes the key nonsurgical management option. Elements of exercise training are reviewed in Chapters 2, 3, and 6.

Disorders of the Rotator Cuff

An extremely wide range of rotator cuff disorders exists, from uncomplicated inflammatory conditions to full thickness tears. In addition, age-related changes of the cuff tendons and weakness of the rotator cuff markedly affect both glenohumeral stability and shoulder function. It is important to carefully study the cuff anatomy as presented in this text. The fiber orientation, muscle cross section, and relationships to the fascial elements are of considerable importance.

It also is helpful to visualize the intimate relationship that the cuff tendons have with the coracoacromial arch and how motion of the humerus results in a gliding of the cuff tendons under this arch (Figure 1-14) (see Chapter 4). There are numerous exercises for the shoulder, but many can compromise the cuff tendons by subjecting them to excessive compression, shear, or tension. You must consider the health and overall integrity of the rotator cuff tendons when prescribing exercises; you need to envision the different stresses that are placed on the tendons with any shoulder exercise (see Chapters 3 and 6).

Disorders of the Biceps Tendon

The two heads of the biceps tendon are unique in their relationship to other shoulder structures. For example, carefully note how the short head of the biceps contributes to the anterior aspect of the coracoacromial arch (see Chapter 4). By comparison, also follow the relatively complex course of the long head of the biceps tendon. The long head is of great clinical importance and a prime culprit in impingement conditions. When studying the long head of the biceps, follow the tendon superiorly over the proximal shaft and head of the humerus, through the capsule and into the glenoid labrum, and observe its

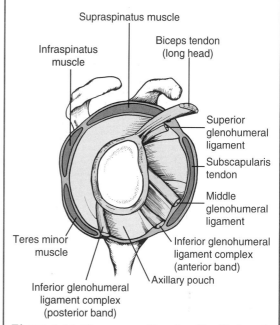

Figure 1-14. The rotator cuff tendons blend intimately with the joint capsule, and this tissue blending is in close relationship with the undersurface of the coracoacromial arch.

unique position between the supraspinatus and subscapularis muscle attachments. This position places it immediately deep to the coracohumeral ligament, the portion of the capsule referred to as the *rotator interval*, and the superior glenohumeral ligament (Figure 1-15).

In reality, the long head of the biceps tendon presents as two different tendinous components: a more fibrous component of the tendon in the region of the bicipital groove that reduces the shear stress as the groove slides back and forth under the tendon, and a more typical tendinous component designed to dissipate the tension associated with its attachment to the glenoid labrum and supraglenoid tubercle. Disorders of the tendon are variable and include uncomplicated tendonitis, tenosynovitis (inflammation of the sheath covering the biceps tendon), mechanical compromise of the tendon under the arch, and tendon rupture. Review the anatomy of the biceps tendon presented here in the context of both painful syndromes and the potential loss of stability as a result of tendon compromise.

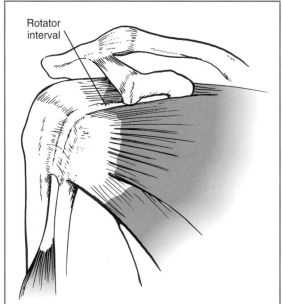

Figure 1-15. The long head of the biceps tendon is a unique structure. Note how the biceps tendon travels over the head of the humerus between the subscapularis and the supraspinatus tendons. These tissues lie inferior to the coracohumeral ligament. This area is referred to as the *rotator interval*.

Arthritis of the Glenohumeral Joint

Articular cartilage is a highly specialized class of connective tissue with very high tensile strength and resistance to compressive and shearing forces. At the same time, it possesses some resilience and elasticity. The surface of articular cartilage is extremely smooth and relatively wear resistant, and when combined with synovial fluid, it provides an exceptionally low coefficient of friction between articulating surfaces. As seen in the other classes of connective tissue, it is the arrangement and types of specific proteoglycans, collagens, and cells, in association with water, that determine the properties of cartilage. A change in one of the structural components will alter articular cartilage function and thus its capacity to accept the various stresses placed on it.

Proteoglycans contribute between 30% and 35% of the dry weight of cartilage[31] and form the major macromolecule of the cartilage ground substance. The type of proteoglycans and the manner in which they are aggregated are important to the structural

rigidity of the extracellular matrix. In addition, the viscoelastic properties of cartilage depend on the concentration of proteoglycans in solution.[54]

There is now good evidence that the structure and composition of the proteoglycans in articular cartilage change with age.[8] Because proteoglycans are important for maintaining cartilage stiffness, especially in regard to compression, and also contribute to the resilience of cartilage, an alteration in proteoglycan composition reduces these qualities.[24] This in turn alters the biomechanics of articular cartilage. It is the cyclic loading and unloading of the synovial joints that squeezes water out of and back into the cartilage, whereas the removal of pressure rehydrates it.[22]

This rehydration phenomenon contributes to cartilage nutrition due to fluid changeover. Although cartilage is described as an avascular structure, this is not entirely correct. What is actually meant is that the chondrocytes are located at a greater distance from the circulation as compared with other tissues.[53] Because of this vascular limitation, the contribution by rehydration is important in maintaining the health of the chondrocyte.

The degenerative changes associated with the articular cartilage affect its smoothness of movement and result in the loss of stability of the glenohumeral joint (see Chapter 4). Degeneration of articular cartilage in the humeral head typically manifests as central denudation surrounded by a rim of peripheral cartilage and osteophytes. As a result of these cartilaginous changes, the head of the humerus looks flat on radiographs and cartilage debris can often be found within the capsular recesses (Figure 1-16). The more common anatomical findings associated with degenerative joint disease of the glenohumeral joint are contracture of the anterior aspect of the capsule, posterior glenohumeral subluxation, and central and posterior wear of the articular cartilage of the humeral head.[12] Table 1-2 lists a number of the important anatomical changes in the tissue associated with the glenohumeral joint as a result of degenerative joint disease. As you review the anatomy of the glenohumeral joint in this text, give special consideration to the alteration in function that might result as a consequence of articular cartilage degeneration.

SUMMARY

We have briefly reviewed the science of connective tissues and suggested how age, injury, and adaptive change alter the capacity of specialized connective

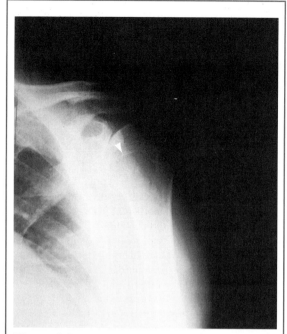

Figure 1-16. Radiograph of glenohumeral joint with degenerative joint disease. Because of the excessive thinning of the articular cartilage in the central region of the humeral head, and the development of a peripheral rim of cartilage and osteophytes, the humeral head takes on a more "flattened" appearance. (Courtesy Rob Bell, MD, Crystal Clinic, Akron, Ohio.)

Table 1-2. Pathoanatomy of Arthritis of the Glenohumeral Joint

Changes Associated With the Humeral Head
Central cartilage erosion with flattening
Central and superior sclerosis
Peripheral osteophytes, especially inferiorly
Subchondral bone cysts

Changes Associated With the Glenoid
Cartilage loss, especially centrally and posteriorly
Sclerosis
Peripheral osteophytes, especially along inferior border
Subchondral bone cysts

Resting Joint Position
Posterior joint subluxation

Changes Associated With the Capsule
Anterior contracture
Inferior enlargement

Modified from Cofield RH: Degenerative and arthritic problems of the glenohumeral joint. In Rockwood CA Jr, Matsen FA III, Wirth MA, et al: *The shoulder*, ed 2, Philadelphia, 1998, WB Saunders.

REFERENCES

1. Akeson WH, Ameil D, Abel MF: Effects of immobilization on joints, *Clin Orthop* 219:33,1987.
2. Akeson WH, Ameil D, La Violette D: The connective tissue response to immobility: an accelerated aging response, *Exp Gerentol* 3:239, 1968.
3. Akeson WH, Ameil D, Woo SLY: Immobility effects of synovial joints: the pathomechanics of joint contracture, *Biorheology* 17:95, 1980.
4. Andersson GBJ: Epidemiology of occupational neck and shoulder disorders. In Gordon SL, Sidney J, Blair MD, et al: *Repetitive motion disorders of the upper extremity*, Rosemont, Ill, 1995, American Academy of Orthopaedic Surgeons.
5. Arem AJ, Madden JW: Effects of stress on healing wounds: intermittent non-cyclical tension, *J Surg Res* 20:93, 1976.
6. Bair GR: The effect of early mobilization versus casting on anterior cruciate ligament reconstruction, *Trans Orthop Res Soc* 5:108, 1980.
7. Buckwalter JA, Cruess R: Healing of musculoskeletal tissues. In Rockwood CA, Green D, editors: *Fractures*, Philadelphia, 1991, JB Lippincott.
8. Buckwalter JA, Kuettner KE, Thonar EJM: Age-related changes in articular cartilage proteoglycans: electron microscopic studies, *J Orthop Res* 3:251, 1985.
9. Buckwalter JA, Maynard JA, Vailas AC: Skeletal fibrous tissues: tendon, joint capsule, and ligaments. In Albright JA, Brandt RA, editors: *The scientific basis of orthopaedics*, Norwalk, Conn, 1987, Appleton & Lange.
10. Burt S, Hornung R, Fine LJ: Health hazard evaluation report: National Institute of Occupational Safety and Health, *HETA* 89:250, 1990.
11. Clancy WG: Tendon trauma and overuse injuries. In Leadbetter WB, Buckwalter JA, Gordon SL, editors: *Sports-*

tissue to tolerate the various stresses on the shoulder. Once the integrity of a specialized connective tissue is compromised, that tissue does not regenerate but instead goes through a repair process, which leaves it less able to tolerate stress. The integrity of the connective tissue, coupled with the exquisite functioning of neuromotor elements, allows the shoulder to meet the demands of mobility while simultaneously remaining stable. In the subsequent chapters we discuss the various aspects of functional shoulder anatomy in detail in order to provide an understanding about how the shoulder meets these conflicting demands of mobility and stability. We present a working knowledge of the anatomy of the region, coupled with an understanding of the expected responses of tissue to injury, which is the basis for a logical progression of evaluation and treatment including the formulation of an exercise prescription.

induced inflammation: clinical and basic science concepts, Park Ridge, Ill, 1990, American Academy of Orthopaedic Surgeons.

12. Cofield RH: Degenerative and arthritic problems of the glenohumeral joint. In Rockwood CA, Matsen FA III, editors: *The shoulder*, Philadelphia, 1990, WB Saunders.

13. Cooper RR: Alterations during immobilization and regeneration of skeletal muscle in cats, *J Bone Joint Surg Am* 54(5):919, 1972.

14. Cotton RE, Rideout DF: Tears of the humeral rotator cuff: a radiological and pathological necropsy survey, *J Bone Joint Surg Am* 46:314, 1964.

15. Dehne E, Torp RP: Treatment of joint injuries by immediate mobilization: based on the spinal adaptation concept, *Clin Orthop* 77:218, 1971.

16. DeWitt MT, Handley CJ, Oakes BW, et al: In vitro response of chondrocytes to mechanical loading: the effect of short-term mechanical tension, *Connect Tissue Res* 12:97, 1984.

17. Diamant J, Keller A, Baer E, et al: Collagen ultrastructure and its relation to mechanical properties as a function of ageing, *Proc Roy Soc* (series B) 180:293, 1972.

18. Eyre DR: Collagen: molecular diversity in the body's protein scaffold, *Science* 207:1315, 1980.

19. Frank CB, Hart DA: Cellular responses to loading. In Leadbetter WB, Buckwalter JA, Gordon SL, editors: *Sports induced inflammation: basic science and clinical concepts*, Park Ridge, Ill, 1990, American Academy of Orthopaedic Surgeons.

20. Fry, HJ: Occupational maladies of musicians: their cause and prevention, *Int J Music Educ*, 2:59, 1984.

21. Gelberman RH, Woo SLY, Lothringer K, et al: Effects of early intermittent passive mobilization on healing of canine flexor tendons, *J Hand Surg* 7(2):170, 1982.

22. Gradisar IA, Porterfield JA: Articular cartilage, *Top Geriatr Rehabil* 4:1, 1989.

23. Ham AW, Cormack DH: *Histology*, ed 8, Philadelphia, 1979, JB Lippincott.

24. Harris ED Jr, Parker HG, Radin EL, et al: Effects of proteolytic enzymes on structural and mechanical properties of cartilage, *Arthritis Rheum* 15:497, 1972.

25. Hirsch G: Tensile properties during tendon healing, *Acta Orthop Scand* (suppl) 153:1, 1974.

26. Jenkinson ML, Bliss MR, Brain AT, et al: Peripheral arthritis in the elderly: a hospital study, *Ann Rheum Dis* 48:227, 1989.

27. Kazar B, Relovsky E: Prognosis of primary dislocation of the shoulder, *Acta Orthop Scand* 40:216, 1969.

28. Klebe RJ, Caldwell H, Milam S: Cells transmit spatial information by orienting collagen fibers, *Matrix* 9:451, 1989.

29. Matsen FA III, Fu FH, Hawkins RJ: *The shoulder: a balance of mobility and stability*, Rosemont, Ill, 1993, American Academy of Orthopaedic Surgeons.

30. Mosler E, Folkhard W, Knorzer E, et al: Stress induced molecular rearrangement in tendon collagen, *J Molec Biol* 182:589, 1985.

31. Muir IHM: The chemistry of the ground substance of joint cartilage. In Sokoloff L, editor: *The joints and synovial fluid*, vol 2, New York, 1980, Academic Press.

32. Murphy OB, Bellamy R, Wheeler W, et al: Posttraumatic osteolysis of the distal clavicle, *Clin Orthop* 109:108, 1975.

33. Nevasier RJ: Painful conditions affecting the shoulder, *Clin Orthop* 173:63, 1983.

34. Nordin M, Frankel VH: Biomechanics of collagenous tissues. In Frankel VH, Nordin M, editors: *Basic biomechanics of the skeletal system*, Philadelphia, 1980, Lea and Febiger.

35. Noyes FR: Fundamental properties of knee ligaments and alterations induced by immobilization, *Clin Orthop* 123:210, 1977.

36. O'Hara H, Aoyama H, Itani T: Health hazard among cash register operators and the effects of improved working conditions, *J Hum Ergol* (Tokyo) 5:31, 1976.

37. Omer GE: Osteotomy of the clavicle in surgical reduction of the anterior sternoclavicular dislocation, *J Trauma* 7:584, 1967.

38. Ozaki L, Fujimoto S, Nakagawa Y, et al: Tears of the rotator cuff of the shoulder associated with pathologic changes in the acromion: a cadaver study, *J Bone Joint Surg Am* 70:1224, 1988.

39. Paulos LE, Tibone JE: *Operative techniques in shoulder surgery*, Rockville, Md, 1991, Aspen.

40. Porterfield JA, DeRosa C: *Mechanical low back pain: perspectives in functional anatomy*, ed 2, Philadelphia, 1998, WB Saunders.

41. Porterfield J, DeRosa C: *Mechanical neck pain: perspectives in functional anatomy*, Philadelphia, 1995, WB Saunders.

42. Punnett L, Robins JM, Wegman DH, et al: Soft tissue disorders in the upper limbs of female garment workers, *Scan J Work Environ Health* 11:417, 1985.

43. Rose SH, Melton LJ, Morrey BF: Epidemiologic features of humeral fractures, *Clin Orthop* 168:24, 1982.

44. Shah JS, Jayson MIV, Hampson WGJ: Low tension studies of collagen fibers from ligaments of the human spine, *Ann Rheum Dis* 36:139, 1977.

45. Simon WH: Soft tissue disorders of the shoulder, *Orthop Clin North Am* 6:521, 1975.

46. United States Department of Labor, Bureau of Labor Statistics: *Survey of occupational injuries and illnesses*, Washington, DC, 1994, U.S. Department of Labor.

47. Uitvlugt G, Detrisac DA, Johnson LL, et al: Arthroscopic observations before and after manipulation of the frozen shoulder, *Arthroscopy* 9:181, 1993.

48. van Schaardenburg D, Van den Brande KJ, Ligthart GJ, et al: Musculoskeletal disorders and disability in persons aged 85 and over: a community survey, *Ann Rheum Dis* 53:807, 1994.

49. Videman T: Connective tissue and immobilization: key factors in musculoskeletal degeneration? *Clin Orthop Rel Res* 221:26, 1987.

50. Wahls SM, Renstrom P: Fibrosis in soft-tissue injuries. In Leadbetter WB, Buckwalter JA, Gordon SL, editors: *Sports induced inflammation: clinical and basic science concepts*, Park Ridge, Ill, 1990, American Academy of Orthopaedic Surgeons.

51. Webb PAO, Suchey JMM: Epiphyseal union of the anterior iliac crest and medial clavicle in a modern multiracial sample of American males and females, *Am J Phys Anthropol* 68:457, 1985.

52. Welsh RP, MacNab I, Riley V, et al: Biomechanical studies of rabbit tendon, *Clin Orthop* 81:171, 1971.

53. Williams PL, Warwick R: *Gray's anatomy*, ed 36 (Br), Philadelphia, 1986, WB Saunders.

54. Woo SLY, Buckwalter JA: *Injury and repair of the musculoskeletal soft tissues*, Park Ridge, Ill, 1988, American Academy of Orthopaedic Surgeons.

55. Woo SLY, Debski RE, Boardman ND, et al: Pathophysiology of injury and healing. In Hawkins RJ, Mismore GW, editors: *Shoulder injuries in athletes*, New York, 1996, Churchill Livingstone.

56. Woo SLY, Ritter MA, Amiel D, et al: The biochemical and biomechanical properties of swine tendons: long term effect of exercise on the digital extensors, *Connect Tiss Res* 7:177, 1980.

CHAPTER 2

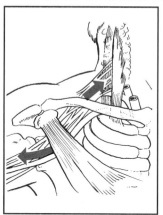

NEUROANATOMICAL AND NEUROMECHANICAL ASPECTS OF THE SHOULDER

INTRODUCTION

Mechanical stresses and loads potentially can injure specialized connective tissues of the shoulder (see Chapter 4). The pain felt at the shoulder as a result of mechanical stresses is often due to the physical distortion of nociceptors that lie within these tissues or is a consequence of chemical activation of the resident nociceptive free nerve endings that are depolarized as a result of damage to the cell walls of the tissues. Nociceptors are the biological transducers that convert physical and chemical energy stimuli into action potentials.

In addition to injury to the specialized connective tissues or damage to the musculotendinous tissues, pain felt within the shoulder may be caused by several other neuroanatomical or neurophysiological factors. These include nerve root irritation of nociceptors that lie within these tissue. It may also be a consequence of chemical activation of the resident degenerative joint disease or spondylosis of the cervical spine, compromise to the brachial plexus along its path through the

axilla, and damage or irritation to the peripheral nerves that supply the various tissues of the region.

In addition to their potential for shoulder pain, nerve root disorders or peripheral nerve injuries are especially complex because these disorders typically change the function of the shoulder. Altered neural input to and from the shoulder girdle as a consequence of nerve root compromise results in abnormal osteokinematics of the humerus on the glenoid, scapula on the clavicle, clavicle on the sternum, or scapula on the thoracic cage. These altered movement patterns further compromise the various innervated tissues of the shoulder region, which results in other tissue sources of pain, potentially confounding the findings in the shoulder examination.

In this chapter we want to provide the reader with an understanding of the relationships between the different components of the nervous system relative to the shoulder rather than provide an exhaustive review of the neuroanatomy and neurophysiology of the upper quarter. Our intent is to discuss the neuroanatomical and neurophysiological implications in a practical, clinical sense. We cover the conditions that refer pain to the shoulder, analyze the peripheral nerves that are key to supplying the shoulder complex and their associated clinical conditions, and finally, explore the integrated role of the sensory and motor systems as both relate to shoulder function and the establishment of treatment regimens for shoulder disorders. Restriction of function, which in

Throughout this chapter you will find small circular icons marked "DVD" (see margin). These icons identify content that is coordinated with a video clip on the DVD accompanying this text. For maximum learning benefit, go to the "Text Reference Section" on the DVD and play the coordinated clip while reading the appropriate section of text. These clips expand on and reinforce the information presented in the text.

reality is neural driven, is the primary reason to treat painful disorders of the shoulder.

In the following sections we discuss shoulder pain that might be due to pathology associated with the cervical spine first. After that we detail the anatomy and clinical implications of the peripheral nerves. Finally, we explain sensorimotor integration as it relates to shoulder function and intervention.

THE CERVICAL SPINE AND SHOULDER PAIN

We limit the involvement of the cervical spine relative to shoulder disorders to two clinical syndromes: pain and dysfunction as a result of the mechanical or chemical irritation of the cervical nerve root, and referred pain from the musculoskeletal tissues of the cervical spine itself. The cervical nerve roots extend from the cervical spinal cord via a series of nerve rootlets (Figure 2-1). The dorsal root is primarily afferent (transmitting information toward the spinal cord), whereas the ventral root is primarily efferent (transmitting information from the spinal cord toward the periphery). Consequently, the dorsal root is considered the sensory nerve root, whereas the ventral root is considered the motor nerve root. The sensory nerve roots of the cervical spine are relatively large and feature an extensive array of nerve rootlets because of the

breadth of the receptor system associated with the upper extremity.

The nerve roots are invested with pia mater, bathed in cerebrospinal fluid, and covered by the arachnoid and dura mater. At approximately the region of the intervertebral foramen, the nerve roots merge to form a very short spinal nerve, after which the spinal nerve immediately breaks into two branches—the dorsal ramus and the ventral ramus (Figure 2-2).

The dorsal ramus branches over the posterior aspect of the neck, supplying the deep muscles of the cervical spine and the skin. The ventral ramus arises from several cervical and thoracic segments and ultimately merges with the dorsal ramus to form the proximal components of the brachial plexus. The brachial plexus is therefore the primary nerve source for the shoulder and upper extremity. It carries both motor and sensory supply to and from the tissues respectively. We will focus on the nerve roots here because they potentially relate to shoulder pain and will discuss the brachial plexus in detail later in the chapter.

The dorsal roots of the cervical and upper thoracic spinal cord levels are responsible for specific regions of the skin (dermatomes), bones (sclerotomes), and muscles (myotomes). The areas of skin innervated by peripheral cutaneous nerves are supplied by the axons stemming from specific cervical and upper thoracic nerve roots, and the representation of these root segments on the skin can be reasonably mapped (Figure 2-3). Note that

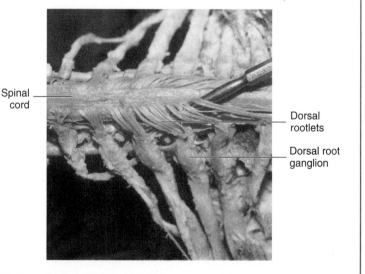

Figure 2-1. The cervical nerve roots are formed from a series of dorsal and ventral rootlets, which are attached to the spinal cord. These rootlets come together and ultimately form the dorsal and ventral roots for each cervical segment.

Spinal cord

Dorsal rootlets

Dorsal root ganglion

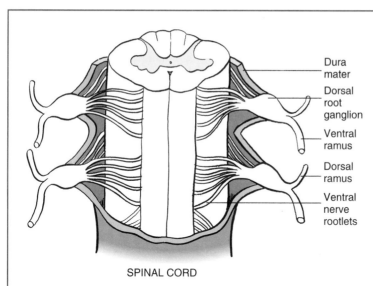

Figure 2-2. The dorsal and ventral nerve roots come together to form the spinal nerve, and almost immediately the spinal nerve divides into its two components: the posterior primary ramus and the ventral primary ramus.

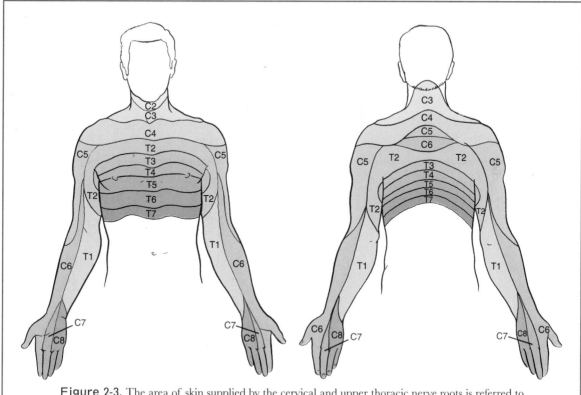

Figure 2-3. The area of skin supplied by the cervical and upper thoracic nerve roots is referred to as the dermatomal distribution of the nerve roots around the shoulder.

in regard to sensory supply, the nerve roots represented in the immediate shoulder region are primarily C4, C5, and C6. The fourth cervical nerve root (C4) is typically limited in distribution to the top of the shoulder (the area surrounding the acromioclavicular joint), whereas the fifth and sixth cervical nerve roots supply the majority of the shoulder area. In addition, the first thoracic dorsal nerve root (T1) is represented in the upper medial aspect of the arm and the axilla. The T1 ventral root is unique because it carries the first spinal cord level of the preganglionic neurons associated with the sympathetic nervous system. After these preganglionic neurons communicate with the sympathetic chain, located immediately adjacent to the spinal nerve, the ventral and dorsal rami of T1 then carry the postganglionic neurons peripherally to the smooth muscle, cardiac muscle, and glands of the upper extremity and face (Figure 2-4).

In the neck, the most common level of nerve root involvement is the middle and lower cervical spine—the C4-C5, C5-C6, and C6-C7 spinal segments. These cervical vertebral levels typically show earlier degenerative changes than the other regions of the cervical spine. The fifth cervical nerve root (C5) exits between the fourth and fifth cervical vertebrae, whereas the sixth cervical nerve root (C6) exits between the fifth and sixth cervical vertebrae (Figure 2-5). It is primarily these two nerve roots (C5 and C6) that are represented in and around the shoulder girdle. These nerve roots are responsible for the largest portion of the sensory feedback from the shoulder to the central nervous system (CNS) and the majority of motor supply to the shoulder musculature.

While several pathoanatomical changes in the cervical spine can compromise the nerve roots, the two most common are intervertebral disc pathology and degenerative joint disease of the apophyseal joints. Because degenerative changes of the disc and the joints are often related to age, it is important that the clinician rule out cervical nerve root involvement in the middle-age or older adult patient who presents with shoulder pain. In such patients a nerve root screen is an essential component of the shoulder evaluation (Table 2-1).

A differential diagnosis may be made based on several features of nerve root pain. The quality of nerve root pain is different from pain from other tissues about

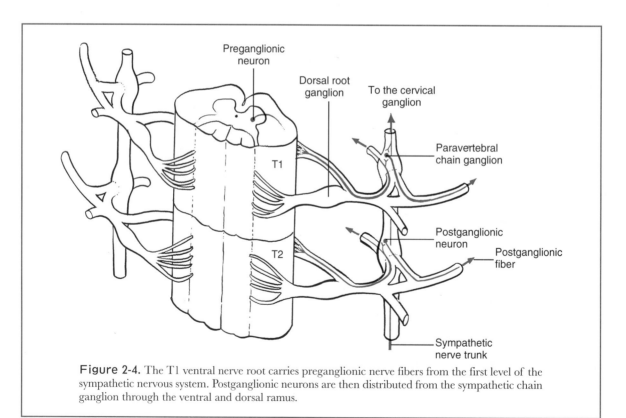

Figure 2-4. The T1 ventral nerve root carries preganglionic nerve fibers from the first level of the sympathetic nervous system. Postganglionic neurons are then distributed from the sympathetic chain ganglion through the ventral and dorsal ramus.

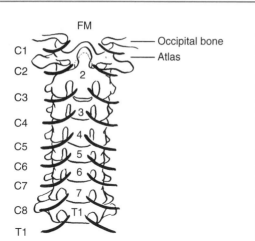

Figure 2-5. Spinal nerves are named for the junction points where the ventral and dorsal roots merge in the cervical spine.

Irritation of the C6 nerve root is associated with pain toward the anterior elbow and paresthesias over the radial aspect of the forearm and thumb.

Whereas nerve root *irritation* may be related to pain within the shoulder region, nerve root *compression* is a more significant disruption of sensory or motor axon function and as such may alter sensation throughout the shoulder region or result in motor changes. Such motor changes are manifested as weakness, atrophy, or altered reflexes. Table 2-2 lists the nerve root segments that are typically represented in the key muscles associated with the shoulder. Note the large distribution of the fifth and sixth cervical nerve roots throughout the musculature of the shoulder. When assessing the integrity of the C5 and C6 nerve roots, testing the muscles is an important part of the clinical examination, especially the shoulder abductors, shoulder external rotators, and the biceps brachii. Reflex testing of the biceps also provides data regarding the status of the nerve roots. Involvement of the C7 nerve root does not typically cause shoulder pain, but if suspected, is best assessed through muscle testing the triceps brachii and its reflex.

The second example of cervical spine involvement that can lead to shoulder pain is referred pain from non–nerve root structures such as the cervical apophyseal joints and the soft tissues related to the cervical spine. Referred pain from the cervical spine to the shoulder is another clinical manifestation that must be considered in the examination of the patients presenting with shoulder pain. The neuroanatomical pathway

the shoulder, typically being sharper, more highly localized, and very disconcerting to the patient. The pain is felt deep throughout the upper extremity, usually in a clearly demarcated zone. Oftentimes the patient presents with shoulder and neck pain, but the extremity pain is typically more distressing than the pain in the cervical spine. The presence of proximal pain and distal paresthesias in the upper extremity is another hallmark of nerve root involvement. For example, C5 nerve root involvement is often manifested by upper arm and shoulder pain and elbow paresthesias.

Table 2-1. Elements of the Nerve Root Screen for the Patient Presenting With Shoulder Pain

1. Quadrant testing of neck: Does this cause radiation into the arm?
2. Foraminal compression test (Spurling's test)
3. Reflex testing of the upper extremity
   a. Biceps: C5
   b. Brachioradialis: C6
   c. Triceps: C7
4. Muscle testing
   a. Shoulder abduction: C5
   b. Elbow flexion: C6
   c. Elbow extension: C7
   d. DIP thumb extension: C8
   e. Abduction-adduction of fingers: T1

Table 2-2. Nerve Root Supply to Muscles of the Shoulder

Muscles	Nerve Roots
Pectoralis major	C5, C6, C7, C8, T1
Pectoralis minor	C7, C8, T1
Deltoid	C5, C6
Supraspinatus	C5, C6
Infraspinatus	C5, C6
Teres minor	C5, C6
Subscapularis	C5, C6
Trapezius	XI, C3, C4
Serratus anterior	C5, C6, C7
Latissimus dorsi	C6, C7, C8
Teres major	C5, C6
Levator scapulae	C3, C4
Rhomboid major	C5
Rhomboid minor	C5
Coracobrachialis	C5, C6, C7
Biceps brachii	C5, C6
Triceps brachii	C6, C7, C8

for referred pain is difficult to precisely define. Cyriax describes referred pain as "pain felt elsewhere than at its true site."[7] Although this definition is adequate as a working clinical description, it only describes the phenomenon as perceived by the patient and observed by the clinician. It is not a neurophysiological description.

The CNS, rather than the peripheral nervous system, is largely responsible for the manifestation and interpretation of referred pain. As stated by Grieve, "pain happens within the CNS, and does not reside in the damaged locality, though it may be perceived so."[18] He is telling us that the subjective experience of pain is the result of processing the afferent impulse at the spinal cord, brainstem, and cerebral cortex levels. The painful stimulus activates many pools of neurons at all levels of the CNS, all of which contribute to the perception of referred pain.

Several tissues of the cervical spine have common referral patterns to the shoulder. For example, the apophyseal joints of the C4-C5 or C5-C6 vertebral segments have a characteristic referral pattern to the

shoulder in addition to the primary complaint of neck pain. Figure 2-6 illustrates the areas of the shoulder typically involved with referred pain from the cervical apophyseal joints.[1,14]

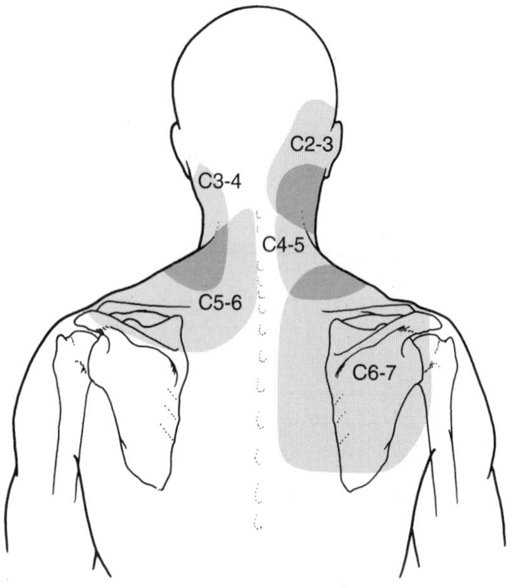

Discogenic pain, thought to arise from the breakdown of the disc at these same levels, may also be a source of referred shoulder pain. Finally, the cervical muscles associated with these same cervical segmental levels have the potential to refer pain into the shoulder region, most commonly over the scapula. We think that referred pain from degenerative joint disease of the apophyseal joints of the cervical spine is the more common mechanism of referred shoulder pain. The palpable changes in muscle tension about the neck and the scapula are reflex responses of the neuromuscular system as a result of injury or degenerative breakdown of the specialized connective tissues of the cervical spine.

As discussed earlier, careful examination of the cervical spine in the middle-age or older adult patient complaining of shoulder pain is important in linking the contribution of the cervical spine to the painful syndrome being examined because primary degenerative joint disease is an age-related phenomenon. A quick screen of the cervical spine to reproduce the pain described typically includes endrange rotation and testing the cervical spine in the extension quadrants (Figure 2-7).

Finally, the clinician should bear in mind that visceral structures also have the potential to refer pain to the shoulder. Pain felt in the shoulder region can be caused by gallbladder disease, disorders of the diaphragm, disorders of the spleen, and pathology of the heart or lungs. Mechanical disorders of the musculoskeletal system, however, often feature a pattern of pain and can be provoked with mechanical stresses, which is atypical of visceral disorders. In the absence of a predictable pain pattern, and when familiar signs or symptoms cannot be elicited through the application of mechanical stresses to the shoulder tissues or cervical spine in the examination (see Chapter 5), additional diagnostic tests are necessary to rule out pain of visceral origin.

Figure 2-6. The cervical apophyseal joints can refer pain toward the shoulder region. This illustration shows the region of the shoulder in which such pain may be perceived by the patient. (Modified from Dwyer A, April C, Bogduk N: Cervical zygapophyseal joint pain patterns I: a study of normal volunteers, *Spine* 15(6):453, 1990.)

THE BRACHIAL PLEXUS

The ventral rami of C5, C6, C7, C8, and T1 interweave to form the brachial plexus, which gives rise to nearly the full complement of sensory and motor nerves associated with the upper extremity (Figure 2-8). The plexus is best studied when divided into its

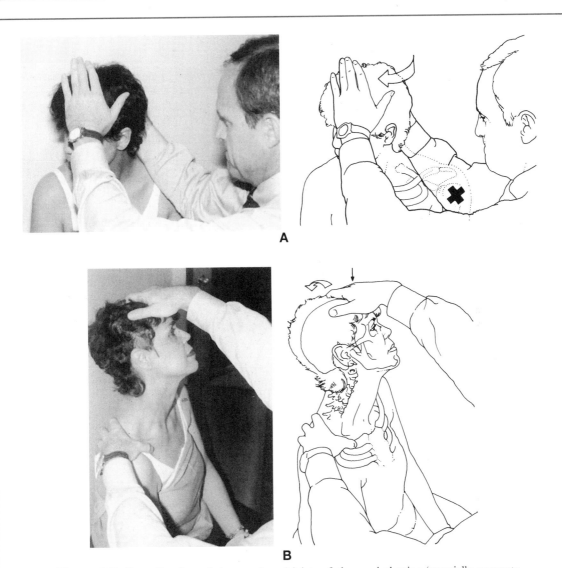

A

B

Figure 2-7. Since disorders of the apophyseal joints of the cervical spine (especially segments C4-C5 and C5-C6) can refer pain to the shoulder, we include a cervical screening in the examination of the patient with shoulder pain, especially middle-age or older adults. In view **A,** the examiner brings the cervical spine to endrange rotation, and in **B,** the examiner brings the cervical spine into the extension quadrant. When the examiner is able to reproduce familiar neck and shoulder pain with these maneuvers, it suggests that the shoulder pain is referred from the cervical spine. (From Porterfield JA, DeRosa C: *Mechanical neck pain: perspectives in functional anatomy,* Philadelphia, 1995, WB Saunders.)

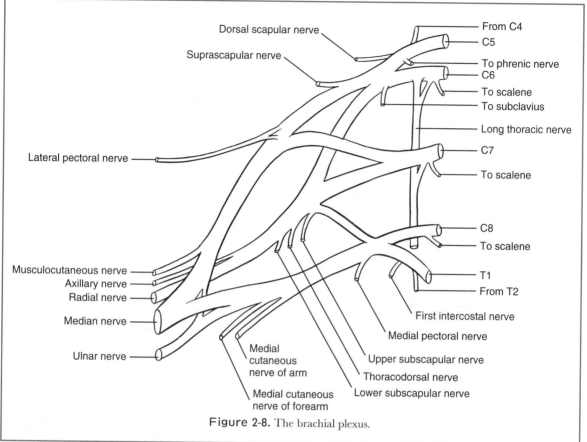

Figure 2-8. The brachial plexus.

component parts: the ventral rami, trunks, divisions, cords, and peripheral nerve branches.

The area of the neck that lies above the clavicle is called the supraclavicular region. It is in this region that the proximal parts of the brachial plexus are located. In addition to the ventral *rami*, there are three *trunks*. The *upper trunk* is formed when the fifth and sixth ventral cervical rami unite. The eighth cervical and first thoracic ventral rami form the *lower trunk* of the brachial plexus, and the ventral ramus of C7 continues as the *middle* trunk.

Injury to the trunks of the brachial plexus can result from trauma. The classic "burner" or "stinger" injury to the shoulder, often seen in athletes who play football or wrestle, usually is a result of a forced depression of the scapula on one side in combination with lateral flexion of the cervical spine to the contralateral side. The combination of these forces to the neck and shoulder girdle results in a stretch injury to the upper trunk

of the brachial plexus (Figure 2-9). While pain from such an injury is often immediate, associated neurological changes in the muscles ultimately supplied by nerve branches of the upper trunk or its continuation might not be evident until several days after injury. As might be expected, injuries to the upper trunk of the brachial plexus can affect deltoid, supraspinatus, infraspinatus, and biceps brachii muscles.[6,9]

Each trunk of the brachial plexus gives rise to anterior and posterior *divisions*. The posterior divisions from the upper, middle, and lower trunks ultimately merge to form the *posterior cord* of the brachial plexus, whereas the anterior divisions of the upper and middle trunk form the *lateral cord*. The anterior division of the lower trunk continues as the *medial cord*. The cords of the brachial plexus are named for their relationship (medial, lateral, or posterior) to the axillary artery (Figure 2-10).

Although some of the peripheral nerves that ultimately supply the skin and muscles of the upper

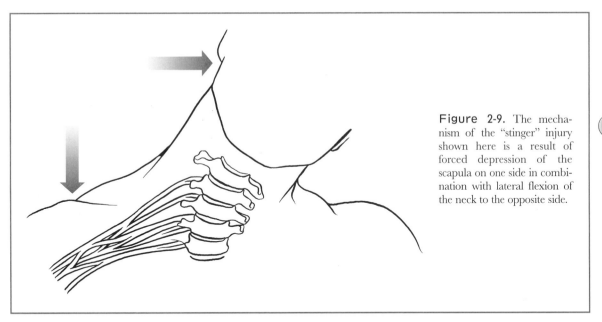

Figure 2-9. The mechanism of the "stinger" injury shown here is a result of forced depression of the scapula on one side in combination with lateral flexion of the neck to the opposite side.

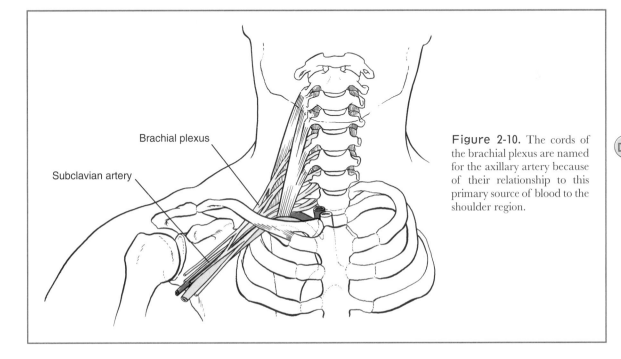

Brachial plexus

Subclavian artery

Figure 2-10. The cords of the brachial plexus are named for the axillary artery because of their relationship to this primary source of blood to the shoulder region.

extremity branch from the trunks and divisions of the plexus, most of the peripheral nerves branch from the cords. Note that the interweaving of the rami, trunks, divisions, and cords results in the potential for many of the peripheral nerves to carry several different nerve root segments ranging from C5 through T1. Figure 2-8 illustrates the peripheral nerves that branch from the brachial plexus.

Physiological Relationships of the Brachial Plexus

The brachial plexus (rami, trunks, divisions, cords, and branches) travels over a fairly complex route in its path from the anterolateral aspect of the cervical spine to the arm. Thus, you need to have a general idea of the relationships of the various components of the brachial plexus to important cervical and shoulder girdle structures. From their position lateral to the nerve roots, the ventral rami lie just outside the intervertebral foramen positioned between the anterior and middle scalene muscles (Figure 2-11). The trunks of the plexus lie anterior to the levator scapulae muscle and course between the anterior and middle scalene muscles toward the upper posterior aspect of the clavicle. At this region, the neural tissue of the brachial plexus is incorporated into the fascial sheath of the scalenes, which allows injections of local anesthetic to be contained within the immediate environs when given as a treatment intervention.

The upper two rami join together to form the upper trunk at Erb's point. This landmark can be visualized as lying 2 to 3 cm above the clavicle immediately posterior to the sternocleidomastoid muscle (Figure 2-12). The lower trunk, in contrast, forms behind the clavicle directly above the pleura of the lung. Thus apical lung tumors can compromise neural function of the lower trunk of the brachial plexus and must be ruled out when evaluating sensory and motor disturbances of the upper extremity of unknown etiology.

Approximately at the level of the clavicle, the trunks split into anterior and posterior divisions. Branches emerging from the anterior division supply the flexors of the upper extremity, whereas branches from the posterior division primarily supply extensors. At this point, however, these components of the brachial plexus lie within the costoclavicular space and pass into the infraclavicular region (Figure 2-13).

After passing between the clavicle and rib and then under the pectoralis minor muscle, the plexus reaches the axilla, where it is thoroughly invested with axillary fascia and protected by the fat, connective tissue, and lymph nodes of the axilla. In this region the cords of

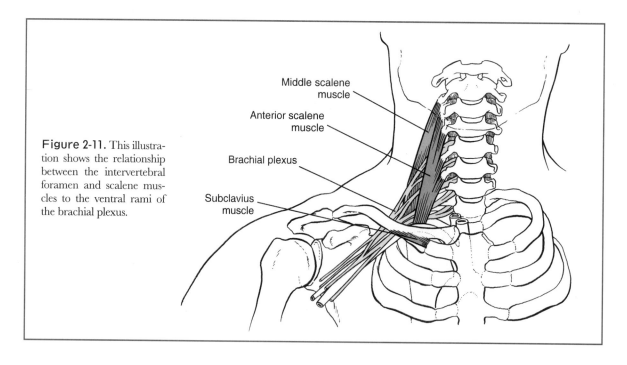

Figure 2-11. This illustration shows the relationship between the intervertebral foramen and scalene muscles to the ventral rami of the brachial plexus.

Middle scalene muscle

Anterior scalene muscle

Brachial plexus

Subclavius muscle

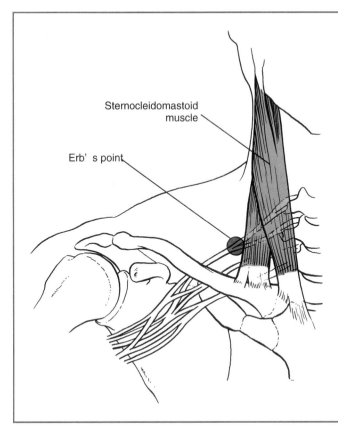

Sternocleidomastoid muscle

Erb' s point

Figure 2-12. Erb's point is the junction of the upper two rami and is typically 2 to 3 cm above the clavicle and immediately posterior to the sternocleidomastoid muscle.

the brachial plexus are formed and lie in close approximation to the axillary artery. The peripheral nerves that carry the alpha and gamma motor neurons that supply the extrafusal and intrafusal muscle fibers respectively, and the sensory nerves that not only carry nociceptive and general sensation but also proprioceptive feedback from the upper extremity to the CNS, emerge from the axillary fascia.

Key Peripheral Nerves of the Brachial Plexus and Related Clinical Syndromes Associated With the Shoulder

Suprascapular Nerve

The suprascapular nerve branches from the upper trunk of the brachial plexus at Erb's point and typically carries the fifth and sixth cervical nerve roots. Its

route toward the two muscles it supplies, the supraspinatus and infraspinatus, is unique because it travels through the suprascapular notch of the scapula, which is bridged by the transverse scapular ligament.[34] The suprascapular artery lies superior to this ligament, whereas the suprascapular nerve travels inferior to it (Figure 2-14). Note that the suprascapular nerve does not move within the notch, but instead, it is the scapular notch that must move relative to the nerve. This scapular motion occurs over the scapulothoracic interface and acromioclavicular joint.

On entering the supraspinous fossa, the nerve supplies the supraspinatus muscle and then courses laterally to supply sensory branches to the acromioclavicular joint and the posterior aspect of the joint capsule. Then the suprascapular nerve swings around the spine of the scapula to enter the infraspinous fossa and supply the infraspinatus muscle. In the supraspinous fossa, branches of the suprascapular nerve supply the acromioclavicular joint and the superior

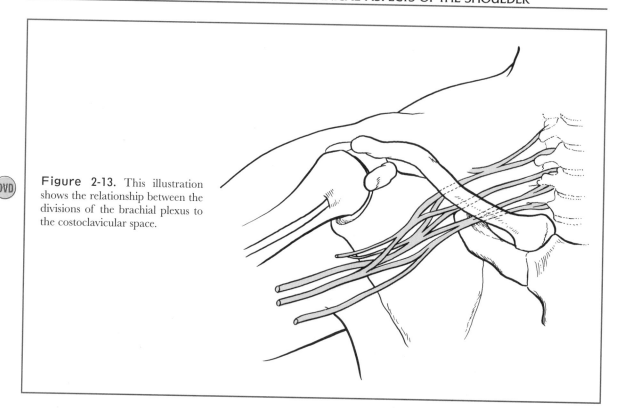

Figure 2-13. This illustration shows the relationship between the divisions of the brachial plexus to the costoclavicular space.

aspect of the glenohumeral joint. In the infraspinous fossa its branches extend to the posterior aspect of the glenohumeral joint.

The suprascapular nerve can be injured or compromised in several ways.[11,13,30] Grade III sprains of the acromioclavicular joint (see Chapter 4) can result in traction to the suprascapular nerve as a result of downward displacement of the scapula and the resultant compression and traction to the nerve by the overlying transverse scapular ligament (Figure 2-15).[34]

Since the suprascapular nerve is relatively fixed at its origin from the upper trunk and at its termination in the infraspinous fossa, it can be injured via tensile stresses, which might occur with excessive range of scapular motions so common in many athletic activities, such as swimming, tennis, and throwing.[5,30] Try to visualize how the distance between the two ends of the nerve increases with scapular motions and how repetitive motion of the scapula continually "rides" the suprascapular notch back and forth under the nerve. Repetitive carrying of heavy loads that forces the scapula into extremes of depression also may result in traction to the nerve.[2,3] The location of the

suprascapular nerve as it crosses the posterior aspect of the glenohumeral joint may render it vulnerable to posterior glenohumeral subluxations and dislocation. Compression by ganglion cysts or neoplasms in the region of the spinoglenoid notch or posterior capsule also may cause pathology.[42]

Although the anatomical course of the nerve and analysis of scapular motion suggest ways in which the suprascapular nerve can be injured, it is often difficult to make a clinical diagnosis. Pain is typically felt posterior and is poorly localized. Depending on the region of the nerve compromised, weakness and atrophy of the supraspinatus and infraspinatus may be present. Compromise at the spinoglenoid notch would affect only the infraspinatus because innervation of the supraspinatus occurs proximal to this point.

Typically, infraspinatus atrophy is easier to detect than supraspinatus atrophy. Weakness of the supraspinatus and infraspinatus muscles has an impact on arm elevation, abduction, and external rotation. Note, however, that weakness of these muscles can be caused by a variety of other conditions, such as rotator cuff tears or cervical nerve root involvement.

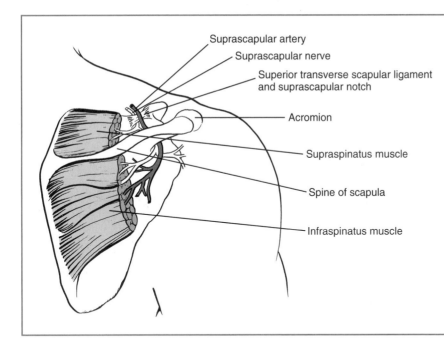

Suprascapular artery
Suprascapular nerve
Superior transverse scapular ligament
and suprascapular notch
Acromion
Supraspinatus muscle
Spine of scapula
Infraspinatus muscle

Figure 2-14. The suprascapular nerve branches from the upper trunk of the brachial plexus and travels posteriorly to run through the suprascapular notch, where it lies under the transverse scapular ligament. After passing through the notch, it supplies the supraspinatus muscle and then swings laterally around the spine of the scapula to supply the infraspinatus muscle. In addition to supplying these two muscles, this nerve also supplies the posterior aspect of the joint capsule and the acromioclavicular joint.

Diagnosis of suprascapular neuritis is therefore very difficult. Electromyography of these two muscles may help confirm the diagnosis. Treatment usually focuses on rest, limiting the range of scapular motion with activity, support of the scapula if possible to avoid it being displaced inferiorly, and scapula elevation exercises in a moderate range.

Finally, the suprascapular nerve is one of the nerves that supply the glenohumeral joint capsule. Stimulation of the suprascapular nerve endings in the joint capsule has demonstrated contractile activity of the biceps, infraspinatus, supraspinatus, and subscapularis muscles in the feline model, implying that reflex arcs exist from the ligaments and joint capsule to their associated muscles.[40] It is reasonable to suspect that motions of the joint, especially those that take the connective tissues to ranges resulting in activation of the nerve endings in the capsule, trigger muscle contractions, which stabilize and keep the humerus centered on the glenoid.

Long Thoracic Nerve

The long thoracic nerve, originating from the C5, C6, and C7 ventral rami at the level of the intervertebral foramen, is one of the few nerves in the body that courses on the external surface of the muscle it innervates (Figure 2-16). The serratus anterior lies superficially on the lateral chest wall, which appears to place the nerve in a fairly vulnerable position but, in fact, the nerve is adequately protected by soft tissues in its course. The common mechanisms of injury are direct trauma to the lateral chest wall or traction stresses to the nerve. Traction of the nerve occurs primarily with scapular retraction and depression since this maneuver stretches the nerve over the first rib. The particular region of the nerve most vulnerable to this stretch is between the upper part of the serratus anterior and the lower border of the middle scalene (Figure 2-17).

The large excursion of scapulothoracic motion seen in numerous sports has been documented as having the potential to injure the long thoracic nerve. Bowling, throwing, discus, football, golf, gymnastics, weightlifting, and wrestling have all been implicated.[16,17,46] Activities in which the arm is vigorously pulled into abnormal positions also may result in the scapula moving in a direction that causes traction to the nerve.[21] Like many of the peripheral nerves, long thoracic nerve palsy can occur as a result of viral infection of the nerve, infections, and lower motor neuron disease.[46]

The serratus anterior is the key upward rotator of the scapula, and weakness caused by long thoracic

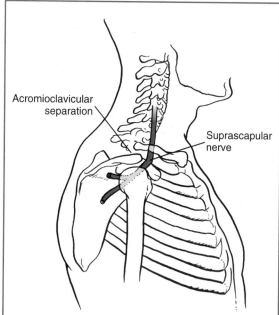

Figure 2-15. When the scapula is subluxed or dislocated from the clavicle at the acromioclavicular joint, it is displaced downward and rides inferiorly, resulting in traction to the suprascapular nerve, and the nerve is compressed against the lower border of the thick transverse scapular ligament.

nerve damage impairs its ability to strongly lift the arm overhead since the scapulothoracic contribution to arm elevation is lost. The strong attachment of this muscle to the medial wall of the scapula will result in the medial border of the scapula losing contact with the chest wall—the classic "winging" scapula—when there is a loss of resting muscle tension as a result of nerve palsy (Figure 2-18).

If traction to the nerve is considered to be the etiological factor, postures that potentiate the nerve tension via stretch of the serratus anterior (marked retraction and downward rotation of the scapula) must be avoided. Stretching of the muscles that are scapular protractors, such as the pectoralis major and pectoralis minor, may also contribute to postural correction. Like most upper quarter problems that have postural mechanics as an etiological factor, strengthening of the scapulothoracic and abdominal muscles is essential for postural balance. Recovery from nerve palsy is typically slow, often taking as long as 2 years.

Axillary Nerve

The axillary nerve carries the C5 and C6 nerve root segments and is one of the terminal branches of the posterior cord of the brachial plexus. It is an often-injured nerve.[22] In addition to supplying the three deltoid heads and the teres minor muscle, it supplies sensory innervation to the shoulder joint capsule and cutaneous sensation about the shoulder. The other terminal branch is the radial nerve.

Once you understand the course of the axillary nerve, you can visualize its potential for injury. From its position on the surface of the subscapularis muscle, it travels posteriorly to the inferior aspect of the shoulder joint capsule[28] (see Figure 2-12). It gains the posterior position of the shoulder by emerging from the quadrilateral space (Figure 2-19), whereupon it branches into anterior and posterior components to supply the deltoid and teres minor muscles and the skin over the region of the lateral arm via its prominent cutaneous branch, the lateral brachial cutaneous nerve. The anterior branch of the axillary nerve is also responsible for the sensory supply to the lower portion of the glenohumeral joint capsule, and on emerging from the quadrilateral space, the posterior branch also contributes to the sensory supply of the glenohumeral joint capsule. These two branches of the axillary nerve constitute the major nerve supply of the glenohumeral joint capsule.[15]

Because of its close relationship to the proximal end of the humerus, the axillary nerve is vulnerable to stretch injuries secondary to dislocations or fractures of the humerus, and its close proximity to the inferior aspect of the joint capsule renders it vulnerable during surgical procedures designed to tighten the joint capsule for glenohumeral joint instability problems.[29a] These articular branches of the axillary nerve have also been found to elicit contractions in the biceps, subscapularis, supraspinatus, and infraspinatus muscles when experimentally stimulated.[20] This implies a synergistic relationship between passive support structures (capsule and ligaments) and the neuromuscular system.

The most common mechanism of injury to the nerve occurs during anterior dislocations of the humerus. Estimates of the incidence of axillary nerve injury following dislocations range from 10% to 18%.[4]

Axillary nerve injury has also been documented in conditions arising from carrying heavy packs on the shoulders, forcing the shoulder girdle into prolonged and excessive depression.[24,36] Signs and symptoms

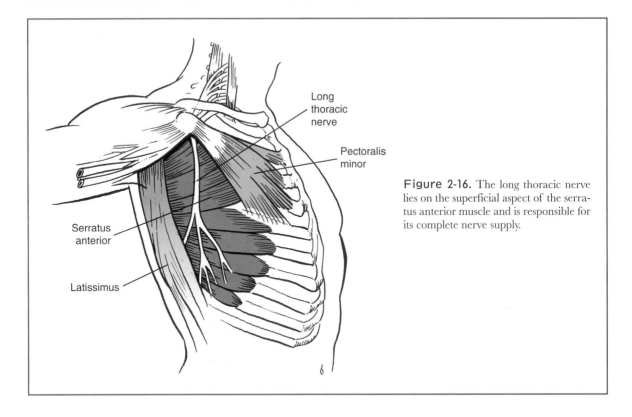

Figure 2-16. The long thoracic nerve lies on the superficial aspect of the serratus anterior muscle and is responsible for its complete nerve supply.

associated with axillary nerve injury include weakness of the deltoid and altered sensation about the shoulder, electromyographic (EMG) changes, pain over the region of the quadrilateral space, and diffuse aching in the shoulder joint especially after use. Because the nerve is relatively short in its course around the humerus, the prognosis for recovery is good. Maintaining strength and range of motion, especially in the rotator cuff and scapulothoracic muscle groups, is important in this recovery phase.

Spinal Accessory Nerve

The spinal accessory nerve is the name for cranial nerve XI with its associated cervical contributions. It is a complex nerve and originates in the cervical spinal cord and medulla. The axons of the cervical cord origin ascend through the foramen magnum to join its counterpart from the medulla in its formation, and the conjoint axons descend to exit through the jugular foramen located at the base of the skull (Figure 2-20). After passing through the sternocleidomastoid muscle that it also innervates, the spinal accessory nerve

travels posteriorly to reach and supply the trapezius muscle on its deep surface (Figure 2-21).

Although the nerve may be injured by trauma to the lateral aspect of the neck, or as a result of traction forces that reach the nerve because of excessive scapular depression, the most common mechanism of injury occurs as a result of surgery within the posterior triangle of the neck. Examples include biopsy or resection of the lymph node or radical neck dissection. The trapezius alone holds up the lateral point of the shoulder, so dropping of the lateral aspect of the shoulder is one of the most common signs.[12,27] In addition, shoulder function can be compromised because of the loss of trapezius contribution to scapulothoracic elevation and upward rotation.

Thoracic Outlet Syndrome

No discussion of the brachial plexus or its components is complete without reference to thoracic outlet syndrome. The thoracic outlet syndrome remains a highly controversial topic in musculoskeletal medicine, with viewpoints that range from skepticism about its

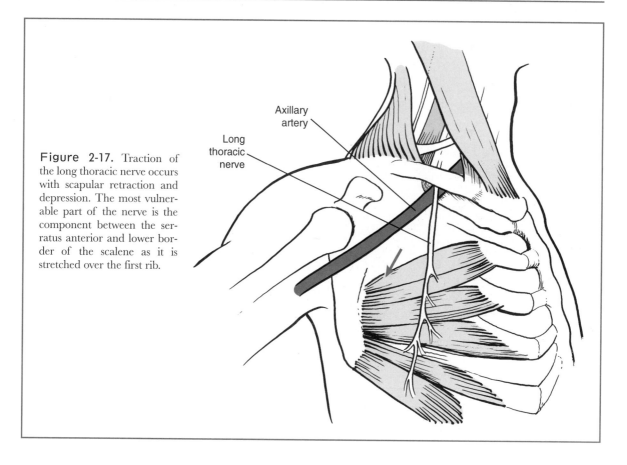

Figure 2-17. Traction of the long thoracic nerve occurs with scapular retraction and depression. The most vulnerable part of the nerve is the component between the serratus anterior and lower border of the scalene as it is stretched over the first rib.

existence to elaborate descriptions of its signs and symptoms. The syndrome is generally considered to arise from mechanical compromise to the brachial plexus and associated vasculature, particularly the subclavian vessels. Its wide spectrum of signs and symptoms have vascular or neurological characteristics that include any combination of pain, paresthesias, weakness, vascular disturbances, sensory loss, and reflex changes related to the upper extremity. We find that the diagnosis of thoracic outlet is often vague and in many cases is used as a diagnosis of exclusion when other causes related to such signs and symptoms have been ruled out.

Some of the earliest descriptions of neurovascular compromise in the lateral aspect of the neck were made in the 1700s when Hunald reported on cases of neurovascular compromise as a result of an anomalous rib associated with the last cervical vertebrae.[44] Decompression of the neurovascular bundle by removal of the cervical rib was, and still is, a method of treatment when the neurovascular bundle appears

to be excessively "arched" over this rib or stretched over an elongated cervical transverse process. This course results in traction to the neurovascular bundle.

Since that time, the course that the neurovascular bundle takes from the neck to the axilla has been carefully studied in order to better understand potential entrapment sites. The subclavian veins that typically drain into the brachiocephalic veins lie on the first rib between the anterior scalene and the subclavius muscles (Figure 2-22). The right subclavian artery that branches off the brachiocephalic artery and the left subclavian artery that typically arises from the arch of the aorta travel with the lower trunk of the brachial plexus to lie between the anterior and middle scalene muscles (Figure 2-23). The space through which these vessels and nerves travel from the neck through the upper lateral chest and into the axilla is referred to as the thoracic outlet. Several specific anatomical locations within this region can be the sites of mechanical compromise (Figure 2-24). These sites include the

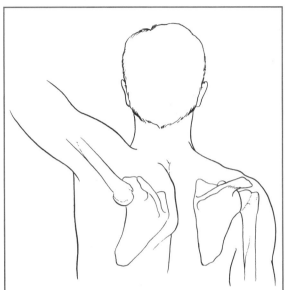

Figure 2-18. The "winging" of the scapula occurs when the medial border of the scapula loses contact with the chest wall because of loss of resting muscle tension of the serratus anterior.

interscalene triangle, or space between the anterior and middle scalenes; the substance of the muscle bellies themselves; over the cervical transverse processes; in the costoclavicular space; and the coracopectoral tunnel, which is found under the pectoralis minor muscle.

The neurovascular bundle must cross over the top of the first rib. The axons contributing to the formation of the T1 ventral ramus and the lower trunk of the brachial plexus have an especially arched pathway resembling an inverted "U" over the first rib. During full shoulder elevation, the clavicle rotates on its longitudinal axis (see Chapter 4), and therefore the space between the first rib and the clavicle is further narrowed.[41]

It is important to note that various arm and scapula movements have the potential to alter the architecture of the spaces that the neurovascular bundle traverses. Space occupying conditions such as cervical ribs, bony callus from old fractures of the clavicle or ribs, and apical lung tumors, or the presence of fibrous bands, can also compromise the plexus and vasculature by altering the dimensions within the thoracic outlet.

Whereas anatomical variants and congenital anomalies can result in signs and symptoms of thoracic

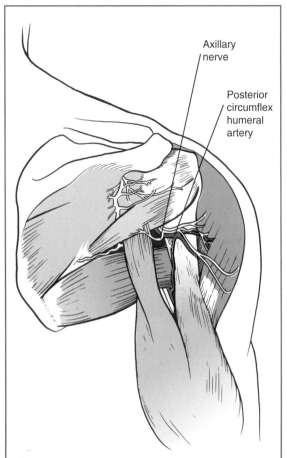

Axillary nerve

Posterior circumflex humeral artery

Figure 2-19. The axillary nerve in the shoulder runs over the posterior and inferior aspect of the shoulder joint capsule and then emerges from the quadrilateral space to supply the deltoid and teres minor muscles. The quadrilateral space is bounded by the teres minor superiorly, the long head of the triceps medially, the humeral laterally, and the teres major inferiorly. In its course around the humerus, the nerve travels with the posterior humeral circumflex artery.

outlet syndrome, the majority of nonsurgical presentations in the clinic are due to altered mechanics of the shoulder girdle or upper back and neck.[23] Typically, the age of onset is between 20 and 40, and it is more common in women than men. Poor posture and weak shoulder girdle and scapular muscles often accompany such presentations.

Thoracic outlet syndrome can be classified into two types: neurological and vascular.[35] Various tests have

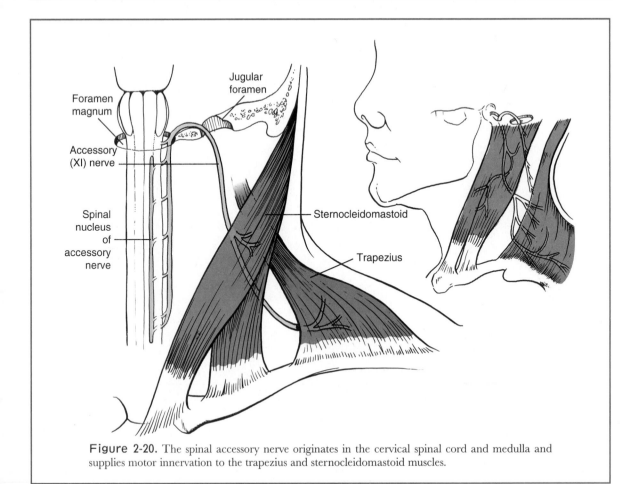

Figure 2-20. The spinal accessory nerve originates in the cervical spinal cord and medulla and supplies motor innervation to the trapezius and sternocleidomastoid muscles.

been described that are intended to mechanically stress the neurovascular bundle or alter the space it travels in order to reproduce the patient's symptoms (Figure 2-25). These tests have a high incidence of false-positive results and therefore cannot be relied on as diagnostic in and of themselves. Objective signs such as EMG changes, temperature or color changes in the hand that are vascular in nature, or neurological signs such as muscle weakness, weakness of grasp and loss of hand coordination, and reflex changes provide more meaningful information. In addition to pain, patients may also complain of paresthesias in the upper extremity, a feeling of heaviness of the arm, arm fatigue, and swelling in the hand.

Nonsurgical management focuses on analysis of upper quarter mechanics in order to alleviate compression to the neurovascular bundle. We prefer to use a program designed to influence the potential stress points from the neck to the axilla. It includes specific stretches to the scalene musculature, specific stretches for the pectoralis minor muscle, strengthening of the abdominal mechanism (since the abdominal muscles are primarily responsible for maintaining the postural relationships of the abdomen, thorax and shoulder girdle, and cervical spine), and strengthening of the scapula retractors, scapula upward rotators (serratus anterior and trapezius), and the posterior rotator cuff (see Chapter 6).[33] It is important to review sitting and sleeping postures with the patient in order to design the optimal positions that will help to decrease any mechanical stress to the neurovascular bundle along its complete course from the neck to the axilla. Also, the patient should be carefully instructed in the optimal postural positioning of the shoulder girdle, thorax, and abdomen, in addition to that of the cervical spine.

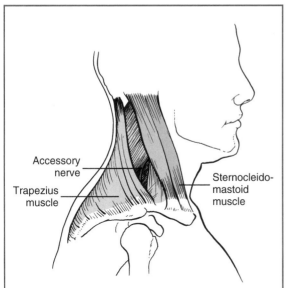

Figure 2-21. The spinal accessory nerve travels through the sternocleidomastoid muscle and posterior triangle of the neck to reach the trapezius muscle. This nerve is vulnerable to compression and traction injuries because of its superficial location.

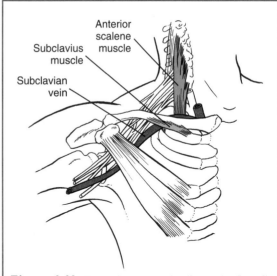

Figure 2-22. The subclavian veins lie on the first rib between the anterior scalene and subclavius muscles.

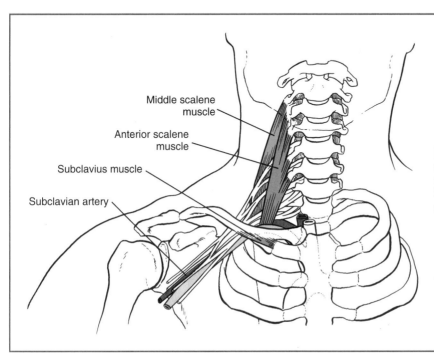

Figure 2-23. The subclavian arteries travel with the lower trunk of the brachial plexus to lie between the anterior and middle scalene muscles.

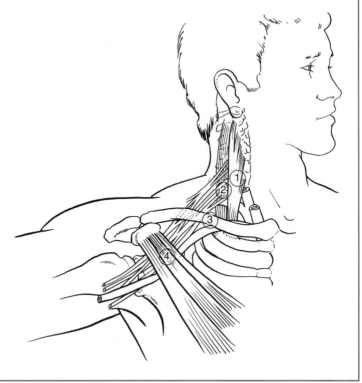

Figure 2-24. The thoracic outlet is the space through which the neurovascular bundle travels and a site of potential nerve entrapment. It is located between the (1) anterior and middle scalenes, at the region of the (2) cervical transverse process, between the (3) clavicle and first rib, and under the (4) pectoralis minor muscle.

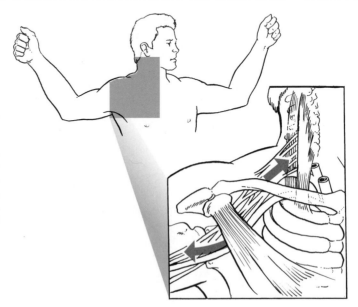

Figure 2-25. Tests used to assess for thoracic outlet syndrome are designed to mechanically compromise the neurovascular bundle between the scalene muscles, in the costoclavicular space, or under the pectoralis minor. The examiner who understands this anatomy can place the arm and shoulder in positions and observe whether vascular or neurological signs can be reproduced. Always remember that such tests have a high incidence of false-positive and false-negative results and therefore will not render a diagnosis in and of themselves.

Articular Neurology of the Shoulder

Nerve fibers that supply the joints of the body follow Hilton's law, which states that the nerves to the muscles that act on the joint also supply branches to the joint itself and the skin over the muscle. Thus the neural supply to the key joints of the shoulder region include (Figure 2-26):

- The glenohumeral joint supplied primarily by the axillary, musculocutaneous, suprascapular, and subscapular nerves
- The acromioclavicular joint supplied by the lateral supraclavicular nerves that arise from the cervical plexus and the suprascapular nerve
- The sternoclavicular joint supplied from the medial supraclavicular nerve branching from the cervical plexus and the small subclavian nerve that arises from the early part of the brachial plexus

These nerves integrate sensory afferents with motor efferents. They carry sensory afferents from the joint and the muscle-tendon units, motor supply to the extrafusal and intrafusal muscle fibers, and vasomotor efferents for the vasculature associated with the joint.

Nociceptive sensory nerve endings are distributed among the joint capsule and ligaments and recognize painful sensations that occur when the joint capsule or supporting ligaments are mechanically or chemically stressed. These sensory afferents are largely free nerve endings. Ruffini and Pacinian afferents, as well as undifferentiated encapsulated nerve endings, all of which are types of mechanoreceptor sensory nerve endings, have also been found within the glenohumeral joint capsule and supporting ligaments.[45]

Whereas the Ruffini endings respond to stretch, the Pacinian endings respond to compressive and tensile forces. These peripheral receptors and other encapsulated mechanoreceptors and free nerve endings are essentially biological transducers that have the unique ability to convert physical, chemical, and thermal energy into an action potential in the neuron associated with that particular receptor. The resulting action potential reaches the CNS, whereupon it produces reflex responses at the spinal cord and brainstem levels, or conscious awareness of the stimuli at the cerebral cortex level.[19] At the spinal cord level local reflexes ensue and the input is further modulated through descending cortical or brainstem tracts. Additionally, input from these mechanoreceptors and nociceptors ultimately ascends via multisynaptic pathways to converge on brainstem nuclei, the cerebellum, and the cerebral cortex.

Since much of the glenohumeral joint capsule is typically lax in the resting position, very little mechanical stress is placed on the mechanoreceptors. The tightening of specific regions of the capsule and ligaments that occurs with motion results in deformation of the mechanoreceptors. For example, the inferior glenohumeral ligament (see Chapter 4) is most lax with the arm at its side, but in external rotation and in the high-five position, there is a marked increase in ligament tension, which activates the capsular and ligament mechanoreceptors. The middle glenohumeral ligament becomes taut between 45 and 75 degrees of external rotation, again potentially increasing the activation of the joint mechanoreceptors. Although there is a wide distribution of mechanoreceptors within most of the glenohumeral joint capsular tissues, no mechanoreceptors appear in the glenoid labrum or subacromial bursa.

The presence of mechanoreceptors in the joint implies several functions, the most notable of which is synergistic linkage with the musculature of the shoulder joint and shoulder proprioception. The synergistic connection between ligaments and musculature was first described in the knee.[38,39] This important concept has now been extended to the shoulder joint.[20] Specifically, reflex arcs are present between the mechanoreceptors of the joint capsule and the muscles that cross the joint. Shoulder joint stability is thus more than the passive restraining ability of the specialized connective tissues of the shoulder. Stimulation of the articular mechanoreceptors associated with branches of the axillary nerve results in immediate and systematic reflex muscle contractions from the subscapularis, supraspinatus, and infraspinatus muscles. Such direct reflex connections between the mechanoreceptors of the joint and the cuff muscles suggest a neuromotoric contribution to joint stability. Joint stability is the sum total of the contribution of the musculature and the capsular restraints linked to the nervous system as a result of afferent mechanoreceptor input and efferent motor output.

In addition to the mechanoreceptors associated with the joint capsules and ligaments, a sophisticated receptor system is also associated with the muscles and tendons surrounding the joints. Golgi tendon organs and muscle spindles are essential components of the musculature of the shoulder joint.[19] It is particularly relevant to consider the presence of Golgi tendon organs, highly sensitive tension receptors located in

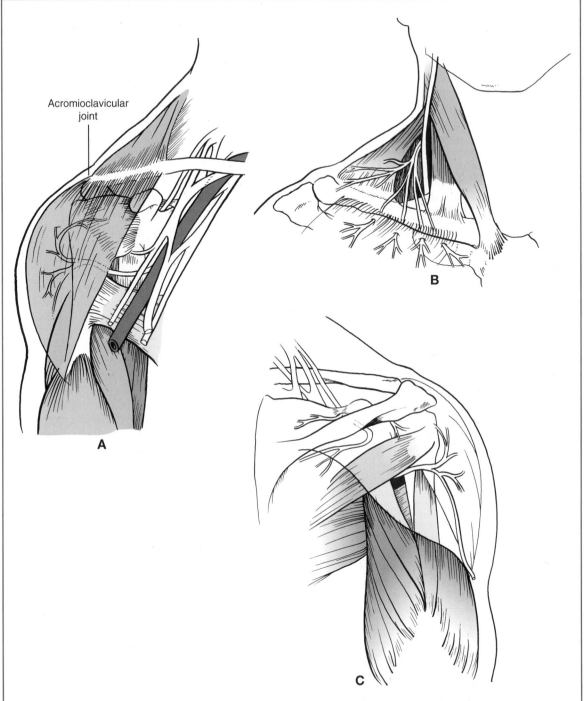

Figure 2-26. Innervation of the glenohumeral joint is supplied primarily by the axillary, musculocutaneous, suprascapular, and subscapular nerves. Views **A** and **C** show the anterior and posterior views of this rich neural supply to the glenohumeral joint and surrounding tissues respectively, whereas view **B** illustrates the neural supply to the anterior structures, including the acromioclavicular (supplied by the lateral supraclavicular nerves that arise from the cervical plexus and the suprascapular nerve) and sternoclavicular joints (supplied by the medial supraclavicular nerve branching from the cervical plexus and the small subclavian nerve arising from the early part of the brachial plexus).

the rotator cuff tendons, because of the intimate relationship of the tendons to the shoulder joint capsule (see Chapter 4). An intricate feedback mechanism relaying proprioceptive input from the capsular connective tissues to the CNS exists: contraction of the rotator cuff muscles stimulates the Golgi tendon organs and the joint capsule mechanoreceptors, providing immediate feedback on joint activity to the CNS. When you consider the partial thickness rotator cuff tendon tear (or complete thickness tear) in combination with a lax, damaged glenohumeral joint capsule, input from the Golgi tendon organs and mechanoreceptors of the joint is diluted and the important link between afferent input and efferent output is marginal at best.

As noted earlier, this complex of mechanoreceptors located within the joint structures themselves, as well as the surrounding muscles and tendons, is largely responsible for communicating proprioceptive information to all parts of the CNS, including the spinal cord, cerebellum, and cerebral cortex. Proprioception includes the awareness of joint movement (kinesthesia or rate of movement) and joint position sense (extent of movement). Input from the muscles to the CNS via the muscle spindles also assists in the analysis of the resistance to movement, and tension within a muscle results from continuous feedback and feed-forward loops of afferents and efferents that are associated with the muscle spindle.

In addition to these proprioceptive functions, the mechanoreceptors are responsible for controlling the resting tension of the muscle and generating reflex responses.[31] Input from the mechanoreceptors ultimately affects the state of muscle contraction via influence on the motor neurons responsible for extrafusal muscle fiber contraction (the skeletal muscle) and intrafusal muscle fiber contraction (the muscle spindle).

Because the shoulder has such a wide range of motion over the different joints and articulations, mechanoreceptors associated with the joint are activated through an extraordinarily wide range, and the CNS is subjected to a barrage of information from the receptor system. This input converges on the spinal cord, where simple local reflexes, subcortical influences, or cortical override results in the coordination and synergy between the glenohumeral, scapulothoracic, and cervical spine muscles.

Later (see Chapters 3 and 4) we will refer to factors that contribute to glenohumeral stability. One of the most important but least understood of these factors is the contribution of the nervous system to shoulder stability. A continuous interplay between the sensory afferents coming from the joint capsule and its supporting ligaments, muscles, and tendons and the motor efferents of the alpha and gamma motor neurons provides for the essential balance of motor activity to allow the joint with the greatest mobility in the body to simultaneously remain stable. Loss of this key interplay may be one of the primary problems with the unstable glenohumeral joint. The mechanoreceptors of the capsule are stretch sensitive; therefore lengthened capsular and ligamentous tissue as a result of injury most likely decreases mechanoreceptor input to the CNS. Several studies have demonstrated that patients who have had glenohumeral dislocations have proprioceptive deficits, most likely as a result of capsular and ligamentous damage.[25,26,37,43] Conversely, it has been suggested that improved proprioception of the glenohumeral joint may occur after radio frequency assisted thermal capsular shift in multidirectional instability because of a mechanical tightening of lax capsular tissues.[10]

In essence, it is the unconscious activation of the dynamic stabilizers coupled with the properly timed and synchronized co-activation of musculature associated with the scapulothoracic articulation and the acromioclavicular, sternoclavicular, and glenohumeral joints that are the essential pieces of rehabilitation for mechanical shoulder disorders. While oftentimes a rehabilitation plan focuses on restoration of range of motion and strength of the shoulder as measured by maximum weight lifted, torque generated, or endurance as determined by repetitions to failure, these measure only a fraction of total shoulder function. We have previously discussed the concept of muscles resembling mechanical springs with varying "set points" of resting tension and the potential of muscles' stiffness (the muscles' inherent resistance to deformation) contributing to joint stability.[32] The comparison to mechanical springs allows us to consider the benefit of muscle stiffness—the resting tension or turgor of the muscle—and the inherent contribution to joint stability (Figure 2-27). As demonstrated in the lower extremity, this enhanced state of muscle readiness prepares the muscle, and consequently the joint, for external loads by heightening the sensitivity of the muscle spindle and quickens the reflexive response of the muscle.[8,29b]

This neural influence suggests several important considerations in regard to the rehabilitation process. Chapters 3 and 6 describe various resistance exercises used in training the musculature of the shoulder girdle

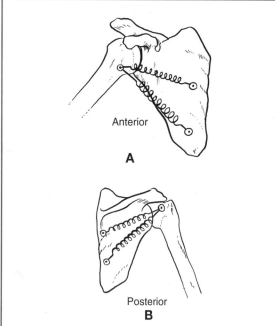

Anterior

A

Posterior

B

Figure 2-27. It is useful to consider muscles as mechanical springs with a resting tension associated with the spring. Views **A** and **B** show the anterior and posterior aspects of the rotator cuff as springs. An increase in resting muscle tension results in increased capsular tension and more compression to the joint, both of which enhance glenohumeral stability.

cuff and the orientation of the major extrinsic muscles of the shoulder are understood.

2. Varying the middle segment (elbow motion) regardless of the pattern direction. All too often the diagonal is used with the elbow kept in the extended position. These shoulder patterns are of neuromotoric value only when the clinician varies the technique to allow the elbow to move from flexion to extension or extension to flexion, and not simply remain in flexion or remain in extension during any pattern direction. Applying the technique in this manner begins to more closely reproduce the sensorimotor demands of the upper extremity in work, sport, and activities of daily living. Furthermore, it is an important consideration that acknowledges the important roles the biceps and triceps play in concert with other shoulder musculature.

3. Proper use of rhythmic stabilization. This technique requires the clinician to maintain keen sensory awareness of the patient's attempt at movement within the pattern. It is far more than simply an isometric hold in different ranges. If properly executed, this technique incorporates the essential rotary component and elbow component and discretely and subtly alters the rotary or diagonal resistance at different points of the range. The clinician can thus position the joint in weak or vulnerable ranges and begin the process of gradually challenging the extremity for neuromotoric control.

Another technique to help establish neuromuscular control uses controlled plyometrics. Plyometrics refers to exercises that challenge the neuromuscular system to produce the maximal force output in the shortest possible time. The key to a plyometric exercise is the *time* it takes for the muscle to reverse from a lengthening phase to a shortening phase. This implies that the rate, not the magnitude, of the stretch determines the storage of elastic energy and the subsequent rapid implementation of this stored energy into work.

Plyometric exercises endeavor to rapidly store energy in the muscles and then dissipate the energy in a manner that allows the elastic properties of the muscle to be combined with the active contraction of the muscle. Consequently, this type of training has the added benefit of enhancing the tolerance and capacity of the muscle for increased stretch loads. This is particularly important for activities in which the glenohumeral joint will be placed in positions vulnerable for subluxation or dislocation.

and trunk. Wilk has described the importance of neuromuscular control of the shoulder complex and its importance to the patient in developing and improving neuromotoric control of the shoulder complex during the rehabilitation process.[47,48,49] We agree that this aspect of rehabilitation is critical and use several variations of such training in the clinical setting to help develop neuromuscular control.

One of the first methods used is proprioceptive neuromuscular facilitation (PNF) technique. This technique is more involved than simply moving the extremity through a pattern, and three of its aspects are especially relevant to shoulder rehabilitation. These include:

1. Emphasis on the rotary component of the motion regardless of whether the pattern is one of full range movement or static holds. This rotary component is the essential element of the pattern in shoulder rehabilitation when the role of the rotator

This type of training program requires that the sensory system—the stretch to the muscle spindle and the Golgi tendon organs and the stretch or compression to the mechanoreceptors of the joint—ultimately drive the resultant desired muscle contraction. Therefore plyometric exercises are useful for training the sensorimotor system. Many plyometric exercises have been described for the lower extremity (box jumps, squats, bounding). These exercises can also be effective in shoulder rehabilitation if carefully adapted to the specific patient needs. Examples using medicine balls of varying weights and circumferences with an emphasis on the rate of reversing the muscle action from the lengthening phase to the shortening phase include:

- Medicine ball "presses" from the bench press position or medicine ball presses from the incline bench position
- Two-handed soccer throws
- Underhand two-handed side throws, single-arm catch and throws, or push-ups (with knees on floor) to 4-inch block (being very aware of the potential for posterior shear at the glenohumeral joint (see Chapter 4)
- Push-ups (with knees on floor) from a 4-inch block to floor and back up to 4-inch block (again, aware of the posterior shear at the glenohumeral joint)
- Modifications of the plyometric push-ups with the patient "falling" toward a wall (as in a wall pectoralis major stretch) and pushing away quickly
- Plyometric sit-ups using elastic energy of muscles involved in push pressing activities or plyometric sit-ups using elastic energy from shoulder extensors

The last two exercises offer excellent ways to incorporate training of the shoulder girdle and abdominal mechanism.

The key to the exercises is that the impact is quickly absorbed (fast eccentric phase—stimulus to the mechanoreceptors of the joint and the muscle), which is followed by as "explosive" a contraction as possible (powerful concentric phase—rapid conversion of sensory input into motor action).

SUMMARY

We have examined several aspects of nervous system function and dysfunction in the shoulder complex. We described disorders of neural tissue that can give rise to the perception of shoulder pain, such as nerve root disorders, peripheral nerve injuries, and pain referred from structures outside the shoulder region. In addition, we considered the poorly understood phenomenon of sensorimotor integration over the shoulder.

Very often shoulder pain is analyzed simply on the basis of a suspected mechanical etiology. The cause of shoulder dysfunction is much more complex than simply joint laxity of the glenohumeral joint capsule or compression of the subacromial bursa or rotator cuff tendons under the coracoacromial arch. There is an increased reliance on the precise functioning of the neuromuscular system in meeting both stability and mobility demands because the shoulder joint does not have exceptional bony stability. The unique interplay of the cervical spine, scapulothoracic articulation, and sternoclavicular, acromioclavicular, and glenohumeral joints is the result of a continuous interaction between afferent and efferent (sensory and motor) neuron loops that regulate shoulder function at the reflex, subcortical, and cortical levels. This suggests the important influence of the nervous system for optimal function. An early and safe return to activity after injury is just as important in maintaining CNS health as it is in maintaining musculoskeletal health. We suggest that restoration of function includes integration of the neuromusculoskeletal system, just as it does with the cervical spine, low back, and other peripheral joints.

REFERENCES

1. April C, Dwyer A, Bogduk N: Cervical zygapophyseal joint pain patterns II: a clinical evaluation, *Spine* 15:458, 1990.
2. Arboleya L, Garcia A: Suprascapular nerve entrapment of occupational etiology: clinical and electrophysiological characteristics, *Clin Exp Rheumatol* 11:665, 1993.
3. Asami A, Sonohata M: Bilateral suprascapular nerve entrapment syndrome associated with rotator cuff tear, *J Shoulder Elbow Surg* 9:70, 2000.
4. Blom S, Dahlback LO: Nerve injuries in dislocations of the shoulder joint and fractures of the neck of the humerus: a clinical and electromyographic study, *Acta Chir Scand* 136:461, 1970.
5. Bryan WJ, Wild JJ Jr: Isolated infraspinatus atrophy: a common cause of posterior shoulder pain and weakness in throwing athletes? *Am J Sports Med* 17:130, 1989.
6. Clancy W, Brand R, Bergfeld J: Upper trunk brachial plexus injuries in contact sports, *Am J Sports Med* 5:209, 1977.
7. Cyriax J: *Textbook of orthopaedic medicine*, vol 1, London, 1978, Bailliere Tindall.
8. DeMont RG, Riemann BL, Ryu KH, et al: The influence of foot position, knee joint angle, and gender on knee muscle joint complex stiffness, *J Athl Train* 34:115, 1999.
9. DiBenedetto M, Markey K: Electrodiagnostic localization of traumatic upper trunk brachial plexopathy, *Arch Phys Med Rehabil* 65:15, 1984.
10. Dodenhoff R, Reilly P, Ilk A, et al: Shoulder proprioception after radiofrequency assisted thermal capsular shift.

Presented at the American Academy of Orthopedics 67th Annual Meeting, Orlando, Fla, March 2000.

11. Drez D Jr: Suprascapular neuropathy in the differential diagnosis of rotator cuff injuries, *Am J Sports Med* 4:43, 1976.

12. Dunn AW: Trapezius paralysis after minor surgical procedures in the posterior clavicle triangle, *South Med J* 67:312, 1974.

13. Duralde XA: Neurologic injuries in the athlete's shoulder, *J Athlet Training* 3:316, 2000.

14. Dwyer A, April C, Bogduk N: Cervical zygapophyseal joint pain patterns I: a study of normal volunteers, *Spine* 15:453, 1990.

15. Gardner E: The innervation of the shoulder joint, *Anat Rec* 102:1, 1948.

16. Goodman CE, Kenrick MM, Blum MV: Long thoracic nerve palsy: a follow-up study, *Arch Phys Med Rehabil* 56:352, 1975.

17. Gregg JR, Lobosky D, Harty M, et al: Serratus anterior paralysis in the young athlete, *J Bone Joint Surg Am* 61:825, 1979.

18. Grieve G: Referred pain. In Grieve G, editor: *Modern manual therapy of the vertebral column.* Edinburgh, 1986, Churchill Livingstone.

19. Grigg P: Peripheral neural mechanism in proprioception, *J Sports Rehabil* 3:2, 1994.

20. Guanche C, Knatt T, Solomonow M, et al: The synergistic action of the capsule and shoulder muscles, *Am J Sports Med* 23:301, 1995.

21. Hester P, David N, Caborn M, et al: Cause of long thoracic nerve palsy: a possible dynamic fascial sling cause, *J Shoulder Elbow Surg* 9(1):31, 2000.

22. Hirasawa Y: Injuries to peripheral nerve in sport, *Semin Orthop* 3:240, 1988.

23. Karas SE: Thoracic outlet syndrome, *Clin Sports Med* 9:297, 1990.

24. Katzman BM, Bozentka DJ: Peripheral nerve injuries secondary to missiles, *Hand Clin* 15:233, 1999.

25. Lephart SM, Henry TJ: The physiological basis for open and closed kinetic chain rehabilitation for the upper extremity, *J Sport Rehabil* 5:71, 1996.

26. Lephart SM, Warner JP, Borsa PA, et al: Proprioception of the shoulder joint in healthy, unstable, and surgically repaired shoulders, *J Shoulder Elbow Surg* 3(6):371, 1994.

27. Logigian EL, McInnes JM, Berger AR, et al: Stretch induced spinal accessory nerve palsy, *Muscle Nerve* 2:146, 1988.

28. Loomer R, Graham B: Anatomy of the axillary nerve and its relation to the inferior capsular shift, *Clin Orthop* 243:100, 1989.

29a.Matsen FA, Thomas SC, Rockwood CS, et al: Glenohumeral instability. In Rockwood CA, Matsen FA, editors: *The Shoulder,* ed 2, Philadelphia, 1998, WB Saunders.

29b.McNair PJ, Wood GA, Marshall RN: Stiffness of the hamstring muscles and its relationship to function in anterior cruciate deficient individuals, *Clin Biomech* 7:131, 1992.

30. Mestdagh M, Drizenko A, Ghestem P: Anatomical basis of suprascapular nerve syndrome, *Anat Clin* 3:67, 1981.

31. Michelson JD, Hutchins C: Mechanoreceptors in human ankle ligaments, *J Bone Joint Surg Am* 77(2):219, 1995.

32. Porterfield JA, DeRosa C: *Mechanical low back pain: perspectives in functional anatomy,* ed 2, Philadelphia, 1998, WB Saunders.

33. Porterfield JA, DeRosa C: *Mechanical neck pain: perspectives in functional anatomy,* Philadelphia, 1995, WB Saunders.

34. Rengachary SS, Burr D, Lucas S, et al: Suprascapular nerve entrapment neuropathy: a clinical, anatomical, and comparative study, part II, *Neurosurgery* 5:447, 1979.

35. Royan G: Thoracic outlet syndrome, *J Shoulder Elbow Surg* 7:440, 1988.

36. Sicuranza MJ, McCue FC III: Compressive neuropathies in the upper extremity of athletes, *Hand Clin* 8:263, 1992.

37. Smith RH, Brunolti J: Shoulder kinesthesia after anterior glenohumeral joint dislocation, *Phys Ther* 69:106, 1989.

38. Solomonow M, Baratta R, Zhou BH, et al: The synergistic action of the anterior cruciate ligament and thigh muscles in maintaining joint stability, *Am J Sports Med* 15:207, 1987.

39. Solomonow M, D'Ambrosia RD: Neural reflex arcs and muscle control of knee stability and motion. In Scott WN, editor: *The knee,* St. Louis, 1994, Mosby.

40. Solomonow M, Guanche C, Wink C, et al: Mechanoreceptors and reflex arc in the feline shoulder, *J Shoulder Elbow Surg* 5:139, 1996.

41. Telford E, Mottershead S: Pressure at the cervical brachial junction: an operative and anatomical study, *J Bone Joint Surg (Br)* 30B:249, 1948.

42. Thompson RC Jr, Schneider W, Kennedy T: Entrapment neuropathy of the inferior branch of the suprascapular nerve by ganglia, *Clin Orthop* 166:185, 1982.

43. Tibone JE, Fletcher J, Kao JT: Evaluation of a proprioception pathway in patients with stable and unstable shoulders with somatosensory cortical evoked potentials, *J Shoulder Elbow Surg* 6:440, 1997.

44. Tyson RR, Kaplan GF: Modern concepts of diagnosis and treatment of the thoracic outlet syndrome, *Orthop Clin North Am* 6:507, 1975.

45. Vangsness CT Jr, Ennis M, Taylor JG, et al: Neural anatomy of the glenohumeral ligaments, labrum, and subacromial bursa, *Arthroscopy* 11:180, 1995.

46. Vastamaki M, Kauppila LI: Etiological factors in isolated paralysis of the serratus anterior muscle: a report of 197 cases, *J Shoulder Elbow Surg* 2:240, 1993.

47. Wilk KE, Arrigo CA: An integrated approach to upper extremity exercises, *Orthop Phys Ther Clin North Am* 9:337, 1992.

48. Wilk KE, Arrigo CA: Current concepts in the rehabilitation of the athletic shoulder, *J Orthop Sports Phys Ther* 18:365, 1993.

49. Wilk KE, Arrigo CA, Andrews JR: Current concepts: the stabilizing structures of the glenohumeral joint, *J Orthop Sports Phys Ther* 25(6):364, 1997.

CHAPTER 3

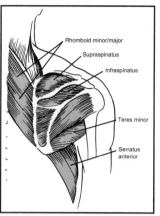

Rhomboid minor/major
Supraspinatus
Infraspinatus
Teres minor
Serratus anterior

MUSCULATURE OF THE SHOULDER COMPLEX

INTRODUCTION

The highly mobile shoulder complex represents a marvelous and fairly unique example of the way in which multiple joints and articulations are precisely controlled by extremely diverse musculature via the central and peripheral nervous systems. Whereas Chapter 2 reviewed the pertinent afferent and efferent neurology of the system and Chapter 4 will detail joint structure and function of the articulations, this chapter provides us with the framework needed to examine the roles that individual muscles and groups of muscles play in meeting the simultaneous demands of stability and mobility.

The purpose of this chapter is to assist you in gaining a three-dimensional understanding of the shoulder girdle musculature. This knowledge, when coupled with an understanding of glenohumeral, scapulothoracic, and trunk mechanics, provides the basis for the evaluation and treatment of shoulder disorders. The synergistic interplay among muscles, tendons, capsules, fascia, and bone gives us the ability to move in a coordinated

manner. This interplay is readily apparent in a study of the shoulder, which, not being a weight-bearing joint, relies heavily on the spine, trunk, and even the lower extremities to create a stable yet immediately adaptable platform from which to function. The scapulothoracic articulation in particular must quickly get into position to serve as a platform for glenohumeral motion. Such interrelationships between different regions of the musculoskeletal system is unparalleled in the human body and speaks to the complexity of analyzing shoulder disorders and then addressing them in as holistic a manner as possible. Throughout this chapter, identification of anatomical and mechanical linkages between individual muscles of the shoulder girdle and between the trunk and shoulder girdle is illustrated and discussed with the intent being to assist the clinician in the decision making processes associated with the analysis of normal and abnormal function.

We also examine muscle structure here as it relates to shoulder girdle functions and carefully consider the interconnections and mechanical linkages between different muscles. This allows us to better determine the relationship of muscle structure to function. Clinically applicable observations and suggestions are included throughout the chapter to assist you in understanding interrelationships between the anatomy and biomechanics as a foundation for use in solving problems of mechanical disorders related to the shoulder girdle complex. When muscle structure is reviewed in this manner,

 Throughout this chapter you will find small circular icons marked "DVD" (see margin). These icons identify content that is coordinated with a video clip on the DVD accompanying this text. For maximum learning benefit, go to the "Text Reference Section" on the DVD and play the coordinated clip while reading the appropriate section of text. These clips expand on and reinforce the information presented in the text.

the importance of maintaining muscular mass and strength in order to ensure coordinated movement and painless performance becomes increasingly apparent.

MUSCLE STRUCTURE

Among the many characteristics of muscle, there are four that are important to consider when studying its function and relationship to force transmission: structure, attachment considerations, relationship of the muscle to the joint, and crossing relationships between different muscles (Table 3-1). Each characteristic in turn has important clinical implications. The first characteristic is the structure of the muscle. This includes not only the cross-sectional area of the muscle, but also the relationship of the muscle fiber to the tendinous attachment. Typically, the physiological cross section of a muscle is directly related to its tension generating ability. In most instances, the larger the cross-sectional area of the muscle, the greater ability it has to generate force. Increases in the cross-sectional area of skeletal muscle via strength training is a biological adaptation resulting from increased workload placed on the muscle, which is an important principle to understand when developing exercise programs. Overload is the essential ingredient for influencing increased hypertrophic changes in the muscle.

The adaptation of increased muscle size leads to an increase in the muscle's capacity to generate tension. Muscle hypertrophy in response to overload training occurs primarily as a result of the enlargement of individual muscle fibers. This process of hypertrophy is directly related to the synthesis of cellular matrix, which is primarily protein and forms the contractile elements.[13] It is important to remember, however, that increases in strength, as they are typically measured in a clinical or laboratory environment, also occur as a result of neurological changes (e.g., alteration of inhibitory and facilitatory pathways) and psychological influences.

The force of a muscle contraction from a muscle with an oblique or spiral orientation can be resolved into several component vectors in addition to a force parallel to that muscle's tendon. Note, for example, the different structural arrangement of the levator scapulae (a spiral arrangement of fibers), the infraspinatus (three heads converging centrally in a tendon and encased in a fascial envelope), and the deltoid muscle (three heads converging distally in a tendon). When viewed in this manner, you can begin to appreciate that muscle function over a complex region such as the shoulder is more than merely moving the insertion toward the origin. What appears to be a simple contraction of a muscle results in unique consequences to the various tissues the muscle interfaces with. A clinician explores several of these examples when he examines individual muscles of the shoulder. Nearly every muscle in the shoulder girdle has a unique structure and muscle fiber orientation, suggesting a unique contribution to the wide scope of motion potential over a platform of stability.

The range of muscle contraction is dependent on muscle fiber length. Simply put, a muscle with long muscle fibers is designed for speed or excursion. This does not necessarily mean that a joint moves "faster" because it has muscles with long fibers associated with it. The point at which the muscle attaches to the bony lever and the manner in which the muscle-tendon unit approaches the attachment ultimately determine the speed at which the articulation moves, which is a much different concept than the speed at which a muscle shortens. Again, you see that the relationship between the muscle and its tendinous endpoints helps determine this range of contraction. Longitudinally oriented muscle fiber arrangements generate rapid muscle shortening or speed, whereas obliquely oriented muscle fibers, such as those arrangements that occur with unipennate, bipennate, or multipennate patterns, permit more muscle cells to be included in the same volume, resulting in greater tension generating ability but less potential for extensive excursions of the bony levers. The potential force of muscle contraction and the resultant range of motion are thus markedly influenced by the fiber arrangement.

Tendinous Attachment to Bone

A second consideration that influences muscle function relates to the type of tendinous attachment of the muscle to the bony levers, such as the humerus, scapula, and clavicle. Several muscles of the shoulder girdle,

---

Table 3-1. Characteristics of Muscle Influencing Function

1. Structure of the muscle
2. Attachment of the muscle to the bony lever
3. Relationship of the muscle to the joint structure
4. Crossing relationships of muscles

including the supraspinatus, infraspinatus, and teres minor, blend together to form a conjoint tendon, whereas other muscles, such as the long head of the biceps brachii, direct their effect to the labrum via a single robust tendon. Still others have a twisting or spiral course as the muscle links the two bony ends. In several key muscles of the shoulder complex, there is a twisting and spiral course. These muscles include the intricate trilaminar fiber arrangement of the pectoralis major tendon, the latissimus dorsi tendon, the muscle fibers of the levator scapulae, and the weaving of the muscle fibers of the infraspinatus. No muscle acts in isolation. Rather, a coordinated series of muscle contractions creates loads on all tissues in the region throughout the range of movement. Simply stated, the continuum of load transference between tissues results from muscle contraction.

Anatomical Relationship of Muscle to Joint

In addition to the cross-sectional area of the muscle, the fiber arrangement and orientation of the muscle fibers as well as the location of the tendon attachment in relation to the bony lever, influence the types of loads to which the articulations are subject. The differences in muscle fiber arrangement and tendinous attachments ultimately allow for a wider range of possibilities regarding the line of pull of the muscle, the speed of bony lever movement, the muscle tension generated over the related articulation, and the compression between the joint surfaces. Thus the third biomechanical and physiological consideration for each muscle is the relationship that the contractile unit has to the joint structures. When muscles act to stabilize and move the arm, they generate forces that must be weakened by the specialized connective tissues of the joint. These forces are generally torque, compression, and shear.

Torque is the force that drives one of the bony levers around an axis of motion, resulting in an arc of motion by the bony lever. This arc of motion is typical for the synovial joints of the body. Since the bony lever is moving around an axis, the distance the muscle attaches from this axis (the moment arm) determines not only the speed at which the articulation moves, but also the relative efficiency of the muscle acting to generate torque over that particular joint. Torque is important to understand because the closer that a muscle attaches to the axis of motion, the greater potential range of motion for the bony levers. This comes with an expense, however, of having a less than optimal mechanical advantage. Conversely, if a muscle is attached at a significant distance from the axis of motion, it has an excellent mechanical advantage to contribute to torque generation, but the speed at which the bony levers move is lessened.

It is also important to remember that the axis of motion is not fixed, but changes as movement occurs. This is one of the difficulties in using resistance exercise machines, which essentially have a fixed axis of motion. Such machines are commonly used when strengthening interventions are applied to the shoulder. Selectorized weight machines for muscles associated with the shoulder girdle, such as the lateral shoulder raise, incline press, overhead press, shoulder dip, elbow curl, and elbow extension machines, for example, have a fixed axis of movement, which unfortunately cannot be instantaneously aligned with the moving axes of the shoulder girdle during the exercise. When you align the axis of the glenohumeral joint with such an exercise machine to start the exercise, the instantaneous axis of motion for the glenohumeral joint assumes different positions as the bony levers move through a range, which results in misalignment between the axis of the glenohumeral joint and the axis of the exercise unit.

The articulations are also subjected to compressive loads as the muscle contracts. *Compression* as it might relate to joint structure refers to a force that is directed toward the center of the joint or perpendicular to the plane of the joint surface. Compressive loads can contribute to joint stability over the various articulations of the shoulder complex because such forces help seat the humeral head into the glenoid socket or squeeze the bones of the acromioclavicular or sternoclavicular joint together, resulting in increased joint stability.

Muscle contraction can also result in compression to subjacent tissues. When a muscle contracts, it broadens, and the broadening effect can load an underlying tissue in compression. For example, contraction of the serratus anterior muscle exerts a compressive force to the underlying subscapular bursa. Contraction of the latissimus dorsi muscle as it crosses the inferior corner of the scapula "presses" the scapula against the rib cage, which results in increased scapulothoracic stability.

Shear forces are those forces parallel to the reference joint surface that can result in a translation or sliding of one bone on the joint surface. Shear forces challenge the specialized connective tissues of the synovial joint because shear results in frictional loading, which can contribute to erosion of the two joint surfaces that are in contact with each other. This is the case with the superior surface of the rotator cuff tendons under the coracoacromial arch, the humeral head over the glenoid labrum, or the undersurface (articular surface) of the supraspinatus tendon over the posterosuperior aspect of the glenoid rim.[12,42]

The line of force of muscle contraction can often be resolved into component forces, which can then be analyzed to understand their effects over the joint structures (Figure 3-1). The combination of muscle contractions about the joint generates the sum total of forces, which ultimately determines the manner in which associated structures are stressed. Uncoordinated muscle action and muscle fatigue alter the loading pattern of the tissues. This is problematic if such loads exceed the physiological loading capacity of the tissue (see Chapter 1). For example, in the presence of damaged anterior glenohumeral ligaments, contraction of the pectoralis major can result in excessive anterior translation of the humeral head over the glenoid rim.

Crossing Relationship of Overlapping Muscles

Finally, an important anatomical arrangement of the shoulder girdle musculature that we describe and discuss throughout this chapter is the overlapping or crossing relationships of muscles that are in immediate proximity to each other, often with muscle fiber orientations being 90 degrees perpendicular to each other (Table 3-2). Our premise is that the crossing relationship increases stability and strength in that specific region, especially in regard to the development of the exercise prescription for rehabilitation, and therefore should represent the focus of strengthening exercises. This suggestion, which we couple with exploring the anatomical and biomechanical relationships between the shoulder girdle and the trunk, constitutes the essential focus in the development of strength training interventions. This concept is continually referred to throughout this chapter.

We describe the pertinent characteristics of structure, function, and clinical biomechanics for each muscle in this chapter. This review of the musculature allows you to gain different perspectives of the functional anatomy of the shoulder complex, which we will apply in the design of practical examination methods that lead to the implementation of successful interventions.

We group muscles and their relationships to surrounding structures in six sections: 1) superficial musculature, 2) scapular layer, 3) posterior scapular layer, 4) subscapular region, 5) anterior shoulder, and 6) abdominal musculature. A short list of representative exercises is included with each section to reinforce some of the actions that are inherent in the different muscles described therein. Chapter 6 focuses on the setup and technique for such exercises, as well as how they might be incorporated into the scheme of rehabilitation for mechanical shoulder disorders.

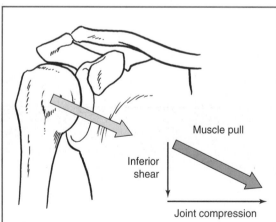

Figure 3-1. The resultant force is a single force that is the combination or sum effect of all forces directed to a joint structure. Here we see the resultant force at the glenohumeral joint at 45 degrees of abduction.

Table 3-2. Crossing Arrangements in Muscles of the Shoulder Complex

1. Latissimus dorsi and serratus anterior, posterior and lateral
2. Latissimus dorsi and gluteus maximus, posterior and central
3. Serratus anterior across the abdominal wall bilaterally (serape effect), anterior and central
4. Trapezius and rhomboids, posterior and superior
5. Pectoralis major bilaterally, anterior and superior
6. Long head of the triceps and the teres major across the infraspinatus, posterior glenohumeral joint
7. Coracobrachialis across the short head of the biceps brachii and the subscapularis, anterior glenohumeral joint

THE SUPERFICIAL MUSCULATURE

Three muscles are discussed in this section: 1) the latissimus dorsi, 2) the teres major, and 3) the trapezius. During dissection, the latissimus dorsi and trapezius muscles are readily seen on removal of the skin and superficial fat, whereas the teres major, although superficial, is not as immediately apparent. The superficial nature of each of these muscles can easily be appreciated in the living body through direct palpation and observation of muscle lines during activity.

Latissimus Dorsi

The latissimus dorsi is a large and powerful extrinsic muscle of the shoulder girdle and superficial layer of the back that contributes to the stability of the lower thoracic and lumbar spine and has essential roles in the function of the scapula and the glenohumeral joint. It is an extensive, broad, fan-shaped muscle that exerts several distinct lines of force: inferior and medial in relationship to the humerus, and superior and lateral through the thoracolumbar fascia relative to the lumbar spine and iliac crest. From its extensive attachment to the iliac crest, thoracolumbar fascia, and thoracic spinous processes, the muscle courses toward the medial lip of the bicipital groove, and as it approaches the humerus, the muscle tendon complex spirals on itself approximately 180 degrees (Figure 3-2). Here it blends with the teres major at its insertion on the humerus and controls humeral motion directly and shoulder girdle motion indirectly from several different vantage points: the pelvis, the thoracolumbar fascia, and the thoracic spine.

In addition, the course and attachments of the latissimus dorsi allow it to control the position and motion of the scapula because of its superficial position to the inferior border of the scapula. Contraction of the latissimus dorsi results in compression of the scapula on the rib cage.

When the superior border of the latissimus dorsi muscle is lifted away from the rib cage, you can also view the mechanical linkage it has with the serratus anterior muscle. Figure 3-3, *A* and *B*, demonstrates an inferior attachment of the serratus anterior to the undersurface of the latissimus dorsi. Analyzing the resultant forces of these two muscles suggests that the latissimus dorsi is pulled against the rib cage and over the inferior border of the scapula as a result of

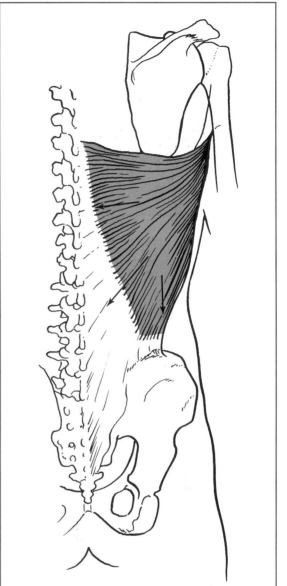

Figure 3-2. Observe the line of attachment of the latissimus dorsi muscle from the medial lip of the intertubercular groove of the humerus to the thoracic spinous processes (horizontal force line), to the thoracolumbar fascia (oblique force line), and to the iliac crest (vertical force line). Note how this muscle courses inferiorly, then passes under the lower trapezius to reach the spinous processes of the thoracic vertebrae, and finally fans out obliquely to attach to the thoracolumbar fascia and iliac crest to cover the entire posterior aspect to the trunk.

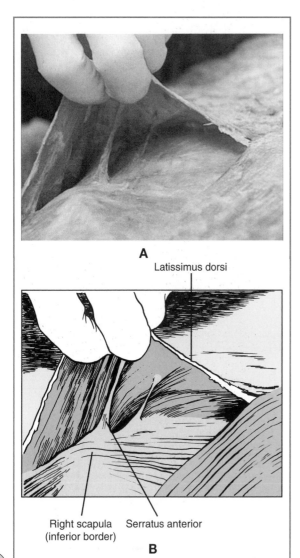

A

Latissimus dorsi

Right scapula   Serratus anterior
(inferior border)

B

Figure 3-3. **A** and **B,** The superior view of the right latissimus dorsi has been lifted off the rib cage to show its linkage to the serratus anterior muscle. This mechanical linkage suggests one muscle working with another to improve its mechanical advantage. Contraction of the serratus anterior pulls the latissimus against the rib cage and the inferior border of the scapula.

serratus anterior muscle contraction. This contributes to forming a semirigid attachment from which the serratus anterior can pull, and such a mechanism also keeps the scapula compressed against the rib cage.

The action of the latissimus dorsi over the humerus is very powerful. It is a strong adductor, extensor, and internal rotator of the humerus. As a result, the latissimus dorsi is a key muscle in the acceleration phase of throwing. The acceleration phase, common in many overhead sports, is considered the phase of throwing during which the arm is propelled forward and a powerful internal rotation motion occurs.[20] Note that this movement is also prevalent with overhead tennis serves and volleyball spikes. The line of force of the muscle also suggests that the glenohumeral joint has an inferior shear force imparted to it as a result of the latissimus muscle contraction. Acting through the glenohumeral joint, the latissimus dorsi depresses and slightly retracts the scapulothoracic articulation, which results in an inferior shear force at the acromioclavicular joint and downward rotation at the sternoclavicular joint. Like most muscles in the neuromuscular system, the latissimus dorsi generates its greatest force closer to the midrange position, as seen when the arms are in a flexed and abducted position.[1] This muscle is especially strong in diagonal motions such as adduction toward the body and adduction and internal rotation, a common component of the proprioceptive neuromuscular facilitation (PNF) diagonal.[7]

There are several crossing relationships among muscles of the shoulder girdle complex that are important to recognize (see Table 3-2). The first is the latissimus dorsi's crossing relationship with the gluteus maximus muscle via the thoracolumbar fascia. The latissimus dorsi tightens or pulls this fascia in a superior and lateral direction. The line of force of the right latissimus dorsi, in conjunction with the inferior and lateral pull on the contralateral side of the thoracolumbar fascia via the left gluteus maximus, forms one line of an **X**. The latissimus dorsi and gluteus maximus of the contralateral side form a second line of the **X** (Figure 3-4). These four lines of pull intersect over the lumbar spine, providing force generation that crosses the midline. The crossing of these lines of force represents an area of required strength and therefore should represent a focus of exercise prescription in the development of therapeutic exercise interventions.

You can best understand the second crossing relationship involving the latissimus dorsi by viewing the musculature in the sagittal plane from humerus to iliac crest (Figure 3-5). From this vantage point the muscle can be seen to connect the shoulder girdle to the pelvis and form one arm of an **X**, with the serratus anterior forming the second arm of this **X**. This muscle

Teres Major

Even though they arise from different regions, several of the actions of the teres major and latissimus dorsi over the glenohumeral joint are similar because of their nearly blended attachments to the humerus. The teres major arises from the middle third of the lateral surface of the scapula and the intermuscular septa that separates the teres major from the teres minor and courses laterally by spiraling upward to end as a flat tendon that attaches to the medial lip of the

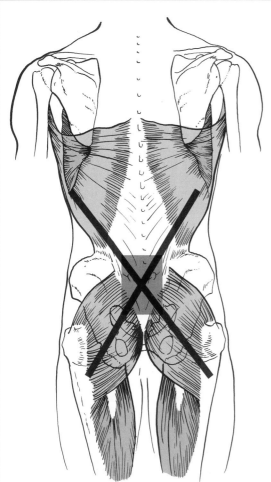

Figure 3-4. The latissimus dorsi and gluteus maximus attachment to the thoracolumbar fascia illustrates their crossing lines of force. This crossing relationship of the muscles suggests the importance of focusing an exercise program to target this and similar regions.

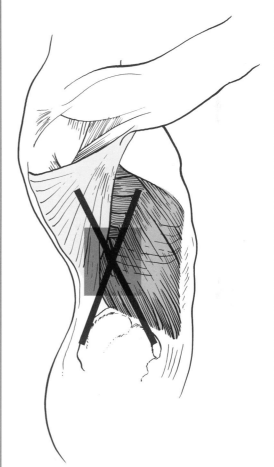

Figure 3-5. This sagittal view shows the relationship between the inferior and posterior direction of the latissimus dorsi and the inferior and anterior direction of the serratus anterior. The focus of therapeutic exercise must be at the point where these opposite vectors cross.

crossing is formed as a result of the latissimus dorsi traveling from its attachment on the humerus in an inferior and posterior direction and the serratus anterior traveling from its attachment on the undersurface of the scapula in an inferior and anterior direction (see Figure 3-5). Again, analyzing the actions of muscles that overlap in perpendicular directions forms the basis for understanding the role of musculature in antigravity postures and the importance of strength for muscle groups contributing to such arrangements.

bicipital groove. The tendons of the large teres major and latissimus dorsi muscles typically intersect, which results in the teres major lying just posterior to the latissimus dorsi at the bicipital groove (Figure 3-6). The tendons of these two muscles are separated by a bursa, and their muscle bellies can be seen to unite for a short period if they are followed proximally from their attachments to the humerus.

The teres major is a stout, thick fusiform muscle, implying exceptional tension generating ability and strength potential. The actions of the teres major over the humerus are adduction, extension, and internal rotation, and like those of the latissimus dorsi are emphasized in the combined diagonal motion in PNF patterns.

Note, however, that the scapula must be effectively fixed in order for the teres major to transmit the force of muscle contraction to the humerus. Exercises for the

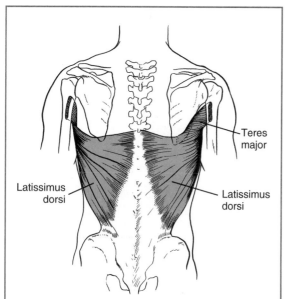

Figure 3-6. The teres major muscle spirals or twists as it travels superiorly and laterally from the middle third of the lateral border of the scapula. It briefly unites with the latissimus dorsi muscle, and the two course superiorly and laterally toward their attachment. These muscles eventually split to form separate tendons. The flat tendon of the teres major attaches to the medial lip of the bicipital groove just posterior to the latissimus dorsi. Although their innervations are different, their functions at the humerus are similar.

teres major by definition require a strong, synchronous contraction of scapular muscles such as the rhomboids and trapezius that serves to fix the medial border of the scapula and prevent it from being pulled laterally by the contraction of the teres major. Always keep this in mind when performing a shoulder adduction muscle test on a patient. Weakness may not be due to an impairment of the teres major but instead may arise because of an inability of the scapular muscle to create a stable platform from which the teres major can pull.

The spiraling structure of muscle is one in which the inferiormost aspect of muscle twists on itself enroute to its opposite attachment. What was the lowest point of the muscle at the region of its "origin" becomes the highest point at the region of the "insertion," or what was originally posterior now faces anterior. The teres major attachment on the lower aspect of the scapula becomes the superior attachment on the humerus. This spiral structure of muscle is seen in several other areas of the body, namely the teres major and latissimus dorsi on the posterior shoulder, the pectoralis major on the anterior shoulder, the levator scapulae at the medial aspect of the scapula and cervical spine, the distal end of the biceps brachii, the deep erector spinae of the low back, and the hamstrings. Each of us can also see similar spiral structural arrangements applied to the steel cables used in suspension bridges and in the twisting of the strands of rope. The spiral nature of such structures increases their ability to reduce tension because as tensile stresses are imparted to a spiral structure, the tensile load also is attenuated via increased compressive loading between the spiraled fibers. The individual fibers of the muscle or steel in the twisted cables "squeeze" together when the ends are pulled apart. A spiral structure withstands greater tensile loads because it is dissipating the force via compression and the fibers become more packed together the greater the tensile force. Spiraling creates an increased potential for tissue strength. Muscles such as the teres major, latissimus dorsi, and pectoralis major are very strong because of their cross-sectional area, as well as this unique fiber orientation.

Exercises designed to strengthen the different muscle groups are listed in Table 3-3 as a point of reference so you can begin to visualize them. Note that many of the exercises for the teres major are also ones that can be effectively used in the training of the latissimus dorsi.

Discussion in Chapter 6 focuses on exercise training descriptions, illustrations, and prescriptions.

Table 3-3. Exercises for the Superficial Musculature

Latissimus and Teres Major
Wide angled pulldowns
One-armed bench rows
Seated cable rows
Bent over rows
Standing high cable rows
Seated dips (scapular depression)
Counter weighted dips and pull-ups
PNF diagonals (extension, adduction, internal rotation)
   against pulleys

Trapezius
Shrugs
Shrug with pre-positioning humerus in external rotation
Seated rows emphasizing scapular motion in retraction
Standing high and mid row emphasizing scapular motion in
   elevation and retraction
One-arm rows
Horizontal adduction on selectorized machines
Bilateral pulley horizontal adductions

PNF, Proprioceptive neuromuscular facilitation.

Trapezius

The final muscle to be described in this superficial layer is the trapezius muscle. This large, expansive muscle with its superior, middle, and inferior heads covers the upper back and has at its center a diamond-shaped tendinous tissue often referred to as the *trapezius aponeurosis*. The connective tissue of this thick aponeurosis affords strength at the important cervicothoracic junction and acts as the base for the strong superior, horizontal, and inferior pull of the muscle. The shape of this aponeurosis also suggests that one of this muscle's main functions is to assist in the maintenance of a retracted position of the scapula (Figure 3-7).

Close examination of all three portions of this expansive muscle suggests that each region has different fiber orientation and that the varying thickness of the muscle points to histological differences. The lower portion of the trapezius that courses from the thoracic spinous processes to the medial border of the scapula appears to be composed primarily of Type I

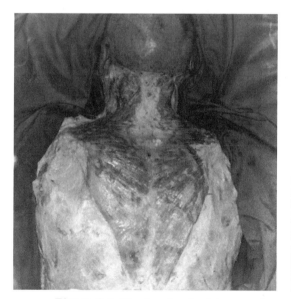
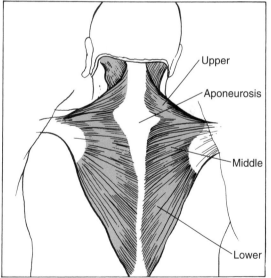

Figure 3-7. The three heads of the trapezius muscle show its central tendinous aponeurosis. The differences in structure between the upper, middle, and lower portions of the trapezius can also be appreciated. The position of the aponeurosis suggests that it serves as the foundation for the backward directed pull of the trapezius, helping to keep the scapula back toward retraction. (From Porterfield JA, DeRosa C: *Mechanical neck pain: perspectives in functional anatomy,* Philadelphia, 1994, WB Saunders.)

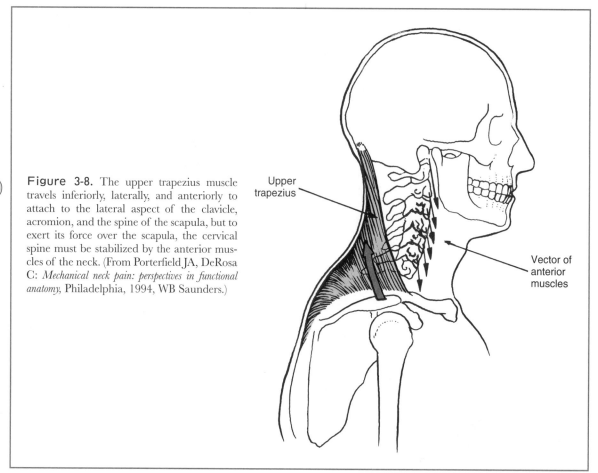

Figure 3-8. The upper trapezius muscle travels inferiorly, laterally, and anteriorly to attach to the lateral aspect of the clavicle, acromion, and the spine of the scapula, but to exert its force over the scapula, the cervical spine must be stabilized by the anterior muscles of the neck. (From Porterfield JA, DeRosa C: *Mechanical neck pain: perspectives in functional anatomy,* Philadelphia, 1994, WB Saunders.)

Upper trapezius

Vector of anterior muscles

fibers, whereas the upper portion reaching from the occiput to the lateral portion of the clavicle has a higher percentage of Type II fibers.[24,25] This may suggest that the lower portion of the trapezius is primarily involved with the maintenance of a stable scapular platform rather than being the primary muscle force responsible for the generation of torque to the scapula.[21] By comparison, upper trapezius function is primarily the generation of more dynamic, explosive, or rapid movements.

If the upper portion of the trapezius reaches the occiput (occasionally it does not), it is attached by a thin, fibrous lamina to the medial third of the superior nuchal line. Over the cervical spine it is attached to the ligamentum nuchae and the spinous processes.[52] These muscle fibers typically angle inferiorly, laterally, and anteriorly to reach the lateral third of the clavicle, the

acromion, and the spine of the scapula. This directly corresponds to the same bony areas from which the deltoid muscle originates. The primary actions of this portion of the upper trapezius muscle are scapular elevation and strong retraction. In order for the trapezius to exert its force over the scapula, the cervical spine must be stabilized by the anterior neck flexors to allow a fixed point of origin (Figure 3-8). By virtue of its clavicular and acromion attachment, the upper trapezius, like the anterior deltoid, is an extremely important stabilizer of the acromioclavicular joint because these muscles completely span the joint.[26,50] The upper trapezius muscle attachment allows the upper trapezius to literally serve as a dynamic suspensory "cable" for the upper extremity.

The middle trapezius is a much thicker portion of the muscle when compared with the upper trapezius.

The fibers are laced with connective tissue as it courses laterally from the spinous processes and the middle portion of the trapezius aponeurosis toward the spine of the scapula. Because of the inclination of the spine of the scapula, the direction of pull is not oriented parallel to the spine of the scapula. This is an important point to remember when visualizing the scapula moving or fixated in varying degrees of upward or downward rotation.

The coarse structure and the thick tendinous insertion at the spine of the scapula and at its attachment into the thickest portion of the aponeurosis suggest strength and the importance of maintaining scapular retraction. There is a direct relationship between the forces at the glenohumeral joint, the forces at suprahumeral space, and the position of the scapula.[19,41] Increasing and maintaining strength, power, and endurance in this part of the upper back is paramount to painless function and enhanced performance of the shoulder girdle. Learning to move the scapula irrespective of the humerus and visualizing the direction of muscle pull represent key considerations in training the shoulder complex.

The lower portion of the trapezius is a long, thick muscle, traveling inferior and medial from the spine of the scapula and the fascia covering the infraspinatus muscle to the thoracic spinous processes (Figure 3-9). Because of the similarity of angles in the anatomical position, the muscle fiber orientation of the lower portion of the trapezius and the spine of the scapula forms a nearly continuous line that begins at the acromion and terminates in the lower thoracic spine. The attachment of the trapezius to the spine of the scapulae is very tendinous, which suggests the convergence of significant forces. You can appreciate this by viewing the deep surface of the lower trapezius as it is reflected superiorly (Figure 3-10).

Keeping in mind that no muscle works in isolation and that any motion of the scapula requires synergistic muscle activity to stabilize the occiput, cervical spine,

Figure 3-9. The attachments of the lower trapezius show how the muscle is also attached to the superficial surface of the infraspinatus fascia.

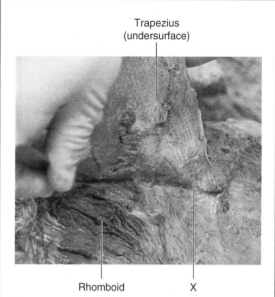
Figure 3-10. Note the deep surface of the trapezius in this photograph of the thick tendinous attachments of the lower trapezius to the spine of the scapula (marked by the **X**).

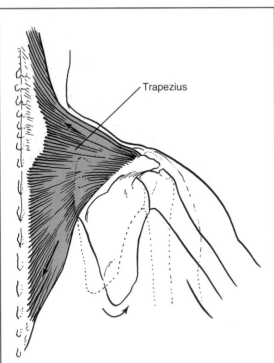

Trapezius

Figure 3-11. The synchronous action of the upper trapezius as it pulls up and back on the distal ⅓ of the clavicle and acromion, and the inferior and medial pull of the lower trapezius at the medial aspect of the spine of the scapula, create an upward rotation of the scapula.

acromioclavicular and sternoclavicular joints (Figure 3-11). Also the scapula is pivoted over the rib cage, with the lower trapezius fixing the medial aspect of the spine of the scapula and the upper trapezius pulling upward on the acromion and the lateral aspect of the clavicle. The middle trapezius works with the lower trapezius to provide a strong stabilizing force by holding the scapula against the rib cage, which helps to create a pivot point. In addition, the lower serratus anterior contributes to scapular rotation especially during the early phase of humeral elevation.[8,49] This upward rotation is essential for complete elevation of the arm. Loss of any two of the four muscles considered critical for arm elevation, the trapezius, serratus anterior, deltoid, or supraspinatus, renders it impossible to actively elevate the arm.[23]

Often the exercises of choice for the trapezius muscles are shoulder shrugs against resistance. It must be noted, however, that the upper trapezius has a greater propensity toward type II fibers, implying more dynamic rather than postural function. We typically have the patient perform a more vertical motion of the scapula initially and then gradually change the angle of cervical and thoracic flexion during subsequent bouts of the exercise. This, combined with the introduction of slight external rotation of the humerus to encourage the patient to retract the scapula, permits the recruitment of different components of the upper and middle trapezius muscles (see Table 3-3). Changing the angle and direction of movement during resistance exercises is advantageous because it directs the training effect (strength, power, and endurance) to different components of the desired muscle groups (see Chapter 6).

For patients with altered shoulder mechanics and impingement problems, strong shrugging exercises may compound their shoulder problem. Better tolerated exercises might include those that strengthen and increase the endurance capabilities of the lower and middle trapezius, such as strong scapular retraction combined with extension and external rotation of the glenohumeral joint using free weights, mid-rows against resistance, standing pulls from a power rack, and the classic "clean" component of the clean and jerk weightlifting maneuver.

THE SCAPULAR LAYER

We define the scapular layer as the levator scapulae, rhomboid major, rhomboid minor, and serratus anterior muscles. All of these muscles converge on the

and thoracic spine, you will understand that the upper fibers of the trapezius assist with elevation of the shoulder girdle, the middle fibers assist with retraction, and the lower trapezius assists with depression. The three heads of the trapezius muscle work in conjunction with all other muscles that attach to the scapula to allow it to serve as a stable but moving platform.

In addition to these actions, upward rotation of the scapula occurs as a result of the combined activity of the upper and lower trapezius and the serratus anterior. Because the lower portion of the trapezius is attached to the spine of the scapula and the upper trapezius is attached to the lateral third of the clavicle and acromion, the combined action of those two portions of the trapezius contributes a force coupled to the scapula that results in an upward rotary movement of the scapula on the thorax. Note also that any movement of the scapula results in motion at the medial border of the scapula. Each of these muscles plays key roles in scapular mobility and stability, and an increased knowledge of their roles results in greater attention toward them when designing therapeutic interventions for shoulder disorders.[22,30,38]

Levator Scapulae

The levator scapulae muscle, a muscle with a surprisingly large cross-sectional area, attaches at the superior medial corner of the scapula, and from this broad, thick attachment it courses superior and medial to attach to the first three or four cervical transverse processes. The cross-sectional area of this muscle is actually greater than that of the upper trapezius,

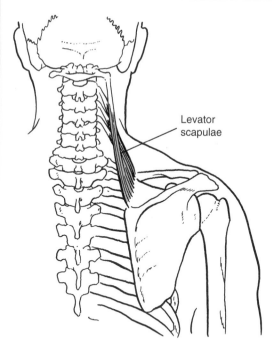

Figure 3-12. Note the attachments of the levator scapulae as they travel superior from the vertebral border of the scapulae and "twist" to attach to the transverse processes of C1 to C4. Recognize that contraction of this muscle creates forces to both mobile attachments, which makes stabilizing one attachment before moving the other an important teaching point during exercise instruction.

which implies significant tension generating ability. The twisting of the muscle as it spirals up from the medial border of the scapula toward the transverse processes results in fibers that attach to the inferiormost aspect of the vertebral border of the scapula and insert on the superiormost cervical transverse processes. Conversely, the superiormost attachment of the levator scapulae to the top of the superior medial border of the scapula attaches to the lowest cervical transverse processes (Figure 3-12). Similar to the structure of a braided rope, as the musculotendinous unit twists, it can withstand a greater tensile load as it stabilizes and elevates the scapula.

The levator scapulae muscle elevates the scapula and provides strong stability to the cervical spine. Indeed, its cross-sectional area and spiral nature suggests that it is quite effective in carrying out these actions. In addition, it fixes the superomedial corner of the scapula, which allows the lower portion of the serratus anterior to strongly and upwardly rotate the scapula.[32]

Like many muscles of the shoulder girdle, the levator scapulae is attached to moveable segments at both ends of the muscle, in this case, the scapula and the cervical spine. For motion to occur, one of the movable attachments must become stabilized. Elevation of the left scapula via the left levator scapulae muscle, for example, results in backward bending, left rotation, and left side bending forces being placed over the cervical spine as a result of levator scapulae activity. The clinician must consider this when exercising the shoulder girdle when injuries or degenerative changes are present in the cervical spine, especially if the scapulothoracic muscles are exercised against resistance. The neck may need to be prepositioned in order to prepare partial unloading of injured tissues in that region.

Tenderness to palpation over the superomedial region of the scapula is common in the examination of patients with neck pain or rotator cuff injuries. Because the levator scapulae is oriented to dynamically check anterior shear of the cervical spine, the tenderness over the superomedial aspect of the scapula may be the result of reflex muscle guarding and increased, prolonged muscle activity. This muscle guarding occurs because the cervical spine is unable to tolerate the anterior shear stress that occurs as a result of gravitational force over the cervical lordosis.

This same corner of the scapula is often a source of pain in patients with rotator cuff injuries. The superomedial corner of the scapula is the juncture of the scapular attachment of the levator scapulae and the medial end of the supraspinatus. Pain with palpation

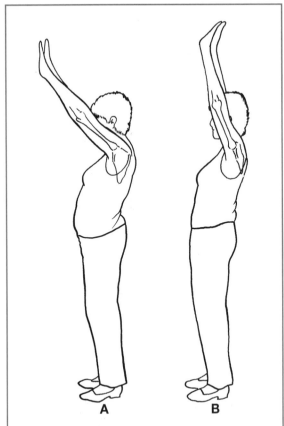

Figure 3-13. An example of the changes in active humeral forward elevation with different positions of the scapula. **A,** Notice the less active humeral forward elevation with the scapula in a protracted position. **B,** An unimpeded humeral forward elevation occurs with a retracted scapula.

over the medial border of the scapula may be referred from the degenerative changes of or injury to the supraspinatus muscle, or it may be a phenomenon associated with the anatomical linkage between the inferior aspect of the levator scapulae muscle and the medial aspect of the supraspinatus muscle.

Obviously, the levator scapulae muscle has no direct attachment to the humerus. Its action over the scapula, however, ultimately affects the mechanics and loads to the glenohumeral joint. For example, if we sit with the trunk slumped in a forward head, rounded shoulder posture and then attempt to elevate our arms, less humeral elevation is possible when compared with forward elevation of the arm with the scapulae in a slightly elevated and retracted position (Figure 3-13). Given a

retracted scapula, the range of arm elevation is greater and the compressive loading of the suprahumeral region is minimized. When the scapula is protracted and elevated as in a forward head posture, the range is less and the force to the anterior shoulder progressively increases to endrange. The important point here is that scapular position affects the compression and shear forces generated in the articulation of the shoulder complex. As discussed in Chapter 1, supporting structures break down by either a rapid endrange movement or a gradual, progressive overload. Teaching the patient with a shoulder compression or shear problem to refrain from allowing the scapula to migrate forward during activity is an important consideration in rehabilitation programs for the injured shoulder.

The Rhomboids: Major and Minor

The next muscles we consider in the scapular layer are the rhomboid major and rhomboid minor. These companion muscles travel superior and medial from the vertebral border of the scapula to attach to the

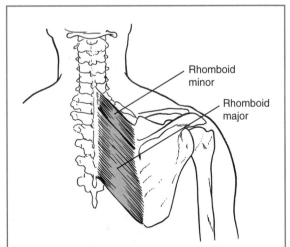

Rhomboid minor

Rhomboid major

Figure 3-14. The rhomboid major and rhomboid minor muscles travel inferior and lateral to attach to the vertebral border of the scapulae. The muscles do not feature the connective tissue matrix found in muscles like the middle trapezius and the latissimus dorsi, which have greater force capabilities. These muscles remain tendinous as they reach the vertebral border of the scapulae, where they blend into the serratus anterior. The rhomboid minor lies just caudal to the levator scapulae. The rhomboid major is larger but remains flat and tendinous at its attachment to the spinous processes (T2 to T5).

spinous processes of the thoracic spine (T2-5 and C7/T1 levels, respectively) (Figure 3-14). The rhomboid minor attaches to the vertebral border of the scapulae just caudal to the levator scapulae, whereas the rhomboid major covers the entire vertebral border of the scapula.

The rhomboid muscles are quite tendinous and flat at their attachments to the spinous processes and then become thicker as they course toward the scapula. At the medial border of the scapula they blend with the serratus anterior. The serratus anterior then courses anteriorly and inferiorly from this medial scapular attachment to encircle the thoracic cage and ultimately end over the anterolateral abdominal wall. We describe the relationship of the rhomboids and the serratus anterior further in the next section.

The most inferior attachment of the rhomboid major is at the inferior border of the scapulae, where the muscle is thick and quite tendinous. The rhomboid major is one of several muscles converging to this bony region on the scapula. The primary concentric muscle activity of the rhomboids is scapular retraction, and because of their inferior inclination from the spinous processes, they contribute slightly to downward rotation and elevation of the scapula. During the acceleration phase of overhead sports in which the arm is propelled forward and accompanied by strong internal rotation, the rhomboids contract eccentrically to control the rate at which the scapula moves laterally from the spinous processes and around the rib cage.[6]

The fiber orientation of the rhomboid major and lower trapezius provides another example of a crossing (**X**) relationship of muscles. This overlap of perpendicular fibers, the inferior and laterally directed rhomboid major and the inferior and medially directed lower trapezius, occurs in the space between the vertebral border of the scapula and the spinous processes (Figure 3-15, *A* and *B*). Rowing exercises are considered one of the most effective types of exercises for strengthening the rhomboids.[29] As mentioned previously, give primary consideration in strengthening programs to muscles oriented in this manner. Table 3-4 lists several exercises that focus on this important scapular layer of muscles.

Serratus Anterior

We describe the serratus anterior muscle last in this scapular layer. From its attachment to the entire vertebral border of the ventral surface of the scapula, the serratus anterior travels anteriorly and inferiorly to

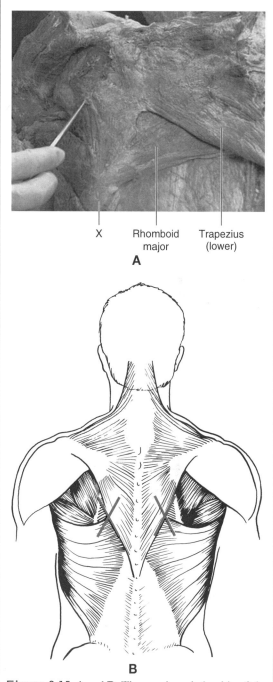

A

X   Rhomboid   Trapezius
    major   (lower)

B

Figure 3-15. A and **B,** The crossing relationship of the lower trapezius and the rhomboid major suggests the importance of stability and strength and represents a focus for strengthening exercises. In view **A,** the inferior border of the left scapula is marked by the **X**.

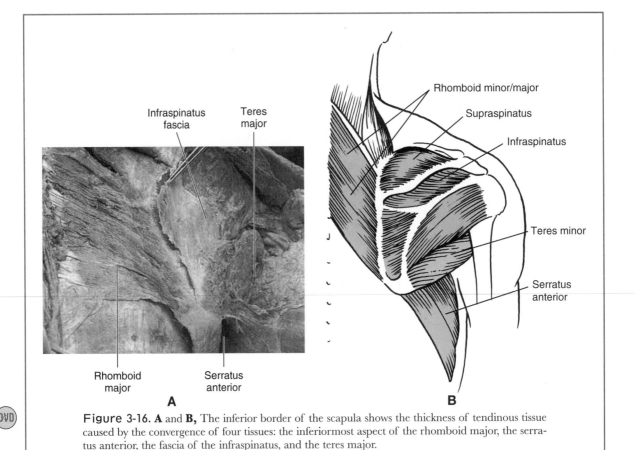

Figure 3-16. **A** and **B,** The inferior border of the scapula shows the thickness of tendinous tissue caused by the convergence of four tissues: the inferiormost aspect of the rhomboid major, the serratus anterior, the fascia of the infraspinatus, and the teres major.

Table 3-4. Exercises for the Scapular Layer

Levator Scapulae
Shrugs: standing straight and slightly forward bent
Low rows: one foot forward, emphasis on scapular elevation and retraction

Rhomboids
Pull-ups: counter weighted
High rows with a rope
Seated rows with flexed starting position
Standing resisted trunk extensions starting with scapular protraction: lift with head first and shrug and retract at end of range

Serratus Anterior
Push-ups (wall, floor, bench, gymnastic ball) emphasizing scapular protraction
Bench, dumbbell, cable presses
Pulley protractions
Supine pullovers
Overhead presses
Supine flys

attach to the first 10 ribs via a series of muscular interdigitations. The lower four interdigitations converge fanlike to blend with the muscular interdigitations of the external abdominal oblique.[52]

The attachment of the serratus anterior at the vertebral border of the scapula is also continuous with the rhomboid major and minor muscles. At the vertebral border of the scapula, the rhomboid groups, the levator scapulae, and the serratus anterior are devoid of the typical tendinous attachment, but instead, the thick muscle bellies of the rhomboids and levator scapulae converge to blend with the extensive musculature of the serratus anterior.

At the inferior border of the scapula, the serratus anterior has a thickened accumulation of connective tissue, suggesting that significant muscle forces are generated in this region (Figure 3-16, *A* and *B*). This tendinous convergence over the inferior border of the scapulae is an amalgamation of four specific tissues: the inferiormost aspect of the rhomboid major, the serratus anterior, the fascia of the infraspinatus, and the teres major. The latissimus dorsi lies superficial to this intersection of tissues as it courses medially from the humerus toward the spinous processes of the thoracic vertebrae.

The posterior and inferior aspect of the serratus anterior also attaches to the undersurface of the latissimus dorsi muscle (see Figure 3-3). The latissimus dorsi thus serves as a dynamically stable base from which the serratus anterior can pull. One of the advantages of such an arrangement is to extend or broaden the attachment of the serratus anterior. This suggests that as this portion of the serratus anterior contracts, it pulls the latissimus dorsi down against the rib cage and over the inferior border of the scapula, creating a compressive,

stabilizing force to the scapula. The result of such complex activity of the serratus anterior is that it works to stabilize the scapula, as well as contribute in guiding scapular movement during pushing or pulling activities. Exercises such as supine protraction, push-ups, wall push-ups, and cable crossover emphasizing humeral adduction and scapular protraction emphasize this function because they concentrate on moving the scapula irrespective of the humerus (see Table 3-4 and Chapter 6).

The serratus courses anteriorly around the rib cage to attach to the ribs and interdigitates with the external oblique muscle. The fiber line of the external oblique then becomes continuous with the internal oblique and adductor muscles of the thigh on the contralateral side. This has been referred to as the "serape effect."[27] A

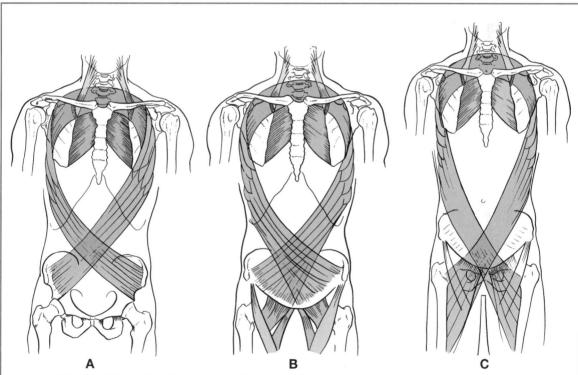

Figure 3-17. A, Note the continuous flow of muscles from the neck and thoracic spine via the levator scapulae and rhomboid major to the serratus anterior that interdigitates with the external oblique and illustrates the "serape effect." The external oblique muscle fiber line can be followed to the contralateral side toward the iliac crest. **B,** The lower aspect of the serratus–external oblique linkage can be tracked below the umbilicus toward the contralateral femoral adductors. Coming from both sides as a wrap of muscle (the serape effect), muscular contribution to the antigravity posture is ensured. **C,** This view emphasizes the muscle fiber line from the levator scapulae toward the contralateral lower extremity.

serape refers to a brightly colored woolen blanket, which was used as an outer garment by men in Hispanic cultures. The significance is not the cloak itself, but rather the way in which it is draped around the shoulders and across the front of the body. This shape is similar to the orientation of these muscles, anatomically linking the neck, thoracic spine, and shoulder girdle to the pelvis and legs (Figure 3-17, *A-C*).

We describe the serape of muscles as follows:

A. The levator scapulae travels inferiorly and posteriorly to the superior medial border of the scapula, where it merges with the upper serratus anterior on the undersurface of the scapula.

B. The rhomboid major and minor anchor the scapula to the spine from the cervicothoracic junction and upper thoracic spinous process; these muscles merge with the serratus anterior at the vertebral border of the scapula, and the serratus anterior then blends with the external oblique, which results in the external oblique being:

   • Oriented along the same line of muscle fiber

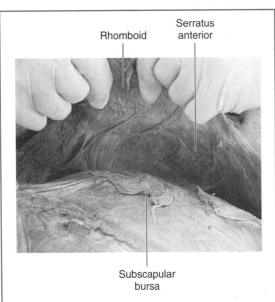

Figure 3-18. When the rhomboids and scapula are reflected, the costal surface of the scapula is visualized blending the rhomboids with the serratus anterior. Note the lack of tendinous tissue where these tissues blend into one another, suggesting a mechanical linkage between the associated groups, and also the size of the subscapular bursa.

direction as the contralateral internal oblique and iliac crest

   • Aligned across the midline below the umbilicus, with the contralateral femoral adductors terminating into the femur

The blending of the levator scapulae and rhomboids into the serratus anterior can be seen in Figure 3-18, where the medial costal surface of the scapula serves as a bony transition between the muscles. The maintenance of the strength, power, and endurance of these muscles plays a significant role in the maintenance of the erect antigravity posture, which is important in controlling loading and function of the base of the neck and the low back and at the suprahumeral space in the shoulder (Figure 3-19).

Patients with impingement symptoms may demonstrate altered scapular mechanics.[49] Electromyographic studies suggest that decreased muscle activity in the serratus anterior and increased activity in the upper and lower trapezius above 90 degrees of humeral flexion may contribute to impingement syndrome and increased glenohumeral forces.[28] Underloaded conditions, and increased anterior tipping of the scapula above 90 degrees may also contribute to increased compression to the suprahumeral tissues at the subacromial space.[35]

Scapulohumeral rhythm (see Chapter 4) varies depending on the arm position, the plane of movement, whether the motion is resisted or unresisted, and the integrity of the glenohumeral capsule. Scapular rotators provide an example of the important force couples that control motion and position of the scapula on the thorax. The serratus anterior generates a downward pull of the scapula toward the axilla, the upper trapezius pulls upward on the scapula toward the occiput, and the lower trapezius pulls downward on the scapula toward the lumbar spine (Figure 3-20).

THE POSTERIOR SCAPULAR LAYER

Muscles of this group attach the humerus to the scapula. They are thick and fibrous muscles built for power, and they work together with muscles outside this layer to stabilize the position of the humeral head. The muscles described in this section are the infraspinatus, teres minor, supraspinatus, deltoid, and the long head of the triceps.

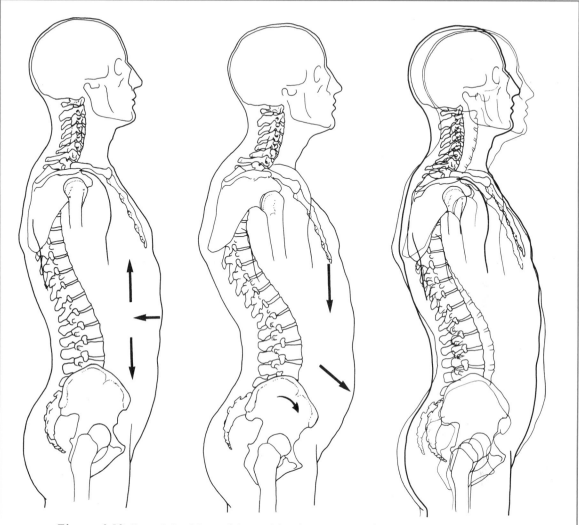

Figure 3-19. Round shoulder and forward head posture place increased stress on three main areas: the base of the neck, the lumbosacral junction, and the suprahumeral space. All are affected by a loss of strength of the musculature that stabilizes the antigravity posture. (From Porterfield JA, DeRosa C: *Mechanical neck pain: perspectives in functional anatomy,* Philadelphia, 1994, WB Saunders.)

Infraspinatus

The infraspinatus is a thick, triangular-shaped muscle consisting of superior, middle, and inferior heads that fill the infraspinous fossa of the scapula. At approximately the middle region of the muscle, a fibrous tendon centralizes and directs the pull of the

three heads of the infraspinatus muscle (Figure 3-21). The three heads join to wrap around the posterior aspect of the head of the humerus and then blend into the superior and posterior aspect of the glenohumeral joint capsule.

The superior head of the infraspinatus muscle attaches to the upper and medial vertebral border of the

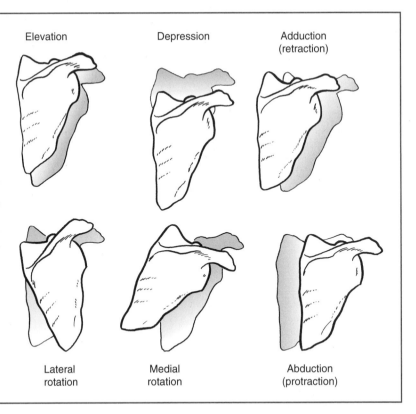

Elevation   Depression   Adduction (retraction)

Lateral rotation   Medial rotation   Abduction (protraction)

Figure 3-20. Note the high degree of scapular mobility on the thorax and the musculature that must work in concert synergistically to permit smooth and timely motion. Also, recognize that the loads and forces generated to the glenohumeral joint vary depending on the position of the scapula.

infraspinous fossa and to the inferior surface of the spine of the scapula. These fibers travel laterally to contribute to the formation of a broad, flat tendon that attaches to the posterior and superior aspect of the greater tubercle of the humerus. The middle head is more fan shaped and terminates primarily into the central thickened tendon. The inferior head of the infraspinatus muscle is attached to the inferior border of the scapula, and its fibers are directed toward the central thickening. It too converges into the flat tendon that wraps around the posterior and superior aspect of the head of the humerus. This characteristic attachment of the muscle to the humeral head allows it to contribute to glenohumeral stability in a unique manner. Because of the manner in which the infraspinatus tendon wraps around the head of the humerus, it serves as a passive connective tissue restraint to posterior subluxation and a dynamic restraint to anterior subluxation of the humeral head on the glenoid.

The dynamic restraint to anterior translation of the humeral head is especially important to consider. In the presence of anterior glenohumeral joint instability, attention is often paid to the strength and mass of the anterior glenohumeral muscles. It is the infraspinatus muscle, however, with its unique attachment method of wrapping around the head of the humerus, coupled with its interplay with its investing fascia, that plays a greater role in the dynamic restraint to anterior subluxation.[4]

The infraspinatus muscle has a greater cross-sectional area than is commonly appreciated (Figure 3-22, *A* and *B*). This suggests the muscle's importance in generating the forces required to center the humeral head and assist in checking the forward and superior migration of the head of the humerus. It is also covered by the dense infraspinatus fascia, which serves as an anchor for the muscle to attach to, augmenting the mechanics of this important muscle (see Figure 3-22). Fascial coverings are typically strategically placed in areas where control and stability are essential. The thoracolumbar fascia, the fascia lata in our thighs, and the abdominal fascia are examples of key fascial units in the body that encase muscles and provide them a place to attach. Thus contraction of

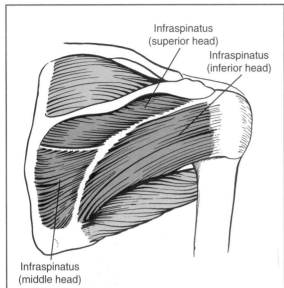

Figure 3-21. The infraspinatus muscle has three heads: superior, middle, and inferior. Note the central tendon that serves as an attachment of the angled fibers of the superior and inferior heads and as a tendon of the fan shaped middle head. These three heads terminate into a flat tendon that covers the posterior aspect of the head of the humerus.

muscles attached to the fascia increase fascial tension and muscles contracting within the fascial envelope also increase tension via the broadening effect of the muscle's contraction. These musculofascial relationships protect areas of the skeleton that are particularly vulnerable to overuse.

Muscles contained within a fascial covering use the tight fascial covering to improve the mechanical advantage of the contraction. As the muscle contracts within the fascial covering, it pushes against the inner walls, which immediately directs tensile forces through the tendon to the bone. A system with these mechanics loses its efficiency as the muscle atrophies. The loss of mass of the infraspinatus muscle, either by aging or injury, decreases the efficiency at which the muscle works to appropriately direct the force of muscle contraction to the skeleton. When this atrophy is coupled with muscular fatigue, the muscular contribution to posture and movement is even further compromised. In the case of the infraspinatus muscle, the ability to strongly center the head of the humerus on the

glenoid may be compromised and result in compression of the suprahumeral tissues between the head of the humerus and coracoacromial arch.

At the glenohumeral joint the infraspinatus muscle functions with the other rotator cuff muscles to center the head of the humerus into the glenoid.[36] The supraspinatus muscle is very important because it is the only muscle that is more active than the infraspinatus muscle in shoulder motions.[32] Acting alone, the infraspinatus becomes an external rotator and humeral head depressor creating a posterior and inferior shear of the humerus on the glenoid. The infraspinatus is also one of the primary decelerators of the throwing arm. This deceleration function is often one of the reasons for breakdown on the undersurface (articular surface) of the infraspinatus tendon. The tensile stress imparted to the tendon during deceleration, coupled with the frictional force of the tendon over the rim of the glenoid, renders the tendon vulnerable to disruption of its fibers.[37] In addition, there is an extreme distraction force between the humerus and the glenoid near the instant of ball release in throwing and throughout the deceleration phase. This distraction is resisted by the strong eccentric contraction of the infraspinatus and renders this muscle susceptible to tensile overload.[51]

Like most muscles associated with the shoulder complex, as the position of the humerus changes, the function of the muscle changes. For example, as the humerus is elevated to 120 degrees in the scaption plane, the infraspinatus muscle is now best aligned to exert an active compressive force between the head of the humerus and the glenoid fossa along with the combined motion of horizontal abduction and external rotation. This is an optimal position to consider using when designing resistance exercises for the infraspinatus muscle. When the arm is at the side, the infraspinatus muscle fibers are more aligned to produce posterior translation, inferior translation, and lateral rotation of the humerus on the glenoid. Even though this is often the position to begin external rotation exercises in postsurgical conditions of the shoulder, it is not the position that optimally aligns the fibers of the infraspinatus muscle.

Teres Minor

The teres minor muscle is slightly fusiform in shape and attaches to the lateral border of the scapula just below the inferior head of the infraspinatus. Because

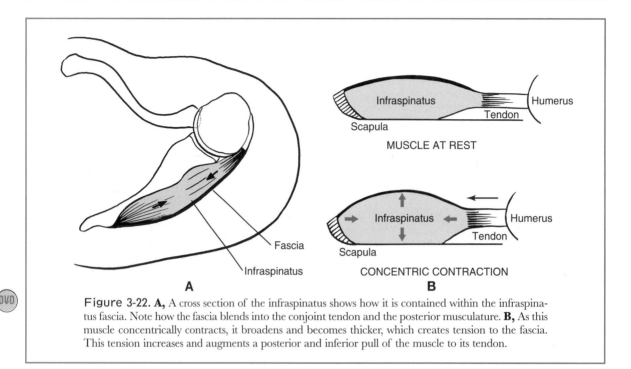

Figure 3-22. A, A cross section of the infraspinatus shows how it is contained within the infraspinatus fascia. Note how the fascia blends into the conjoint tendon and the posterior musculature. **B,** As this muscle concentrically contracts, it broadens and becomes thicker, which creates tension to the fascia. This tension increases and augments a posterior and inferior pull of the muscle to its tendon.

of its location, the narrow medial attachment is also attached to the infraspinatus fascia. From these points it courses laterally and flattens as it attaches to the head and neck of the humerus (Figure 3-23, *A* and *B*). It spreads to cover the inferior extent of the posterior glenohumeral joint capsule. Although supplied with a different peripheral nerve (the axillary nerve) than the infraspinatus muscle (suprascapular nerve), its unopposed actions are similar: to depress and externally rotate the humerus. The muscle also functions with its anterior counterparts to center the head of the humerus in the glenoid. Acting eccentrically, the teres minor serves to decelerate the humerus during throwing activities and stabilizes the head of the humerus against anterior subluxation.

Supraspinatus

The supraspinatus muscle arises from the supraspinous fossa and supraspinatus fascia. Although the medial attachment is thin, owing to the decreased depth of the medial aspect of the supraspinous fossa, the muscle becomes thicker as it travels laterally below the acromion.[16] In this region the muscle gives rise to a flat tendon that attaches to the superior facet of the greater tubercle of the humerus and blends with the capsule of the glenohumeral joint. The coracoacromial ligament lies anterior to the supraspinatus tendon, and the infraspinatus muscle tendon lies posterior.

Three different muscular heads, structured like a braided rope, can be seen on close inspection (Figure 3-24). The anterior head travels posteriorly, the middle head directly laterally, and the posterior head, which arises from the spine of the scapula, courses anteriorly, forming a type of helical weave. The tendon of the posterior head, thinner in cross section compared with the middle and anterior sections, overlaps the tendon of the anterior head. The intertwining of the anterior, middle, and posterior heads of the muscle results in an enhanced ability to dilute tensile stresses. The tensile capabilities are such that the posterior fibers are the weakest whereas the anterior are the strongest and most elastic.[16] The primary roles of this muscle are to initiate and contribute to glenohumeral abduction and to increase compression between the head of the humerus and the glenoid. It is the most active of any of the rotator cuff muscles and is involved with any motion that elevates the arm.[15]

The supraspinatus, infraspinatus, and teres minor muscles together form an expansive, domelike tendon that blends directly into the joint capsule covering the superior and posterior aspect of the head of the humerus.[2,43,45] The actions of these three muscles, in concert with the subscapularis muscle, center and stabilize the head of the humerus in the glenoid by counterbalancing the superior directed force the deltoid has on the humerus during elevation and check translations of the head of the humerus that might occur when other muscles attached to the humerus contract. For example, contraction of the latissimus dorsi would pull the head of the humerus inferiorly and posteriorly, whereas contraction of the sternocostal portion of the pectoralis major would pull the head of the humerus inferiorly and anteriorly. In order for these muscles to carry out their actions, the humeral head must be fixated in the glenoid socket via these rotator cuff muscles. The infraspinatus and teres minor also function to pull the head of the humerus inferiorly, away from the acromion and coracoacromial ligament (suprahumeral hood) (Figure 3-25).

Within the glenohumeral joint capsule, the long head of the biceps brachii is positioned between the supraspinatus and subscapularis tendons. This route across the top of the head of the humerus allows it to contribute to stabilization of the humeral head with the rotator cuff (Figure 3-26). Because of its location, however, the biceps tendon, like the adjacent supraspinatus tendon, is often involved in impingement syndromes in the shoulder.[40]

The intricate arrangement of converging tendons and capsular tissue of the glenohumeral joint contributes to control of the relationship between the head of the humerus and glenoid throughout all ranges of motion (Figure 3-27). The microscopic anatomy of this conjoint tendon is just as complex. Clark and colleagues have described five microscopic layers of this conjoint tendon, which essentially fills the suprahumeral space (Figure 3-28).[5] The most superficial layer is primarily ligamentous tissue of the acromioclavicular ligament. The second layer consists of closely packed tendinous tissue that connects the muscle belly to the bone. Layer three of the rotator cuff tendon is also composed of tendinous tissue made up of smaller fascicles. The fiber orientation of this layer is less compactly arranged. Layer four is composed of collagen fibers in loose connective tissues that run perpendicular to one another. This layer incorporates the deep portion of the coracohumeral ligament. The fifth and deepest layer of the rotator cuff tendon

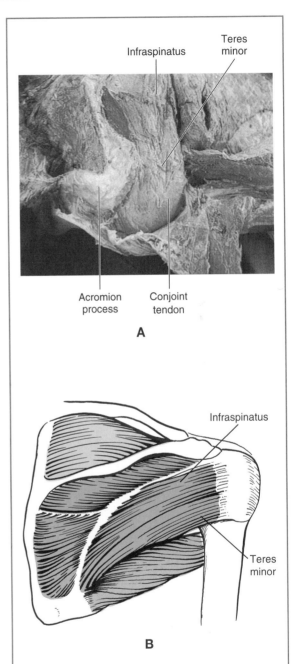

Figure 3-23. **A** and **B,** A posterior view of the attachments of the infraspinatus and teres minor to the head of the humerus shows the absence of a distinct separation between the tendons. Instead the tendons blend together to unite with the joint capsule and to cover the posterior aspect of the humerus.

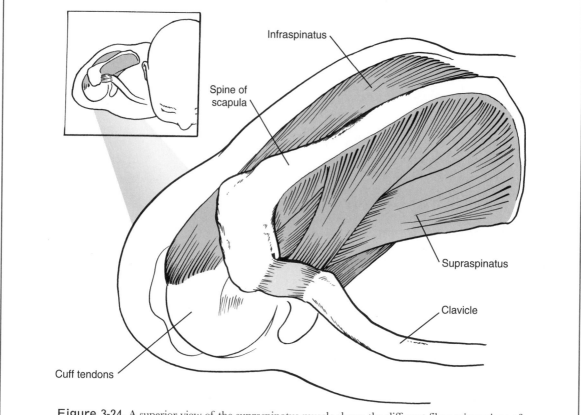

Infraspinatus

Spine of
scapula

Supraspinatus

Clavicle

Cuff tendons

Figure 3-24. A superior view of the supraspinatus muscle shows the different fiber orientations of the anterior, middle, and posterior portions of the muscle.

is randomly organized capsular tissue surrounding the glenohumeral joint.

The superficial (bursal) surface of the tendons is thus different from the deep (articular) surface.[9,10,31,48] Aging of the tendons is progressive, is characterized by decreased cellularity and vascularity, and typically is seen on the undersurface of the cuff tendons first.[44] As the tendon ages, the articular portion of the tendon becomes more rigid and granular and less vascular. Tears to the tendon can either be on the articular side or spread through the midsubstance to the bursal side. Tears are also seen on the bursal surface alone (Figure 3-29, A-C). The articular side of the supraspinatus tendon is more susceptible to mechanical failure than the bursal or midsubstance portions, with partial thickness tears on the joint side being very common. Tears of the rotator cuff tendon are often classified as small (less than 1 cm), containing only the supraspinatus tendon,

to massive (greater than 5 cm), which include the supraspinatus, infraspinatus, and subscapularis tendons (Figure 3-30, A-D).[14]

Partial and full thickness tears are commonly seen as a result of athletic and work activities that involve repetitive overhead motions and contact sports.[3,46] Rotator cuff injuries lead to glenohumeral instability and are contributing factors to impingement syndromes. Prolonged and progressively increased pressure weakens the connective tissues of the coracoacromial arch, stiffens the coracoacromial ligament, causes traction spurs to form on the acromion and coracoid processes, and weakens the cuff tendons, resulting in decreased tissue tolerance.[48] The soft tissues of the coracoacromial arch (see Chapter 4) provide some force attenuation abilities; however, the changes seen at the undersurface of the acromion and the thickening of the coracoacromial ligament suggest

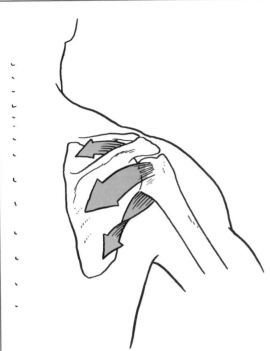

Figure 3-25. The downward pull of the infraspinatus and teres minor muscles can be seen as the humerus is abducted. Without this balance of forces, the chances of excessive compression forces between the head of the humerus and the acromion and coracoacromial ligament are high. (Modified from Kapandji IA: *The physiology of the joints: annotated diagrams of the mechanics of the human joints,* New York, 1982, Churchill Livingstone.)

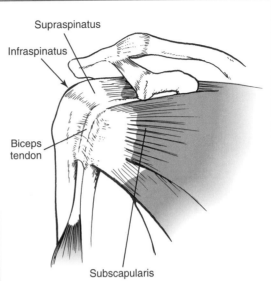

Figure 3-26. Note the route of the long head of the biceps tendon as it passes over the head of the humerus and blends with the conjoint tendon of the supraspinatus and infraspinatus muscles.

that this area is a focus of compression in the glenohumeral joint, thus illustrating the crucial role the cuff tendons play in the centralization of the humeral head in any position.

Instability of the glenohumeral joint is also associated with tears of the rotator cuff tendons. Aberrant motions of the humerus on the glenoid occur as a result of rotator cuff muscle and tendon failure. As in any synovial joint, aberrant motion resulting from injury to supporting structures of the joint predispose the articulation to overload and possible early degeneration.

It is important to remember that degeneration of the rotator cuff tendons is primarily a function of age.[9] Furthermore, because of the wide range of shoulder motion, continual friction between the undersurface of the tendon and the glenoid rim, and the

hypovascularity of the rotator cuff tendons, lesions of the cuff tendons do not heal spontaneously.[54] This highlights the importance of maintaining musculoskeletal health and strength, particularly in those muscles focused over the thoracic spine, trunk, and scapula that maintain our erect posture. Table 3-5 lists several key exercises used in maximizing shoulder function, including those with a strengthening effect to the rotator cuff. Historically, exercise for the supraspinatus was prescribed with the arm in the thumb down ("empty can") position. Placing the glenohumeral joint in this position and then performing resistance exercises significantly compromises the tendon and places the supraspinatus at further risk.[17] We encourage all overhead resistance exercises to be performed with the humerus in the laterally rotated position.

Deltoid

The thick, triangular-shaped deltoid muscle has three heads: anterior, middle, and posterior (Figure 3-31). The anterior, attaching to the lateral third of the clavicle, and the posterior, which attaches to the spine of the scapula, are essentially parallel to each

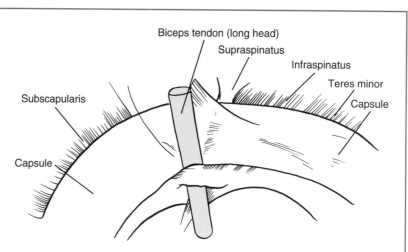

Figure 3-27. The deep structural arrangement of the conjoint tendon of the rotator cuff located at the head of the humerus consists of the biceps tendon and four muscles: the subscapularis, the supraspinatus, the infraspinatus, and the teres minor. (Modified from Clark JM, Harryman DT II: Tendons, ligaments and capsule of the rotator cuff, *J Bone Joint Surg Am* 74(5):717, 1992.)

other and cover the front and back of the shoulder. The middle deltoid is actually composed of four separated multipennate, coarsely structured sections traveling inferior from the acromion. It joins with the anterior and posterior heads to attach via a short

Figure 3-28. Note the layered anatomy of the suprahumeral tissues. (Modified from Clark JM, Harryman DT II: Tendons, ligaments and capsule of the rotator cuff, *J Bone Joint Surg Am* 74(5):723, 1992.)

tendon to the deltoid tuberosity on the lateral distal humerus. The three heads of the deltoid check the inferior migration of the humeral head on the glenoid. Other muscles assisting the deltoid in this function include the long head of the triceps, coracobrachialis, and short head of the biceps brachii. The anterior deltoid is a strong sagittal plane elevator and internal rotator of the humerus, the middle deltoid a frontal plane elevator (abductor) of the humerus. The posterior deltoid extends, hyperextends (being the only muscle with this capability), and externally rotates the humerus.

Figure 3-32 illustrates a horizontal section that demonstrates the differences in structure between the anterior and posterior deltoid. Note the difference in mass between the anterior muscles, such as the anterior deltoid and pectoralis major, and the posterior deltoid and scapular muscles. The posterior muscles are quite substantial by comparison, which suggests the importance of emphasizing the posterior musculature in exercise programs. Exercises emphasizing pulling up and back, and down and back without exacerbating shoulder pain, and learning (teaching) to appropriately direct the force of the exercise toward the intended musculature are essential in designing exercises for the shoulder.

The deltoid tuberosity, serving as the point of humeral attachment, lies approximately halfway down the lateral shaft of the humerus. When the line of muscle pull is analyzed from the acromial end to the humeral end, we can see that the action of the muscle over the lever of the humerus is dependent on the superior translation and an increasing force of glenohumeral compression.

Once the humerus reaches approximately 20 degrees of abduction, the deltoid line of muscle pull begins to be positioned to allow it to serve as a powerful elevator of the humerus in the frontal, sagittal, and scaption planes, but only if the rotator cuff has centralized and fixated the humerus within the shallow glenoid. Note also that the line of pull of the latissimus dorsi and sternocostal portion of the pectoralis major counterbalances the deltoid pull as well (Figure 3-33). Without these counterbalances, the middle deltoid muscle simply drives the head of the humerus superiorly into the acromion, coracoacromial ligament, coracoid process, or tendons of the pectoralis minor, coracobrachialis, and short head of the biceps brachii. Figure 3-34 illustrates the differences in forces at the suprahumeral space below 60 degrees and above 120 degrees with a retracted scapula.

Long Head of the Triceps

The long head of the triceps is the final muscle we discuss in the posterior scapular layer. From its distal attachment at the olecranon of the ulna, the long head travels superiorly and medially to pass between the teres major and teres minor muscles, attaching to the infraglenoid tubercle of the scapula. This intersection with the teres major and minor creates the quadrangular and triangular spaces (Figure 3-35). The axillary nerve and the posterior humeral circumflex vessels travel through the quadrangular space as they course around the neck of the humerus, whereas the triangular space houses the scapular circumflex vessels.

The crossing of the teres group and the triceps muscle provides yet another example of the crossing relationship of muscles potentially adding stability to the area, in this case the posterior and inferior aspect to the glenohumeral joint. A similar crossing relationship lies anterior to the glenohumeral joint, consisting of the crossing relationship between the subscapularis, coracobrachialis, and short head of the biceps. Together the weave of muscles formed by these posterior and anterior crossing relationships adds increased stability to the inherently unstable glenohumeral joint (Figure 3-36).

The long head of the triceps helps minimize inferior translation of the humeral head on the glenoid

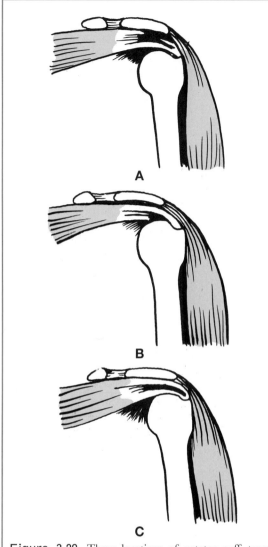

Figure 3-29. Three locations of rotator cuff tears: **A,** Bursal side; **B,** articular side; and **C,** midsubstance. The articular side tears are most commonly seen. (Redrawn from Hawkins RJ, Bell RH, Lippitt SB: *Atlas of shoulder surgery,* St. Louis, 1996, Mosby.)

glenohumeral joint angle. From the resting, anatomical position, the line of deltoid muscle pull on the humerus is primarily superior translation of the humerus. Conversely, it is markedly active between 90 and 180 degrees of elevation.[47] As the arm is raised further in the frontal plane, there is less force of

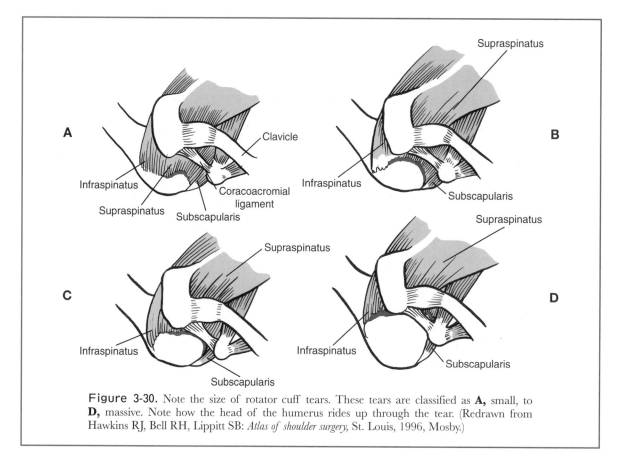

Figure 3-30. Note the size of rotator cuff tears. These tears are classified as **A,** small, to **D,** massive. Note how the head of the humerus rides up through the tear. (Redrawn from Hawkins RJ, Bell RH, Lippitt SB: *Atlas of shoulder surgery,* St. Louis, 1996, Mosby.)

when an inferior shear force is introduced. Contraction of the long head pulls the humerus superiorly, resulting in superior translation of the humeral head at the glenohumeral joint. The patient with a hemiparetic arm or one who has had a radial nerve injury may exhibit inferior subluxation of the

Table 3-5. Exercises for the Posterior Scapular Layer
Superior Cuff, Posterior Cuff, Posterior Deltoid
Low row with external rotation
PNF cable resistance patterns: horizontal abduction and external rotation
Seated row
Reverse fly
Forward elevations and overhead presses
Lateral shoulder raises

*PNF, Proprioceptive neuromuscular facilitation.

humerus because of the loss of this triceps muscle stabilizing function over the glenohumeral joint. Other functions of the long head of the triceps include pulling the humerus back down to the anatomical position from starting points of glenohumeral elevation, such as in "chopping" strokes that extend or adduct the arm. At the elbow, the triceps contributes to elbow extension with its associated lateral and medial heads.

We can see through this discussion that groups of muscles work together to form a system of counterbalances and muscular reinforcements via crossing relationships that work to check the inferior-superior and the anterior-posterior migration of the head of the humerus. Concentric contraction of the long head of the triceps, the short head of the biceps brachii, coracobrachialis, clavicular head of the pectoralis major, and deltoid have a line of muscle force that pulls the humerus superiorly, whereas the eccentric activity of these same muscles controls inferior movement of the

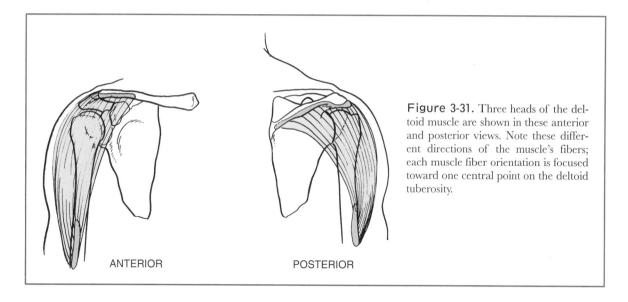

Figure 3-31. Three heads of the deltoid muscle are shown in these anterior and posterior views. Note these different directions of the muscle's fibers; each muscle fiber orientation is focused toward one central point on the deltoid tuberosity.

ANTERIOR   POSTERIOR

humerus (Figure 3-37, *A*). We refer to these muscles as "hanger muscles" because they dynamically suspend the humerus at the glenoid. These muscles are counterbalanced by the line of pull offered by the latissimus dorsi, teres major, teres minor, the inferior head of the infraspinatus, inferior head of the subscapularis, and the costal portion of the pectoralis major, which exert an inferiorly directed line of force over the humeral head (Figure 3-37, *B*). Coordinated muscle activity helps ensure that the forces of gravity and the contractile forces of movement secure the position of the humeral head in the glenoid.

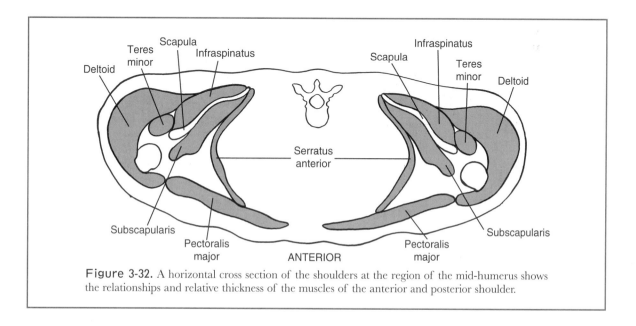

Figure 3-32. A horizontal cross section of the shoulders at the region of the mid-humerus shows the relationships and relative thickness of the muscles of the anterior and posterior shoulder.

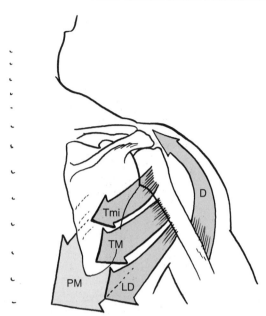

Figure 3-33. This schematic illustration shows the downward pull of the latissimus dorsi (LD), teres major (TM), teres minor (Tmi), and the costal portion of the pectoralis major (PM) to counterbalance the superior migration of the humerus as a result of the contraction of the middle deltoid (D) muscle. (Modified from Kapandji IA: *The physiology of the joints: annotated diagrams of the mechanics of the human joints,* New York, 1982, Churchill Livingstone.)

THE SUBSCAPULAR REGION

The subscapular region includes the serratus anterior and subscapularis muscles and can be approached during dissection in several ways. One of the best approaches, which allows us to better appreciate the movement potential of the scapula on the thorax, is a posterior approach. By reflecting the trapezius and rhomboid muscles from the spine of the scapula, we essentially free the scapula from the spinous processes. From this vantage point, the costal surface of the scapula can then be explored.

Serratus Anterior

One of the first structures encountered during dissection of the subscapular region from a posterior direction is the subscapular bursa. This large and expansive tissue comes into view when the rhomboids have been reflected from the spinous processes, allowing the costal surface of the scapula to be explored. The serratus anterior muscle is easily seen where it attaches to the vertebral border of the scapula. The large subscapular bursa lies between the serratus anterior and the underlying small muscles of respiration consisting of the serratus posterior superior and intercostal muscles. The bursa is quite extensive, typically exceeding the dimensions of the scapula, and it serves to form a relatively friction free environment for these tissues to move relative to one another (see Figure 3-18).

DVD

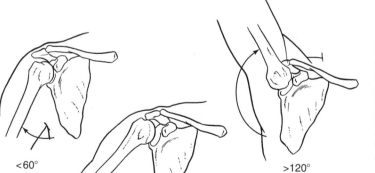

Figure 3-34. Three frontal plane views of the glenohumeral articulation show the shear and compression of the suprahumeral tissues below 60 degrees, between 60 and 120 degrees, and above 120 degrees. Note the importance of scapular position in the analysis of these forces.

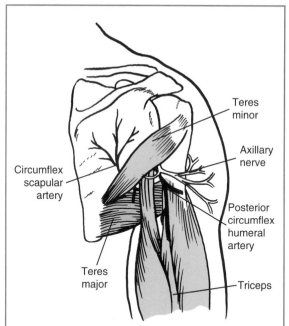

Figure 3-35. A posterior view of the right shoulder shows the relationship of the long head of the triceps, teres major, and teres minor muscles. Note the crossing relationship of the teres major and the long head of the triceps, which forms a quadrilateral space laterally and the triangular space medially. These spaces house the axillary nerve and the posterior humeral and scapular circumflex arteries.

The extremely important role that the serratus anterior plays in concert with the rhomboids, levator scapulae, and external oblique has already been described in previous sections of this chapter. The discussion now focuses on how the shoulder girdle is tied through a system of muscles to the trunk and lower extremities through the serape effect. Acting alone, the serratus anterior line of muscle pull allows for protraction and upward rotation of the scapula.

The upward rotation function of the serratus anterior is extremely important, since it is one of the few muscles capable of this important action, the other being the combined effort of the upper and lower trapezius. Often individuals engaging in upper extremity exercise programs fail to complete the stroke of humeral elevation exercise, meaning that the strong upward rotation of the scapula as they work to elevate their arms against resistance is lacking. Failure to do so leaves the elevated shoulder (arms overhead) in a position of downward scapular rotation, thereby increasing subacromial compression. Therefore it is essential that the scapula be monitored for full and strong upward rotation activity during any shoulder elevation exercise. The anatomy of the serratus anterior suggests how important this upward rotation function is; the heaviest serratus anterior attachment is at the important inferior angle of the scapula.

Likewise, pushing exercises such as bench presses, dumbbell presses, and supine horizontal "fly" exercises (see Chapter 6) must emphasize scapular protraction in

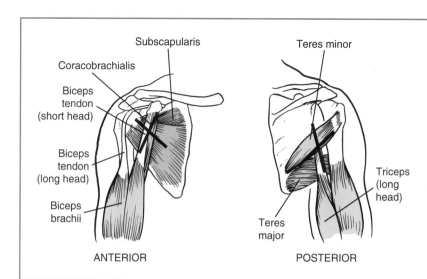

Figure 3-36. The crossing relationship posterior to the glenohumeral joint from the long head of the triceps and the teres muscles forms an X close to the posterior and inferior aspect of the glenohumeral joint. A complement to this X is seen on the anterior side when the coracobrachialis, short head of the biceps brachii, and the subscapularis are viewed.

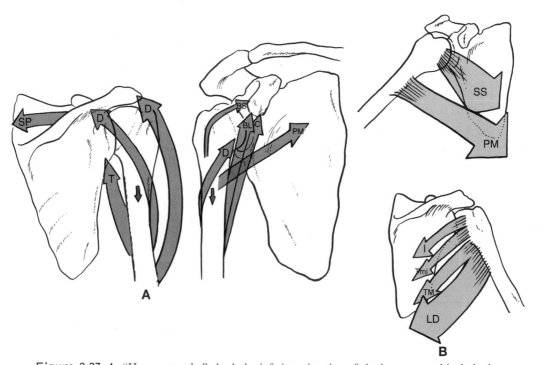

Figure 3-37. A, "Hanger muscles" check the inferior migration of the humerus and include the triceps (T), short (BS) and long (BL) head of the biceps brachii, coracobrachialis (C), clavicular head of the pectoralis major (PM), supraspinatus (SP), and deltoid (D). Their eccentric contraction controls the inferior migration of the humeral head. **B,** Muscles that, during concentric contraction, pull the humerus down place a counter force to the hanger muscles ensuring proper positioning of the head of the humerus. These muscles include the latissimus dorsi (LD), teres major (TM), teres minor (Tmi), the inferior head of the infraspinatus (I) and subscapularis (SS), and the costal portion of the pectoralis major (PM). (Modified from Kapandji IA: *The physiology of the joints: annotated diagrams of the mechanics of the human joints*, New York, 1982, Churchill Livingstone.)

order to be effective. If exercising focuses only on movement of the humerus, we do not benefit from its most important aspects: moving the scapula from a position of retraction to an endrange of protraction. This activity is a function of concentric action of the serratus anterior, whereas the eccentric activity of the muscle allows for a controlled return to a retracted scapular position.

Subscapularis

If the serratus anterior is detached from the vertebral border of the scapula and the scapula lifted away from the thorax, the subscapularis muscle

comes into view where it is positioned between the serratus anterior muscle and the subscapular fossa. The subscapularis has three heads as it lies on the subscapular fossa (Figure 3-38). This muscle is quite thick and like the infraspinatus has muscular fibers converging from a wide medial position toward a central tendon covering the anterior aspect of the glenohumeral joint. The superior head originates from the superior portion of the subscapular fossa and travels slightly inferiorly and laterally, whereas the fan-shaped and thinner middle head travels laterally. The inferior head is thicker and exhibits a stronger looking stature, and the majority of the subscapular tendon appears to be associated with the inferior head.

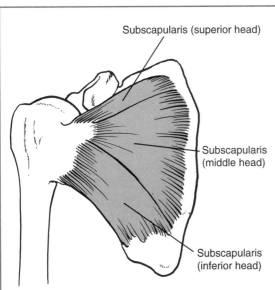

Subscapularis (superior head)

Subscapularis (middle head)

Subscapularis (inferior head)

Figure 3-38. The superior, middle, and inferior heads of the subscapularis muscle show that the inferior head is larger and contributes to the majority of the tendon.

The tendon of the subscapularis has the largest cross section of any tendon in the shoulder (Figure 3-39). This broad tendon covers the anterior shoulder and dynamically reinforces the anterior aspect of the shoulder, including the anterior aspect of the glenoid labrum and the glenohumeral ligaments. Acting unopposed, the subscapularis internally rotates the humerus, and with the arm in the anatomical position, the angled fibers of the inferior head create an inferiorly directed force to the proximal humerus. As the humerus changes position, however, the muscle adopts different functions. For example, as the humerus is abducted and externally rotated, the angle of the fibers of the muscle changes so that contraction of the subscapularis serves to compress the head of the humerus into the glenoid and provide some contribution to glenohumeral adduction. Perhaps most importantly, the subscapularis is the major dynamic restraint to posterior instability of the glenohumeral joint.[39]

As described above, there are always counterbalancing muscular forces that ensure the proper balance between joint mobility and stability. The inferiorly directed fibers of the large, anteriorly placed inferior head of the subscapularis are counterbalanced by the posteriorly placed fibers of the inferior head of the infraspinatus and the teres minor muscles, providing a dynamic restraint to anterior posterior translation. In both muscle groups the anterior subscapularis and

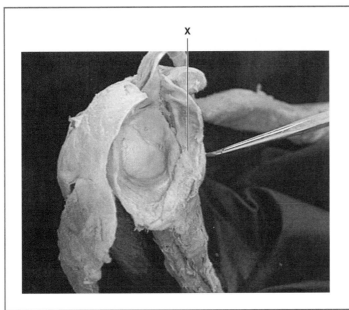

X

Figure 3-39. The cross section of the subscapularis tendon shows the thickness and breadth of its structure (marked by the **X**). It dynamically reinforces the anterior glenohumeral ligaments of the joint capsule.

Table 3-6. Counterbalancing Muscles of the Glenohumeral Joint

Muscles Pulling Humeral Head Superiorly
Triceps (long head)
Biceps brachii (short head)
Coracobrachialis
Clavicular head of the pectoralis major
Deltoid

Muscles Pulling Humeral Head Inferiorly
Latissimus dorsi
Teres major
Teres minor
Infraspinatus (inferior head)
Subscapularis
Pectoralis major (sternocostal head)

posterior infraspinatus provide the counterbalance to the superior translation of the humeral head generated by the deltoid muscle (Table 3-6).

Excellent representative exercises to strengthen muscles associated with the subscapular layer are listed in Table 3-7. Descriptions and details are in Chapter 6.

THE ANTERIOR SHOULDER

In this section we describe the sternocleidomastoid, pectoralis major, anterior deltoid, pectoralis minor, coracobrachialis, and both heads of the biceps brachii. We begin medially at the sternoclavicular joint and move forward laterally toward the glenohumeral joint.

Table 3-7. Exercises for Muscles of the Subscapular Layer

Supine flys: emphasize arc of motion
Pullovers from supine
Push presses emphasizing scapular protraction
Bench presses emphasizing scapular protraction
Upward rotation of scapula with humerus held at 90 degrees elevation and full external rotation
Push-ups with protraction at end
Gymnastic ball push-ups with protraction at end
Overhead presses
PNF pulls across the body with internal rotation and scapular protraction emphasis

*PNF, Proprioceptive neuromuscular facilitation.

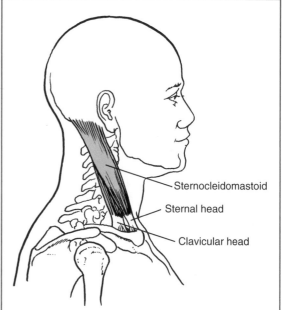

Sternocleidomastoid

Sternal head

Clavicular head

Figure 3-40. The sternocleidomastoid muscle arises from the mastoid process and travels inferiorly and anteriorly to form two heads. The clavicular head attaches to the medial clavicle, and the sternal head attaches to the sternum.

Sternocleidomastoid

The sternocleidomastoid muscle is a superficial muscle arising from the mastoid process. It lies in the same plane as the trapezius muscle and is similarly covered with the investing fascia of the neck. Like the trapezius muscle, it is innervated via the spinal accessory nerve. From the occiput, the muscle angles toward the midline and divides into two heads on reaching the anterior aspect. The smaller sternal head attaches to the manubrium of the sternum, and the broader clavicular head attaches to the medial aspect of the clavicle (Figure 3-40). The anterior costoclavicular ligament is oriented as a continuation of the line of pull of this muscle and serves to transfer the superiorly directed force of the clavicular head of the sternocleidomastoid muscle to the first rib via this ligamentous attachment from the clavicle to the rib.

Because the sternocleidomastoid muscle lies superficially, it is easily seen during the physical examination of the patient. When the head and neck are properly

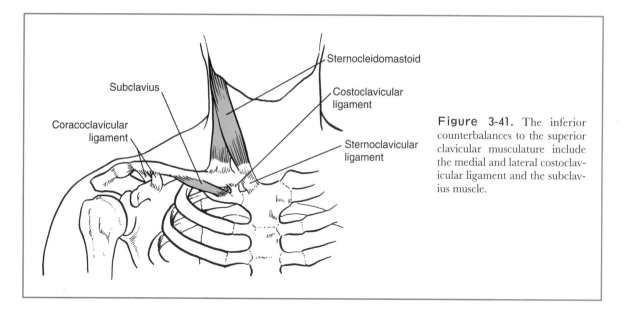

Figure 3-41. The inferior counterbalances to the superior clavicular musculature include the medial and lateral costoclavicular ligament and the subclavius muscle.

aligned over the thoracic spine and shoulder girdle, the muscle can be seen in its normal oblique orientation. If the sternocleidomastoid is oriented more vertically instead of obliquely, it cues us that a forward head posture is present.

The several actions of the sternocleidomastoid muscle include its extension of the occiput on the atlas, flexion of the lower cervical spine, rotation of the cervical spine contralaterally, lateral flexion of the cervical spine, and the ability to bring the head and neck forward. This forward head posture is one that places the sternocleidomastoid muscle in a shortened position and is a posture often assumed following hyperextension injuries of the neck since the posture places the injured musculature in a rest position.

Although not considered part of the anterior shoulder musculature, the position of the subclavius bears mentioning at this point. The small subclavius muscle attaches to the inferior surface of the clavicle and travels inferiorly and anteriorly to attach to the superior surface of the first rib. It assists in providing a check and balance of the forces and loads that are directed into the sternoclavicular joint and ultimately pass through the shoulder complex (Figure 3-41). The inferior pull of the subclavius on the clavicle, in combination with the costoclavicular ligaments, counterbalances the pull of the sternocleidomastoid muscles.

Pectoralis Major

The upper part of the pectoralis major muscle originates from the sternal half of the clavicle and travels directly laterally to attach to the lateral lip of the bicipital groove. The middle or sternocostal aspect of the pectoralis major takes attachment from the manubrium, sternum, and the upper ribs. It courses laterally, and its tendon attaches just posterior to the tendon of the clavicular head. The abdominal head of the muscle takes origin from the lower ribs and the abdominal fascia and courses to the lateral lip of the bicipital groove but does so by twisting on itself. As a result, the lower fibers of this portion of the muscle insert highest on the humerus whereas the upper portion of the abdominal head fibers insert lowest on the humerus. This results in the tendinous insertion of the muscle taking the form of a highly complex amalgamation of connective tissue oriented in a trilaminar complex.

As the pectoralis major tendon approaches the anterior shoulder, it also has important anatomical relationships with other structures. A fascial expansion from the tendon of the abdominal head referred to as the *falciform ligament* combines with the main portion of the tendon to surround the tendon of the long head of the biceps brachii muscle over the intertubercular groove of the humerus. This ligamentous expansion not only attaches to both lips of the bicipital groove

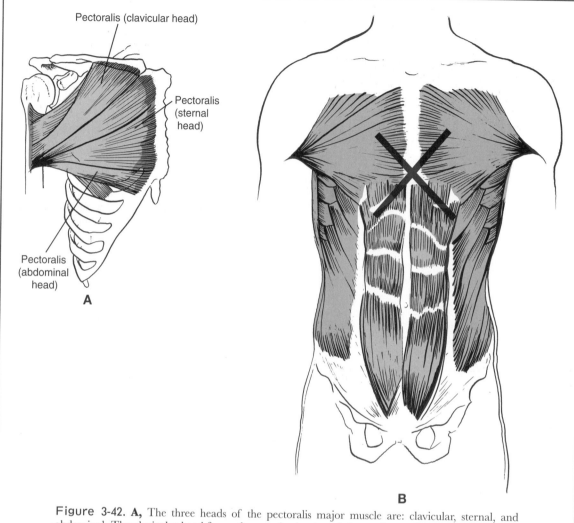

Figure 3-42. A, The three heads of the pectoralis major muscle are: clavicular, sternal, and abdominal. The clavicular head forms the anterior lamina of the tendon and travels inferiorly and laterally to the medial lip of the intertubercular groove. However, the sternal and abdominal heads blend and twist, forming a medial and posterior lamina that attaches to the glenohumeral joint capsule superiorly and surrounds the tendon of the long head of the biceps brachii muscle as it courses through the intertubercular groove. The inferiormost aspect of the abdominal head attaches most superior, and the superiormost aspect of the sternal head attaches most inferior. **B,** Note the crossing relationship of the pectoralis major.

and helps stabilize the long head tendon but also reinforces the glenohumeral joint capsule.

Because of the broad attachments of the pectoralis major, the actions of the muscle are several and are dependent on the starting position of the glenohumeral joint. From the anatomical position, the clavicular head participates in sagittal plane elevation. Once the arm is

overhead, the abdominal and sternocostal heads pull the arm strongly back toward extension and adduction. The strong adduction capabilities of the pectoralis major allow its pull also to result in depression and downward rotation of the scapulothoracic articulation. All of the heads are aligned to contribute to internal rotation, and the combination of the latissimus dorsi, teres major, anterior deltoid, and pectoralis major makes internal rotation a much stronger motion than glenohumeral external rotation. Most of the pectoralis major muscle is oriented to horizontally adduct the humerus across the body.

In the abdominal region, the pectoralis major blends into the abdominal fascia bilaterally to form another crossing relationship over the anterior superior aspect of the trunk. Thus contraction of the pectoralis major muscle pulls up or "cinches" the abdominal fascia much like the latissimus dorsi over the posterior shoulder cinches up the thoracolumbar fascia (Figure 3-42, *A* and *B*).

Anterior Deltoid

Although it was described earlier, the anterior deltoid is mentioned briefly again here because of its muscular attachments to the clavicle. It arises from the lateral third of the clavicle, where it helps reinforce the acromioclavicular joint, and travels posteriorly and laterally to merge with a central tendon that is also associated with the middle and posterior heads of the deltoid. The tendon is thick and fibrous and inserts into

the deltoid tuberosity of the humerus. As previously noted, this tuberosity is located on the lateral surface of the humerus midway down the shaft. Unlike the middle portion of the deltoid, which has several different parts, the anterior head courses obliquely and is thus oriented to flex, internally rotate, and adduct the humerus. The stronger the contraction of the deltoid to move the humerus, the more vigorous the activity of the muscles attached to the clavicle and scapula in order to provide a stable yet moving platform.

Pectoralis Minor

With the pectoralis major and anterior deltoid reflected, we can view three muscles that are attached to the coracoid process. These are the more medially placed pectoralis minor and the laterally placed conjoint tendons of the coracobrachialis and the short head of the biceps brachii (Figure 3-43). The pectoralis minor is a thin, triangular-shaped muscle that lies directly under the pectoralis major. From the coracoid process, it travels inferiorly and medially to attach to the second, third, fourth, and fifth ribs just lateral to the costocartilaginous junction and the aponeurosis that covers the intercostal muscles from ribs 2 through 5. In the region of the anterior axilla, the pectoralis minor covers the neurovascular complex coursing from the neck to the upper extremity (see Chapter 2).

Beginning with the scapula in a starting position of full retraction, the pectoralis minor pulls the scapula forward (protraction). Keep in mind that a position of retraction collapses the pectoralis minor over the neurovascular bundle in the axilla. In the presence of neural or vascular symptoms in the upper extremity, the postural role of the pectoralis minor needs to be carefully evaluated. If the scapula is in an upwardly rotated position, the pectoralis minor pulls down on the coracoid process, resulting in downward rotation at the scapulothoracic articulation. Because of this combined effect of downward rotation and protraction, tightness of the muscle may be a contributing factor in the rounded shoulder posture. Finally, if the scapula is fixated, the muscle may act to raise the rib cage.

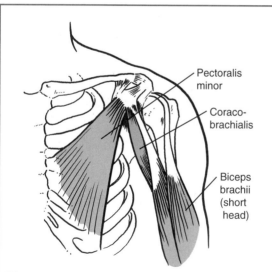

Figure 3-43. The three muscles that attach to the coracoid process are from lateral to medial: the pectoralis minor, the coracobrachialis, and the short head of the biceps brachii.

Coracobrachialis

The coracobrachialis muscle lies medial to but is blended with the short head of the biceps brachii at the coracoid process. From this attachment the long

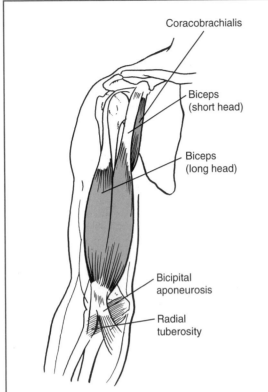

Figure 3-44. The short and long heads of the biceps brachii muscle join to form a thick, round muscle belly that eventually twists to attach on the radial tuberosity. The bicipital aponeurosis arises from the tendon and courses obliquely downward and medially to blend into the fascial covering of the flexor forearm.

straplike muscle actually broadens quite dramatically as it courses inferiorly and laterally to insert on the anteromedial aspect of nearly a third of the humerus in the region between the triceps brachii and the brachialis muscles. The coracobrachialis lies over the top of the subscapularis muscle, and the coracobrachialis bursa is interposed between the two. Note again how a crossing relationship is formed between the more vertically oriented coracobrachialis and the more horizontally oriented subscapularis.

The action of the muscle is primarily elevation of the glenohumeral joint in the sagittal plane, as well as adduction and horizontal adduction of the humerus. When the extent of the coracobrachialis insertion on the humerus is closely inspected, we can see how the muscle strongly contributes to glenohumeral adduction, and this is the primary motion with which the muscle is trained using resistance exercises.

Short Head of Biceps Brachii

The short head of the biceps brachii arises from the tip of the coracoid process as thick, flat tendon in common with and lateral to the coracobrachialis muscle. From the coracoid process it travels inferiorly and laterally to join the long head of the biceps, forming a single muscle belly, which ultimately attaches to the forearm in two distinct ways. The lateral part of the muscle attaches to the radial tuberosity, whereas the medial aspect of the muscle blends in with the forearm fascia as the bicipital aponeurosis (Figure 3-44). The primary actions of the biceps occur at the elbow region and include elbow flexion and forearm supination. Over the shoulder, the muscle can contribute to the initiation of elevation of the humerus, and from the overhead position the muscle helps pull the humerus down to the side of the body. The short head of the biceps and the coracobrachialis form a crossing relationship with the subscapularis muscles, which contributes to the stabilization of the anterior aspect of the glenohumeral joint (see Figure 3-36).

Long Head of Biceps Brachii

The long head of the biceps brachii arises from the supraglenoid tubercle and the posterior-superior glenoid labrum and glenoid rim. It is enclosed in a special synovial sheath within the glenohumeral joint, and the tendon exits through an opening of the capsule. Such an arrangement allows the tendon to be intracapsular yet extrasynovial relative to the glenohumeral joint. It travels over the humeral head and emerges from the capsule to lie within the intertubercular groove.

Several tissues stabilize the long head of the biceps over the head of the humerus and through the bicipital groove. Proximally the tendon is covered by the coracohumeral ligament and superior glenohumeral ligament of the joint capsule, thus stabilizing the tendon in this region. The tendon then exits the capsule and reaches the proximal aspect of the bicipital groove. At this region, the upper portion of the subscapularis tendon and lower aspect of the supraspinatus tendon form the floor of the sheath embracing the biceps tendon.

Another fascial expansion from the supraspinatus combines with the coracohumeral ligament to cover the tendon. Finally, as the tendon enters the main portion of the groove, it is covered by the falciform ligament, which is the fascial expansion of the pectoralis major tendon. The falciform ligament attaches not only to both lips of the bicipital groove but also to the glenohumeral capsule. Thus the long head of the biceps is stabilized at the shoulder joint via a complex array of several important connective tissues.

In order to most effectively design exercise programs in the presence of long head of the biceps tendon involvement, we must realize that the long head of the biceps tendon does not slide in the bicipital groove but rather the humerus moves under a stationary tendon. The sheath that surrounds the biceps tendon helps minimize the friction between the moving humerus and the static tendon. Bicipital tenosynovitis is an inflammation of this tendinous sheath, and it is important to recognize the mechanics of the groove tendon relationship to effectively manage this condition. The clinician must decrease shoulder flexion, both extension and abduction, and adduction activities rather than elbow flexion and extension activities to successfully rest this area. Pulling exercises that require the humerus to move against resistance from flexion to extension potentially aggravate the tenosynovitis problem and exacerbate the condition.

The actions of the biceps over the elbow have been noted previously. The long head has several unique functions. It is a major decelerator of the throwing arm as the elbow rapidly moves from a flexed position in the early stages of throwing to an extended position. In addition, it most likely serves as a weak flexor at the glenohumeral joint. The long head also functions to increase stability of the glenohumeral joint. Its very anatomical position allows it to serve as a static restraint to superior translation of the head of the humerus. Active contraction of the long head only slightly depresses the humeral head, so the tendon's role is primarily a passive one in regard to this function.[53] It is important to note that its normal static contribution is dependent on the positioning of the tendon within the groove, which is a function of the stabilizing mechanisms provided by the supraspinatus and subscapularis tendons. Tears of the rotator cuff can thus affect the positioning of the long head of the biceps tendon, resulting in its inability to contribute to glenohumeral stabilization.

The position of the glenohumeral joint also influences the contribution of the long head of the biceps tendon to shoulder stabilization. When the arm is placed in a position of abduction and external rotation, the long and short heads of the biceps become anterior reinforcements to the anterior glenohumeral ligaments and joint capsule. When there has been injury to the glenohumeral ligaments, the biceps tendons serve to stabilize the humeral head against anterior translation.[18]

Finally, the tendon of the long head of the biceps brachii passes over the head of the humerus in a position that is vulnerable to excessive compression between the head of the humerus and the suprahumeral dome. It is common for the tendon of the long head of the biceps brachii to flatten because of compression, rendering it vulnerable to swelling and possible rupture (see Chapter 4). The tendon is also vulnerable at its attachments to the glenoid labrum, where it can be avulsed away from its attachment especially as resulting sequelae to long term, continuous stress that weakens the tissue. Tears of the glenoid labrum, in particular the SLAP (superior labrum anterior to posterior) lesions discussed in Chapter 4, can be compromised even further when tension is applied through the biceps tendon, which places further stress to an already compromised glenoid labrum. A torn labrum with a split longitudinally in the long head of the biceps is evidence of a very advanced SLAP lesion.[11] We can easily see that traction through the long head of the biceps tendon not only further compromises the tendon but also further avulses the glenoid labrum.

Exercises primarily for training the muscles of the anterior shoulder are listed in Table 3-8 and are illustrated and discussed in Chapter 6.

Table 3-8. Exercises for the Anterior Shoulder Layer
Pectoralis: Major and Minor
Coracobrachialis
Supine flys
Bench presses
Incline bench presses
Weight assisted bar dips
Shoulder elevations in various planes between sagittal and frontal with external rotated humerus
Biceps Brachii
Elbow curls with simultaneous supination
Seated rows with supination
Counter weighted pull-ups with underhand grip

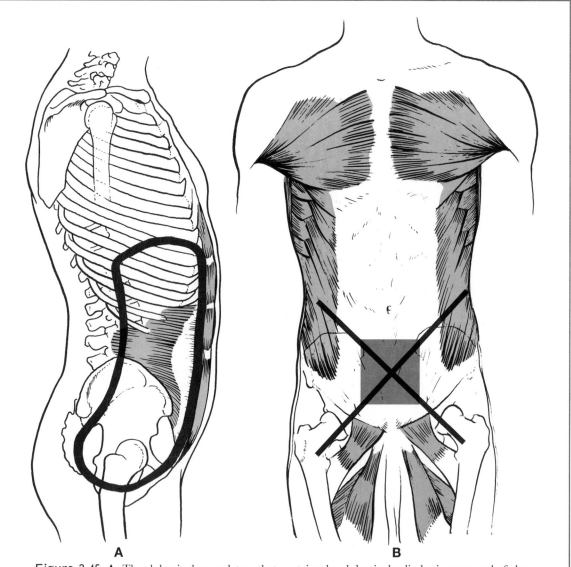

Figure 3-45. A, The abdominal musculature that contains the abdominal cylinder is composed of the abdominal muscles, the diaphragm, the lumbar spine and its related muscles, and the muscles that comprise the pelvic floor. **B,** The abdominal wall also includes a crossing relationship that affords increased stability of the anterior and inferior aspect of our trunk below the umbilicus.

ABDOMINAL MUSCULATURE

The last muscle group that should be described briefly in any textbook about mechanical shoulder disorders includes those of the abdominal wall. We have discussed these muscles in detail in previous texts.[33,34]

The abdominal wall functions to maintain the cylinder of the trunk responsible for the maintenance of an erect posture. It also serves to ensure efficient movement of the appendages.

The abdominal wall has four muscles directly associated with its structure, namely the transversus

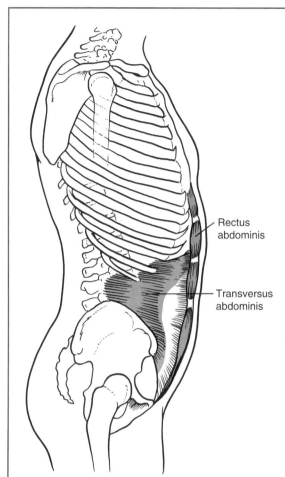

Figure 3-46. A sagittal plane view of the abdominal wall shows the fiber orientation of the transversus abdominis muscle and its importance in alignment of the spine and shoulder girdle with the lumbopelvic region and hips.

Table 3-9. Exercises for the Abdominal Mechanism

Standing high rows with thoracic cage flexion and pelvis tilt
Standing rotary cable crosses
Gymnastic ball stabilization
Keeping abdominal wall toward beltline with concurrent upper extremity and/or lower extremity load challenges
Supine pullovers

are best positioned to pull the abdominal contents straight back, thus effectively aligning the upper spine and shoulder girdle over the lumbopelvic region and hips (Figure 3-46). Indirectly, the rhomboids, pectoralis major, serratus anterior, and femoral adductors can be considered as part of the abdominal mechanism as well (see Figure 3-17, *C*). The pectoralis major's linkage to the abdominal fascia and the serratus anterior's linkage to the external oblique have been described in previous sections of this chapter. These key shoulder muscles are in fact an integral component of what we typically refer to as the "abdominal mechanism." Exercises that can be used to strengthen the abdominal wall, including those that incorporate shoulder girdle activity, are listed in Table 3-9 and described in detail in Chapter 6.

SUMMARY

We have carefully described the clinically relevant aspects of the muscles associated with the shoulder girdle. The explanation of crossing relationships between various muscles gives you additional information about how a region with such great mobility simultaneously remains remarkably stable. In addition, we have emphasized the relationships of muscles to each other and their associated fascial networks. Strengthening the muscles that pull on these thick connective tissues and performing exercises designed to hypertrophy those muscles that are contained within these fascial systems represent primary goals of rehabilitation programs designed to improve performance.

Appropriately maintaining the health of these tissues helps maintain the position of the scapula on the thorax and control the forces directed to the head of the humerus. When we lose the health of shoulder girdle muscles or the anterior strut of the abdominal cylinder, loads to the supporting tissues of the glenohumeral joint are increased. It is logical to conclude

abdominis, internal oblique, external oblique, and rectus abdominis (Figure 3-45, *A* and *B*). These muscles form, connect into, and function via a fascial system referred to as the *abdominal fascia*. This fascial system forms an anterior and lateral strut that contains the abdominal contents and operates as the base from which the upper and lower extremities function. The external oblique, internal oblique, and transversus abdominis attach into the abdominal fascia that surround the rectus abdominis muscle. The fibers of the transversus abdominis muscle travel horizontally and that initiating activities in the area predisposed to increased joint pressures renders the tissues vulnerable to overload. The ability to maintain upright posture is critical to secure scapular position and the successful attenuation of stresses to the entire shoulder complex. Strengthening the musculature of the shoulder girdle has to be complemented by a critical assessment of the trunk and lower extremity strength in order to provide a comprehensive approach to rehabilitation in managing mechanical disorders of the shoulder complex. In Chapters 5 and 6 we will build on the clinical anatomy that has been discussed in the first four chapters as the foundation for the evaluation and treatment of mechanical disorders of the shoulder girdle.

REFERENCES

1. Arwert HJ, de Groot J, Van Woensel WW, et al: Electromyography of shoulder muscles in relation to force direction, *J Shoulder Elbow Surg* 6(4):360, 1997.
2. Blevins FT, Djurasovic M, Flatow EL, et al: Biology of the rotator cuff tendon, *Orthop Clin North Am* 28(1):31, 1997.
3. Blevins FT, Hayes WM, Warren RF: Rotator cuff injuries in contact athletics, *Am J Sports Med* 24:263, 1996.
4. Cain PR, Mutschler TA, Fu FH, et al: Anterior instability of the glenohumeral joint: a dynamic model, *Am J Sports Med* 15:144, 1987.
5. Clark JM, Harryman DT II: Tendons, ligaments and capsule of the rotator cuff, *J Bone Joint Surg Am* 74(5):713, 1992.
6. DiGiovine NM, Jobe FW, Pink M, et al: An electromyographic analysis of the upper extremity in pitching, *J Shoulder Elbow Surg* 1:15, 1992.
7. Elkhorn J, Arborelius UP, Hillered L, et al: Shoulder muscle EMG and resisting movement during diagonal exercise movements resisted by weight and pulley circuit, *Scand J Rehabil Med* 10:179, 1978.
8. Filo J, Furani J, De Freitas B: Electromyographic study of the trapezius muscle in free movement of the shoulder, *Clin Neurophysiol* 31:93, 1991.
9. Frost P, Andersen JH, Lundorf E: Is supraspinatus pathology as defined by magnetic resonance imaging associated with clinical signs of shoulder impingement? *J Shoulder Elbow Surg* 8 (6): 565, 1999.
10. Fukuda H, Hamada K, Yamanaka K: Pathology and pathogenesis of bursal side rotator cuff tears viewed from endblock histologic sections, *Clin Orthop* 254:75, 1990.
11. Gartsman GM, Hammerman SM: Superior labrum, anterior and posterior lesions, *Clinics in Sports Med* 19:115, 2000.
12. Giombini A, Rossi G, Pettrone FA, et al: Posterosuperior glenoid rim impingement as a cause of shoulder pain in top level water polo players, *J Sports Med Phys Fitness* 37:273, 1997.
13. Goldberg AL: Mechanism of work induced hypertrophy in skeletal muscle, *Med Sci Sports* 7:185, 1975.
14. Hawkins RJ, Bell RH, Lippitt SB: *Atlas of shoulder surgery*, St. Louis, 1996, Mosby.
15. Howell SM, Imobersteg AM, Seger DH, et al: Clarification of the role of the supraspinatus muscle in shoulder function, *J Bone Joint Surg Am* 68(A):398, 1986.
16. Itoi E, Bergland LJ, Grabowski JJ, et al: Tensile properties of the supraspinatus tendon, *J Orthop Res* 13:578, 1995.
17. Itoi E, Kido T, Sano A, et al: Which is more useful, the "full can test" or the "empty can test" in detecting the torn supraspinatus tendon? *Am J Sports Med* 27:65, 1999.
18. Itoi E, Kuechle DK, Newman SR, et al: Stabilizing function of the biceps in stable and unstable shoulders, *J Bone Joint Surg Am* 75(B):546, 1993.
19. Jensen BR, Jorgensen K, Huijing PA, et al: Soft tissue architecture and intramuscular pressure in the shoulder region, *European J Morph* 33:205, 1995.
20. Jobe FW, Moynes DR, Tibone JE, et al: An EMG analysis of the shoulder in pitching: a second report, *Am J Sports Med* 12:218, 1984.
21. Johnson G, Bogduk N, Nowitzke A, et al: Anatomy and actions of the trapezius muscle, *Clin Biomech* 9:44, 1994.
22. Kibler WB: The role of the scapula in athletic shoulder function, *Am J Sports Med* 26:325-337, 1998.
23. Laumann U: Kinesiology of the shoulder joint. In Koelbel R, editor, *Shoulder replacement*. Berlin, 1987, Springer Verlag.
24. Lindman R, Eriksson A, Thornell LE: Fiber type composition of the human female trapezius muscle: enzyme-histochemical characteristics, *Am J Anat* 190:385, 1991.
25. Lindman R, Eriksson A, Thornell LE: Fiber type composition of the human male trapezius muscle: enzyme-histochemical characteristics, *Am J Anat* 189:236, 1990.
26. Lizaur A, Marco L, Cebrian R: Acute dislocation of the acromioclavicular joint: traumatic anatomy and the importance of the deltoid and trapezius, *J Bone Joint Surg Am* 76(Br):602, 1994.
27. Logan GA, McKinney WC: The serape effect. In *Kinesiology*, Dubuque, Iowa, 1970, Wm C Brown.
28. Ludewig PM, Cook TM: Alterations in shoulder kinematics and associated muscle activity in people with symptoms of shoulder impingement, *Phys Ther* 80:276, 2000.
29. Mosely BJ, Jobe FW, Pink M, et al: EMG analysis of the scapular muscles during a rehabilitation program, *Am J Sports Med* 20:128, 1992.
30. Mottram SL: Dynamic stability of the scapula, *Man Ther* 2:123, 1997.
31. Nakajima T, Rokuuma N, Hamada K, et al: Histologic and biomechanical considerations of the supraspinatus tendon: reference to rotator cuff tearing, *J Shoulder Elbow Surg* 3:79, 1994.
32. Perry J: Biomechanics of the shoulder. In Bowe C, editor: *The shoulder*, New York, 1988, Churchill Livingstone.
33. Porterfield JA, DeRosa C: *Mechanical low back pain: perspectives in functional anatomy*, ed 2, Philadelphia, 1998, WB Saunders.
34. Porterfield JA, DeRosa C: *Mechanical neck pain: perspectives in functional anatomy*, Philadelphia, 1995, WB Saunders.
35. Reddy AS, Mohr KJ, Pink MM, et al: Electromyographic analysis of the deltoid and rotator cuff in persons with subacromial impingement, *J Shoulder Elbow Surg* 9(6):519, 2000.
36. Saha AK: Dynamic stability of the glenohumeral joint, *Acta Orthop Scand* 42:491, 1971.
37. Scarpinato DF, Bramhall JP, Andrews JR: Arthroscopic management of the throwing athlete's shoulder: indications, techniques, and results, *Clin Sports Med* 10(4):913, 1991.

38. Schmitt L, Snyder-Mackler L: Role of the scapular stabilizers in etiology and treatment of impingement syndrome, *J Orthop Sports Phys Ther* 29:31,1999.

39. Schwartz E, Warren RF, O'Brien SJ, et al: Posterior shoulder instability, *Orthop Clin North Am* 18:409, 1987.

40. Sethi N, Wright R, Yamaguchi K: Disorders of the long head of the biceps tendon, *J Shoulder Elbow Surg* 8:6, 1999.

41. Solem-Bertoft E, Thuomas KA, Westerberg CE: The influence of scapular retraction and protraction on the width of the subacromial space: an MRI study, *Clin Orthop and Rel Res* 296:99, 1993.

42. Sonnery-Cottet B, Edwards B, Noel E, et al: Results of arthroscopic treatment of posterosuperior glenoid impingement in tennis players, *Am J Sports Med* 30:227, 2002.

43. Soslowsky LJ, Carpenter JE, Bucchieri JS, et al: Biomechanics of the rotator cuff, *Orthop Clin North Am* 28:1, 1997.

44. Tempelhof S, Rupp S, Seil R: Age-related prevalence of rotator cuff tears in asymptomatic shoulders, *J Shoulder Elbow Surg* 8:296, 1999.

45. Terry GC, Chopp TM: Functional anatomy of the shoulder, *J Athletic Training* 35(3):248, 2000.

46. Tibone JE, Elrod B, Jobe FW, et al: Surgical treatment of tears of the rotator cuff in athletics, *J Bone Joint Surg Am* 68(A):887, 1986.

47. Townsend H, Jobe FW, Pink M, et al: Electromyographic analysis of the glenohumeral muscles during a baseball rehabilitation program, 19[jb13](3):264,1991.

48. Uhthoff HK, Sano H: Pathology of failure of the rotator cuff tendon, *Orthopedic Clinics North Am* 28:31, 1997.

49. Wadsworth DJS, Bullock-Saxton JE: Recruitment patterns of the scapular rotator muscle in freestyle swimmers with subacromial impingement, *Int J Sports Med* 18:618, 1997.

50. Wagner DB, Swienckowski JJ, Lennox JD: Painful subluxation of the acromioclavicular joint, *Am J Sports Med* 29:513, 2001.

51. Werner SL, Gill TJ, Murray TA, et al: Relationships between throwing mechanics and shoulder distraction in professional baseball pitchers, *Am J Sports Med* 29:354, 2001.

52. Williams PL, Warwick R: *Gray's anatomy*, ed 36, Philadelphia, 1980, WB Saunders.

53. Yamaguchi K, Riew KD, Galatz LM, et al: Biceps function in normal and rotator cuff deficient shoulders: an electromyographic analysis, *Orthop Trans* 18:191, 1994.

54. Yamanaka K, Matsumoto T: The joint side tear of the rotator cuff: a follow-up study by arthrography, *Clin Orthop* 304:68, 1994.

CHAPTER 4

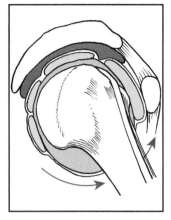

ARTICULATIONS OF THE SHOULDER GIRDLE

INTRODUCTION

The often repeated words "the shoulder is built for mobility rather than stability" can prevent us from fully understanding how this remarkable complex of articulations simultaneously meets the demands of mobility and stability. Indeed, it is perhaps more instructive to consider the shoulder complex as extraordinarily stable when it is viewed in the context of the wide variety of motion possibilities and the numerous torques and linear forces it is subjected to.

Shoulder girdle motion consists of a complex series of moving bony levers, motion of soft tissues over and between bursal interfaces, and an extraordinarily large number of combinations of muscle contractions in the specific segments of muscles associated with the scapula, humerus, clavicle, radius, ulna, spine, and occiput. Bony levers forming these multiple articulations are under control of the neuromuscular system

and must instantaneously assume roles of stability and mobility on demand throughout even the simplest arc of motion.

Such an intricate mechanism presents the clinician with challenges during examination, evaluation, and selection of the most appropriate treatment interventions for the patient with shoulder pain or loss of function related to mechanical problems of the shoulder girdle. The functional interplay of the multiple tissues is closely aligned with the reality of shoulder disorders: most mechanical shoulder problems are not isolated injuries affecting only one structure within the shoulder complex. Instead, most shoulder disorders, whether they occur from isolated injury, overuse syndromes, or simply as a result of the aging process, affect several tissues or structures of the shoulder girdle. In addition, the trunk and hip musculature play a major role in the resting posture and movement patterns of the upper quarter, further increasing an already complex physiology.

In this chapter we detail the articulations of the shoulder girdle and consider the implications of structure and function on selected aspects of the shoulder examination and various interventions used in the management of shoulder disorders. Our emphasis will be on the glenohumeral joint, acromioclavicular joint, and the sternoclavicular joint and on two unique interfaces,

Throughout this chapter you will find small circular icons marked "DVD" (see margin). These icons identify content that is coordinated with a video clip on the DVD accompanying this text. For maximum learning benefit, go to the "Text Reference Section" on the DVD and play the coordinated clip while reading the appropriate section of text. These clips expand on and reinforce the information presented in the text.

the scapulothoracic interface and the suprahumeral-subacromial interface. That said, we approach these structures within a framework of the full shoulder girdle motion that also is dependent on motion of the cervical and thoracic spine and the ultimate ability to stabilize the trunk. For example, complete range of shoulder motion in elevation (lifting the arms completely overhead) requires a significant degree of cervical and thoracic spine extension. To hold a weight overhead, the spine must first move toward extension and then serve as a relatively stiff platform in order to keep the weight stabilized overhead. Shoulder elevation with overpressure is an excellent way to assess the extension and weight-bearing capacity of the apophyseal joints in the cervical and thoracic spines.

THE GLENOHUMERAL JOINT

The Head of the Humerus

The relationship of the head of the humerus to the glenoid fossa has often been likened to the "fit" of a golf ball (head of the humerus) on a golf tee (glenoid fossa). Such a comparison emphasizes the disproportional contact relationship between the articular surfaces of the humeral head and the glenoid fossa. It is a good analogy because the actual contact relationship between the head of the humerus and the glenoid fossa is relatively small. At any given moment of any motion, nearly 70% of the humeral head is not in contact with any part of the glenoid fossa. Despite this mismatch, the connective tissue and neuromuscular stabilizing mechanisms precisely maintain the head of the humerus within a 1 to 2 mm variation throughout an arc of motion.[39,49]

Before more sophisticated analysis of glenohumeral motion was possible, clinicians liberally applied the arthrokinematic rules for concave-convex joint surfaces to the glenohumeral joint.[61] Such rules imply that elevation of the humerus on the glenoid results in the humeral head translating inferiorly on the glenoid. The clinical application of such a rule suggested using inferior glide translations of the humeral head in order to improve glenohumeral elevation (i.e., abduction or flexion). Several studies have now shown that there is very little inferior glide of the humeral head on the glenoid during elevation.[30,31,49] In fact, when the arm begins to elevate, the head of the humerus first translates superiorly approximately 1 to 3 mm and then remains relatively centered within the glenoid fossa. This ability of the head of the humerus to remain centered on the glenoid is largely a function of the rotator cuff musculature, but other passive mech-

anisms that will be discussed later also come into play.[21] Joint mobilization techniques remain excellent treatment tools; however, use of these interventions is primarily to introduce various translations and rotary stresses to the joint in order to maintain or improve generalized capsular mobility and enhance fluid dynamics. Used as a treatment intervention, such techniques result in improved motion in all ranges of the glenohumeral joint, rather than using a particular translation (glide) to improve physiological flexion, abduction, or rotation (see Chapter 6).

In addition to the head of the humerus, the proximal portion of the humerus features several key bony landmarks: the greater tuberosity with its three smooth and flat surfaces for muscle attachments (supraspinatus,

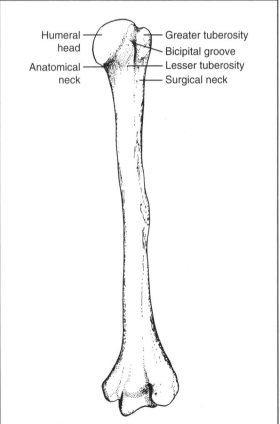

Figure 4-1. Key structures of the proximal portion of the humerus include the humeral head, greater and lesser tuberosities, bicipital or intertubercular groove, the anatomical neck of the humerus, and the surgical neck of the humerus.

infraspinatus, and teres minor); the lesser tuberosity with a flattened surface for the subscapularis attachment, the bicipital or intertubercular groove; and the anatomical and surgical necks of the humerus (Figure 4-1).

The head of the humerus is not a complete sphere, and the smoothest part of its spherical head is covered with hyaline cartilage. This cartilage covered humeral head faces medially and then is oriented upward approximately 130 to 150 degrees and backward (retroverted) approximately 26 to 31 degrees when the arm is by the side.[34] It has also been suggested that high level overhead athletes demonstrate even greater humeral head retroversion on the dominant shoulder when compared with the nondominant side, implying even further bony adaptation as a result of prolonged cumulative stresses.[10]

The cartilage covering the head of the humerus is not uniformly thick but instead is thicker in the central region of the humeral head and then becomes thinner at the peripheral aspect of the head (Figure 4-2). This is exactly opposite to the relationship of the articular cartilage with the glenoid fossa, in which the cartilage is thicker at its periphery but thinner toward the center. The contribution that such a unique cartilaginous interface makes to the stability of the glenohumeral joint is discussed later in the Glenoid Labrum section of this chapter.

There are typically eight ossification centers within the humerus, but only three relate directly to the proximal aspect of the humerus. These three ossification centers are located in the head of the humerus, the greater tuberosity, and the lesser tuberosity. While preliminary epiphyseal closure begins during childhood, it is generally not complete in these three centers until 25 years of age (Figure 4-3).[6] The medial end of this upper epiphyseal line is intracapsular. The clinician needs to remember this especially important consideration when dealing with young athletes who present with shoulder trauma, or shoulder pain as a result of microtrauma and overuse.

The Scapula

The triangular-shaped scapula typically overlies the second to seventh ribs and has three very distinct bony projections: the spine of the scapula, the continuation of this spine of the scapula as the acromion process, and the coracoid process. The upwardly facing glenoid fossa lies on the lateral aspect of the scapula. This fossa articulates with the head of the humerus. In addition, two bony tubercles are associated with the glenoid cavity: the

supraglenoid tubercle and the infraglenoid tubercle (Figure 4-4, *A*).

There are numerous ossification centers in the scapula, including two in the coracoid process, three in the acromion process, one in the scapula body, and one in the rim of the glenoid cavity. The ossification centers of the scapula are typically united between the ages of 20 and 24 years of age. The three ossification centers in the acromion are united by 22 years of age, but if they fail to unite, a condition referred to as *osacromiale* results. This condition is often associated with rotator cuff degeneration.[46] The clinician needs to always keep the presence of these ossification centers in mind when evaluating children, adolescents, and young adults for shoulder pain.

The Glenoid Cavity

The total articular surface of the glenoid fossa is less than a third of the total articular surface of the humeral head (see Figure 4-2). Its relatively small fossa faces backward approximately 4 to 12 degrees relative to the plane of the scapula. Since the plane of the scapula is approximately 30 to 40 degrees anterior to the coronal plane of the body, the glenoid fossa is actually directly facing the posteriorly facing humeral head.

Because the scapula is a relatively flat bone, a scapular "plane" can be described based on the position of the scapula as it moves over the thorax (Figure 4-4, *B*). The reader needs to be able to visualize this plane because the position of the scapula on the thorax ultimately results in the glenoid fossa having a variety of possible orientations relative to the plane of the body. For example, when the shoulder girdle is in complete retraction, the scapular plane more closely parallels the coronal plane of the body. When the shoulder is fully protracted, however, the scapular plane more closely parallels the sagittal plane of the body.

The importance of being able to visualize the plane of the scapula is related to the clinician's ability to analyze forces of the humerus on the glenoid and between the humeral head and the suprahumeral dome with various exercises. The suprahumeral dome consists of the undersurface of the acromion, coracoacromial ligament, coracoid process, and the conjoint tendon of the coracobrachialis and short head of the biceps brachii. Note that with the scapula protracted and the glenohumeral joint in flexion, there is a compressive load of the humerus on the glenoid when a force is applied through the long axis of the humerus. The same force applied through the long axis of the humerus with the same glenohumeral

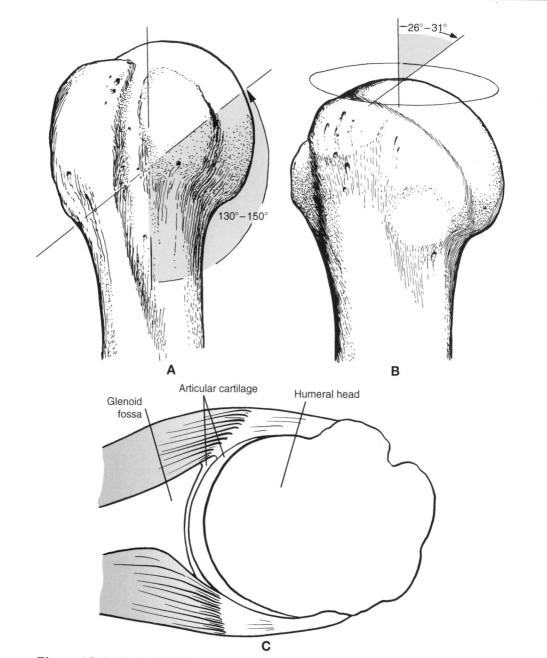

Figure 4-2. A, The head of the humerus is angled upward 130 to 150 degrees, and **B,** backward 26 to 31 degrees. **C,** The articular cartilage, as seen in the superior transverse section, that covers the head of the humerus is thicker in its central region and thinner in the periphery.

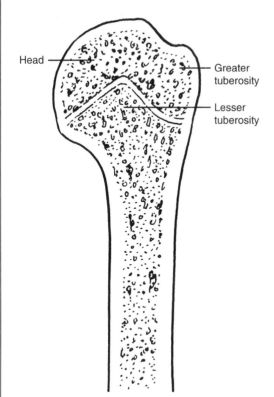

Head

Greater
tuberosity

Lesser
tuberosity

Figure 4-3. A cross section of the right humerus shows the three ossification centers associated with the proximal aspect of the humerus (head, and greater and lesser tuberosity), which typically fuse to form one larger ossification center by the sixth year of life.

analysis can be performed with open kinetic chain exercises such as shoulder elevation. When performed in three different scapular planes—along the sagittal plane of the body, the frontal plane of the body, and midway between the two—differences in the glenohumeral joint reactive forces result.

The clinician working with a patient with any mechanical shoulder disorder must be cognizant of those scapular and humeral positions that result in increased glenohumeral shear or compression. This is true when applying passive joint mobilization techniques, as well as when designing an exercise prescription for resistance exercises for the shoulder. For example, we typically recommend that shoulder elevation exercises, especially when using free weights or pulleys, be performed in a plane midway between the coronal and sagittal planes. This is the approximate plane of the scapula as it rests over the thorax, often referred to as the *scaption plane*. Careful observation or palpation of the scapular motion during the exercise can help verify that plane. Furthermore, it is essential that the clinician note the quality and the quantity of scapular motion during any resisted shoulder elevation exercises. We typically emphasize the scapular protraction, rotation, and elevation components of any lateral or forward arm raise exercises. Ignoring this fundamental shoulder exercise concept—the scapula moving smoothly and strongly into protraction, upward rotation, and elevation during forward or lateral arm raise exercises—results in excessive compression of the soft tissues lying in the suprahumeral space, which we will discuss in detail later. Ludewig and Cook have demonstrated that decreased serratus anterior muscle activity is very common in patients with impingement syndrome and note that attention to the actions of this key muscle is essential in shoulder rehabilitation programs.[37]

It is equally important to analyze the scapular position when performing closed kinetic chain exercises. Most importantly, the clinician must take great care in developing a closed kinetic chain exercise prescription for shoulder strengthening because 1) the glenohumeral joint is not designed to be a weight-bearing joint, and 2) shear loads may be poorly tolerated because of limitations of the specialized connective tissue restraints. The complexity of these mechanisms is one of the reasons why designing an exercise program for the compromised shoulder joint is so difficult.

The above descriptions reinforce the fact that the glenohumeral joint is a multiaxial joint, which is capable of movement in all planes. Only a small portion of

flexion but with the scapula retracted results in a greater posterior shear force between the humerus and scapula and markedly less compression between the humeral head and glenoid.

Consider the application of these mechanics to shoulder girdle exercises. When we do a wall push-up or a floor push-up, the position of the scapula ultimately dictates what the joint reactive force will be at the glenohumeral joint. Weak scapular protractors result in the scapula being positioned in the coronal plane of the body with a significant glenohumeral shear force occurring with the exercise. In the same exercise, strong scapular protractors would align the scapula more closely to the sagittal plane and result in more glenohumeral joint compression and less shear of the humeral head on the glenoid. The same type of

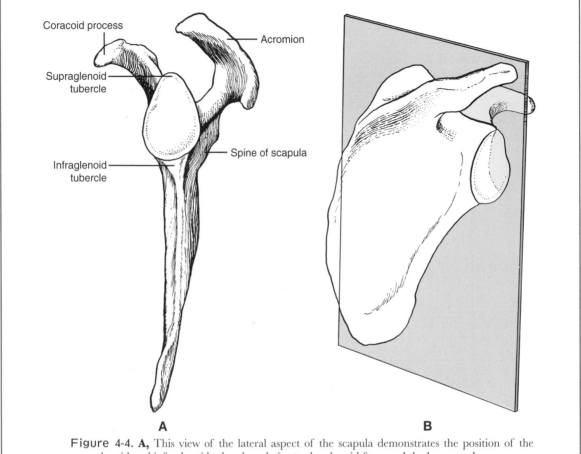

Figure 4-4. A, This view of the lateral aspect of the scapula demonstrates the position of the supraglenoid and infraglenoid tubercles relative to the glenoid fossa and the key scapular processes: the spine of the scapula, acromion process, and coracoid process. **B,** This view shows the plane of the scapula.

the head of the humerus is in contact with the glenoid fossa at any given moment; additionally there are very few positions in which the head of the humerus becomes completely congruent with the surface of the glenoid fossa. Maximal congruency between the bony partners of a synovial joint is referred to as the *close-packed* position of the joint, and the position of maximal congruency for the glenohumeral joint occurs when the humerus is abducted and externally rotated. As expected, this position of abduction and external rotation is also the position in which the highest degree of load-bearing articular pressure between the head of the humerus and the glenoid fossa occurs.[8] This position also places the inferior aspect of the joint

capsule and the inferior glenohumeral ligament under significant tension, and it is a very vulnerable position for dislocation, subluxation, or excessive strain of these specialized connective tissues supporting the joint. In contrast, the loose-packed position of the joint, a position in which there is the least resistance to any translation because of capsular and ligamentous laxity, is a position in which the humerus is placed in approximately the plane of the scapula, namely, 55 degrees abduction and 30 degrees horizontal adduction.

Applying this understanding of the bony levers that form the glenohumeral joint, we can now detail several of the support structures that help maintain the contact relationship between the humerus and the glenoid. Several key specialized connective tissue structures are intimately associated with the bony levers constituting the glenohumeral joint, including the glenoid labrum, long head of the biceps tendon, joint capsule, synovial lining, capsular ligaments, bursal interfaces, and the rotator cuff tendons. The interplay between each of these structures is critical to normal shoulder function, so we will examine several important clinical points related to these structures.

Specialized Connective Tissue Structures Associated With the Glenohumeral Joint

The Glenoid Labrum

The triangular- to round-shaped glenoid labrum is attached around the margins of the glenoid rim and is a composite of fibrous and cartilaginous material.[9] The structure of the labrum is such that the thicker portion of labrum is attached to the glenoid rim, whereas the thinner portion comprises its free edge. The superior aspect of the labrum or "12 o'clock position" on the glenoid face generally has a "looser" attachment to the glenoid than the inferior aspect of the labrum or "6 o'clock position" and is continuous with the long head of the biceps tendon (Figure 4-5). The inferior labrum is also more substantive and has more bulk than the superior aspect.[23] As a result of its peripherally placed position on the glenoid, the labrum effectively deepens the glenoid socket to a depth ranging from 5 mm to 10 mm.[29]

The labrum plays several important roles in shoulder mechanics, but the primary role is its contribution to stability of the glenohumeral joint. As evidence of its contribution to stability, it is estimated that a torn or deficient labrum results in approximately 20% more translatory movement of the humeral head on the glenoid than when the labrum is intact. This clearly results in instability between the humeral head and glenoid.[35]

How do the hyaline cartilage coverings of the glenoid and humerus work in concert with the labrum to contribute to glenohumeral stability? The combination of a thicker hyaline cartilage in the periphery of the glenoid rim in conjunction with the added glenoid rim elevation afforded by the glenoid labrum results in a more closely matching radius of curvature of the head of the humerus with the radius of curvature of

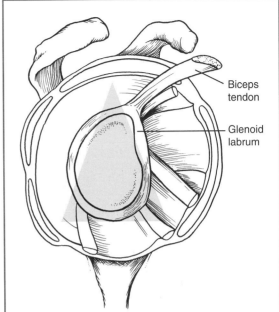

Biceps tendon

Glenoid labrum

Figure 4-5. The glenoid labrum is triangular in cross section and is continuous at its superior surface with the long head of the biceps tendon.

the glenoid. The fossa is functionally deepened by this arrangement. Thus one contribution to stability is simply the increase in the concavity of the glenoid fossa via deformation of the articular cartilage and the mechanics of the labrum.

The thicker cartilage at the periphery, plus the fibrocartilaginous glenoid labrum, contributes to the mechanical stability of the glenohumeral joint in more ways than simply increasing the depth of the fossa. A region in which there is a thick hyaline cartilage "cushion" typically has greater flex or ability to deform (i.e., that region can be more easily compressed and then can spring back to its original shape). The periphery of the glenoid rim exhibits this particular quality of deformability. At the periphery of the glenoid rim the articular cartilage becomes thicker as it blends into the fibrocartilaginous labrum. The combination of the thicker cartilage and fibrous labrum leads to increased flexibility or deformability at the periphery of the glenoid rim, resulting in the humeral head being "sealed" when pressed into the glenoid (Figure 4-6). The compression of the humeral head into the glenoid fossa ultimately creates a functional seal between the peripheral rim of the cartilaginous glenoid and the

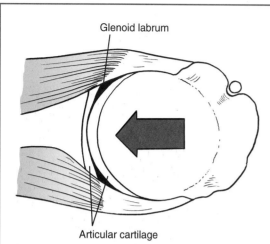

Figure 4-6. The sealing phenomenon of the gleno-humeral joint capsule results from the thicker articular cartilage and the fibrous glenoid labrum, which give the periphery of the glenoid rim greater flexibility. As the head of the humerus is compressed into the glenoid, its ease of deformability on the peripheral aspect of the glenoid allows the creation of a negative pressure within the glenohumeral joint, thereby contributing to glenohumeral stability.

humeral head, much like the outer rim of a toy dart constructed with flexible rubber on its periphery (glenoid) creates a "seal" that would allow the dart to stick to a glass ball (head of humerus).

A slightly negative pressure also is present within the joint cavity. Although the joint surfaces are wet (coated with synovial fluid), very little fluid is actually present in the joint. This is because of the osmotic action of the synoviocytes within the joint synovium. As long as the synovial osmotic pressure (ability of the synoviocytes to remove fluid from the joint environs) remains greater than the osmotic pressure of the colloids within the synovial fluid, a "negative" pressure exists within the joint cavity and the joint is better sealed. This stabilizing or sealing phenomenon brought about by a squeezing together of the wet surfaces of the head of the humerus and the glenoid is further enhanced via contraction of the rotator cuff musculature, which illustrates one of their many roles in contributing to the stability of the glenohumeral joint.

If the joint has an increase in the volume of joint fluid, which might occur as a result of joint effusion or hemarthrosis, a functional seal between the humeral head and glenoid cannot be maintained, in part because of increased joint volume and in part because of a difference in osmotic pressure. The osmotic pressure in the joint cavity exceeds the osmotic pressure in the synovium. This scenario can create an abnormal contact relationship of the humeral head and the glenoid, resulting in joint instability.

When you recognize these labral, cartilage, and joint mechanics, you will more fully understand how instability of the glenohumeral joint might result from defects in the glenoid labrum or from degenerative joint disease associated with the humeral head or glenoid fossa. Although there are several causes of glenohumeral joint instability (Table 4-1), labral or humeral head defects are important factors because when present, they result in the joint losing its ability to maintain the essential functional seal created within the joint cavity. Thus the structural integrity of the very structures that must create this type of seal has been compromised.

Many tests have been described for assessing instability of the glenohumeral joint. Regardless of the name of the test, the intent remains the same: to translate the head of the humerus parallel to the glenoid surface through the application of shear forces in varying degrees of glenohumeral positioning and with the glenohumeral joint placed in high risk positions. The examiner assesses the quantity, quality, and end feel of the translation, all the while noting the effect on the patient's familiar symptoms. Instability is a clinical diagnosis and should not be confused with generalized joint laxity. Although individuals with excessive joint laxity are at risk for instability, the clinical diagnosis typically is made when function is impaired or pain results. Table 4-2 lists clinical tests and evaluation findings that lead us to suspect glenohumeral instability.

Table 4-1. Anatomical Changes Contributing to the Loss of Glenohumeral Stability

1. Defects in the glenoid labrum
2. Irregular, roughened surface of humeral head (DJD)
3. Increased fluid volume within joint cavity
4. Defect in joint capsule
5. Loss of compliance of joint capsule or glenohumeral ligaments

DJD, Degenerative joint disease.

Table 4-2. Tests and Examination Findings Pointing Toward Glenohumeral Instability

1. Positive sulcus sign
   - Excessive space noted at suprahumeral region as a result of inferior translation of humerus
   - Can be assessed for in a neutral position and at 90 degrees abduction
2. Positive drawer test
   - Excessive anterior or posterior translation of humeral head on glenoid
   - Can also be performed with shoulder in varying ranges of elevation or rotation
3. Positive load and shift test
   - Compression of head of humerus into glenoid and then anterior-posterior translation assessed
4. Positive apprehension test (crank test)
   - Shoulder is positioned at 90 degrees abduction and slowly externally rotated
5. Positive relocation test
   - Apprehension position is repeated but with examiner stabilizing anterior aspect of joint
6. "Clunk" test
   - Full overhead flexion and caudal glide from which position the examiner performs a circumduction motion of the humerus, trying to cause a clunk of the humeral head over anterior labrum
7. Anterior glenoid rim tender with palpation
8. Past frequency of dislocations or reductions
9. Does arm transiently "go dead"?
10. Are there associated impingement phenomena?
11. What is the generalized connective tissue "laxity" of the patient?

Labral Defects

Labral defects can occur along any portion of the glenoid, but two in particular have received a great deal of clinical attention: the Bankart lesion and the SLAP (superior labral anterior to posterior) lesion. The Bankart lesion is a detachment of the labrum from the anterior glenoid rim (Figure 4-7, *A*). Forced abduction and external rotation of the glenohumeral joint at endrange loads the anterior-inferior aspect of the joint capsule and the anterior labrum and is the typical position in which the detachment of the labrum and stretch or tear of the inferior glenohumeral ligament complex might occur, resulting in the Bankart lesion.

Trauma, typically forced abduction and external rotation or a force over the back of the humerus driving it anteriorly against the anterior capsular wall, can result in glenohumeral subluxation or dislocation in

addition to a Bankart lesion. A tear of the anterior labrum and capsule renders the joint unstable as a result of this trauma. This type of injury is easily recognized and has resulted in one of the more common classifications of glenohumeral instability, referred to by the acronym *TUBS* (Traumatic Unilateral Bankart Surgery). TUBS means the mechanism of injury was trauma to one shoulder (unilateral), resulting in a Bankart lesion that most likely requires surgery to repair the labrum and avulsed capsular complex in order to restore joint stability (see Chapter 5).

Cumulative stresses may also place excessive stress on this same anterior capsule-labrum complex. A good example is throwing. During the late cocking phase of throwing, the shoulder is in maximal external rotation while the body is moving forward. With the arm going "backward" in external rotation and the body simultaneously coming forward, there is a considerable buildup of tensile stress to the anterior capsule and labrum that renders the region susceptible to damage and a resultant Bankart lesion. Such cumulative stress can result in a continuum of tissue damage in the Bankart lesion from simple fraying of the labrum to detachment and substantial fraying of the labrum.[22]

We want to emphasize the importance of the strength and endurance of the scapular muscles in helping to prevent Bankart lesions now that the mechanisms of injury leading to Bankart lesions are understood (Figure 4-7, *B* and *C*). If the scapular stabilizers cannot position the scapula in the scaption plane, the potential for greater stress to the anterior capsule-labrum complex increases. When the scapula "lags" behind in the frontal plane during the cocking phase of throwing, it results in the anterior capsule and labrum being placed under a significant tensile load. In contrast, scapular muscle control that places and helps maintain the scapula closer to the scaption plane will minimize the stress to the anterior capsule-labrum complex.

The detachment of the superior labrum–long head of the biceps complex is referred to as a SLAP lesion (Figure 4-8). There are several different mechanical derangements of the long head of the biceps tendon that have been described and range from a minor avulsion of only a few fibers to complete separation of the biceps tendon and labrum away from the glenoid so that it resembles the classic bucket handle lesion of the knee joint.[12]

The SLAP lesion typically occurs with shoulder trauma that might occur with glenohumeral

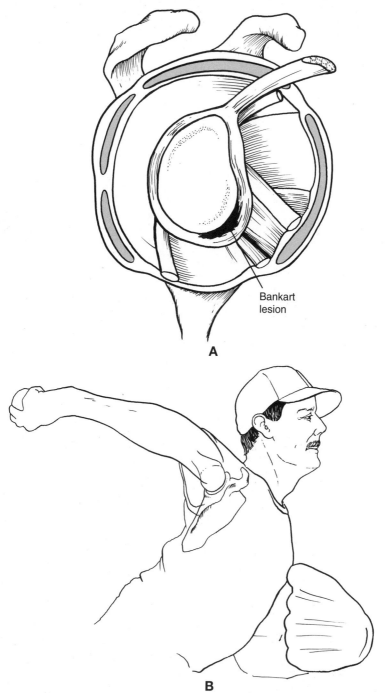

Bankart
lesion

A

B

Figure 4-7. A, This view shows the anatomical location of the Bankart lesion. **B** and **C,** Visualize the stress to the anterior wall of the glenohumeral joint capsule and capsular ligaments during the cocking phase of throwing. In addition, the position of the scapula (protracted versus retracted) also determines whether there is a shear stress or compression stress between the humerus and the glenoid.

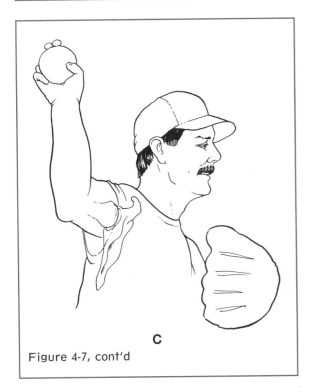

C

Figure 4-7, cont'd

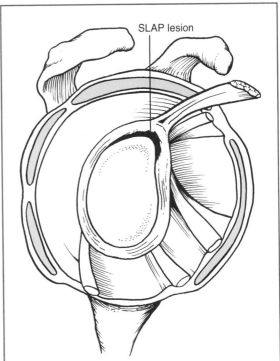

SLAP lesion

Figure 4-8. Note the close relationship of the long head of the biceps tendon and glenohumeral ligaments in this superior aspect of the glenoid labrum. This is also the location of the SLAP lesion.

dislocations or subluxations, with falls on the outstretched arm, and in throwing sports and overhead work.[55] These mechanisms of injury result in several different loading patterns to the labrum–biceps tendon complex. The fall on the outstretched hand drives a force through the long axis of the humerus and ultimately compresses the soft tissues located within the suprahumeral space into the undersurface of the coracoacromial arch. This not only excessively compresses the rotator cuff tendons but also the superiorly positioned glenoid labrum–biceps tendon complex.[54]

Traction through the long head of the biceps tendon associated with the repetitive motion and deceleration requirements of throwing or racquet sports may also result in avulsion of the labrum–biceps tendon complex. The throwing motion is especially complex since considerable stress is applied to the biceps tendon during the deceleration phase of the throwing motion. During this phase of the throwing motion, the elbow is rapidly extending and the biceps is contracting vigorously to control the rate and extent of the elbow extension (Figure 4-9). The tension increase at the attachment of the biceps tendon to the labrum is due to the eccentric contraction of the biceps, as well

as the extension motion of the elbow and arm. Another example of increased tension is the rapid overload to the elbow flexors, such as in catching a falling object or in rapid jerking motions of lifting.

The superior aspect of the glenoid labrum (the region on the glenoid face between 11 and 3 o'clock) is even more complex because the labrum–long head of the biceps tendon complex is also intimately related to the superior and middle glenohumeral ligaments (see Figure 4-8). The anatomical configurations of this confluence of highly specialized connective tissue may take several different variations, and therefore the line between a pathological lesion in this region and a normal variant of the anatomy remains unclear. The clinical picture is further complicated because the superior portion of the glenoid labrum is typically less vascular than the inferior aspect. Thus there may be limitations to the healing capabilities of the superior region in pathological states.[12]

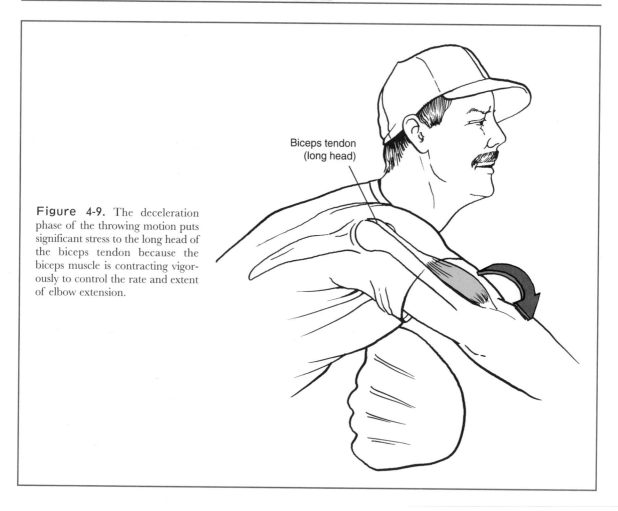

Biceps tendon
(long head)

Figure 4-9. The deceleration phase of the throwing motion puts significant stress to the long head of the biceps tendon because the biceps muscle is contracting vigorously to control the rate and extent of elbow extension.

A clinician should suspect glenohumeral instability whenever the patient's history is suggestive of a defect to any aspect of the glenoid labrum. A few endrange movement tests of the glenohumeral joint have been described in this chapter, but labral defects present an even more formidable rehabilitation challenge. Although labral lesions are difficult to detect with non-invasive tests during the physical examination, there are some symptoms and signs that can lead us to suspect that the labrum is involved. These include sensations of "catching" or "clicking" during specific repetitive shoulder movements and the presence of tenderness to palpation when the soft tissues over the anterior aspect of the glenoid rim are compressed by the examiner's fingers and moved over the anterior glenoid rim (see Chapter 5).

The Joint Capsule and Synovial Membrane

A fibrous capsule lined with a synovial membrane envelops the glenohumeral joint. It is similar to most synovial linings of the joints, and its cells within the synovium synthesize and maintain the major components of the joint fluid. The remarkable feature of the joint fluid is that it adheres to the articular cartilage, enhancing joint lubrication, while simultaneously the fluid-lined articular cartilage surfaces "stick" to each other. This is an important factor that contributes to glenohumeral joint stability. Disease processes such as rheumatoid arthritis, in which the viscosity of the synovial fluid is altered or where the ability of the synovial fluid to adhere to cartilage is diminished, can result in joint instability. This is because of the decrease in the adhesive and cohesive properties of the synovial fluid. In addition, the osmotic pressure equilibrium between joint fluid and the synovial lining is altered.

The joint capsule itself is fairly thin and redundant and makes a minimal contribution to static gleno-humeral joint stability. Medially, the capsule is attached to the complete rim of the glenoid just outside the glenoid labrum. Laterally, the joint capsule is attached to the anatomical neck of the humerus. Most of the connective tissue fibers of the capsule run horizontally, but close inspection of the capsule reveals oblique and transverse fibers as well. One of the unique features of the joint capsule is its laxity. Not only can the scapula and humerus be moved relative to each other, but when the glenohumeral joint is abducted so as to relax the superior portion of the capsule, the joint surfaces can also be slightly "decompressed" as a result of distractive force. When the arm is at the side, the inferior part of the capsule is typically lax with a characteristic redundant "fold." This fold is taken out of the joint capsule as the arm is elevated, and the inferior aspect of the joint capsule becomes increasingly taut.

Another unique feature of the shoulder joint capsule is the additional support it receives on its outer and inner aspects. The external aspect of the fibrous capsule is supported by the four rotator cuff tendons (see Chapter 3): the supraspinatus on the capsule's superior surface, the infraspinatus and teres minor on the posterior surface, and the subscapularis on the anterior surface (Figure 4-10). Although not considered part of the rotator cuff, the long head of the triceps supports the inferior aspect of the joint capsule, particularly when the humerus is in a position of forward elevation.

The relationship of the rotator cuff tendons to the joint capsule is important because the cuff tendons have well defined bony attachments to the humeral tuberosities and completely blending with the fibrous capsule of the glenohumeral joint (see Figure 4-10). As noted in Chapter 3, contraction of the rotator cuff muscles not only results in movement of the humerus on the scapula but also contributes to increasing tension to the glenohumeral joint capsule. The increase in capsular tension results in enhanced stability at the glenohumeral joint through a type of dynamic support to glenohumeral stability as a result of increased muscle action augmenting the connective tissue stiffness of the joint capsule.

This relationship of the rotator cuff tendons to the joint capsule is especially important to consider in the examination of the patient with limited range of

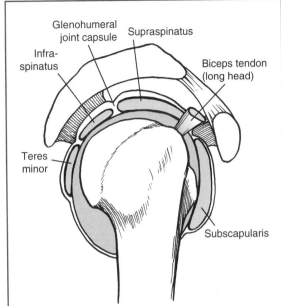

Figure 4-10. A lateral view of the glenohumeral joint capsule shows the relationship of the rotator cuff tendons to the capsule's external aspect.

motion of the glenohumeral joint. Unless the musculature is fully relaxed, passive motion of the humerus on the glenoid will present as limited glenohumeral motion. In addition to considering that the capsule itself might have been subjected to adaptive shortening or has fibrous adhesions, it is also anatomically and neurophysiologically plausible to consider that an increased resting tension or protective guarding of the rotator cuff musculature, in particular the infraspinatus and teres minor, may be contributing to limited motion.

For example, a limitation in glenohumeral internal rotation may be due to tightness of the posterior capsule but might also be a result of increased resting state of muscle contraction of the infraspinatus and teres minor muscles in order to minimize compression within the suprahumeral space. Figure 4-11 demonstrates a patient with limited internal rotation on one side compared with the other. Note that because of the arm position, the internal rotation motion itself results in increased compression of the humeral head into the coracoacromial arch. It is this resultant compression to previously irritated or swollen tissues (impingement syndrome) that may trigger the immediate protective guarding of the shoulder external

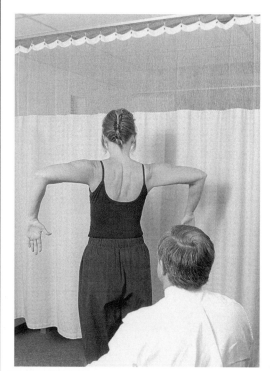

Figure 4-11. The patient has been asked to internally rotate both shoulders from the starting position of 90 degrees abduction. The right shoulder demonstrates limited internal rotation, which might be caused by two different reasons: a tight posterior capsule or protective guarding of the infraspinatus and teres minor as they contract to minimize further compression of the head of the humerus into the coracoacromial arch in the patient with a shoulder impingement lesion.

rotators and minimize any further motion in the direction of internal rotation.

The openings found within the fibrous capsule itself are the final unique anatomical features of the joint capsule. Typically there are two openings, but occasionally three may be seen. One opening is present at the upper region of the intertubercular (bicipital) groove. This opening allows the long head of the biceps tendon to travel along the superior head of the humerus in its course to reach the supraglenoid tubercle and the glenoid labrum of the scapula. At the region in which this opening appears, the fibrous capsule becomes increasingly thick and the fibers of the capsule contribute to the intricate framework of connective tissues that help secure the long head of the biceps in the intertubercular

groove (see Chapter 3). The second opening of the fibrous capsule is anteriorly placed, which permits communication of the synovial membranes of the glenohumeral joint capsule with the synovial bursal sac forming the subscapular bursa. The subscapular bursa lies deep to the subscapularis tendon as it crosses the glenoid neck and travels toward the lesser tuberosity (Figure 4-12). A third opening is often found posteriorly in which the synovial membrane of the joint capsule communicates with the infraspinatus bursa in the same way communication with the subscapularis bursa occurs on the anterior aspect of the joint.

The Capsular Ligaments

In addition to the external reinforcement of the capsule by the rotator cuff tendons, further support is provided on the *inner* surface of the joint capsule by three ligaments: the superior, middle, and inferior

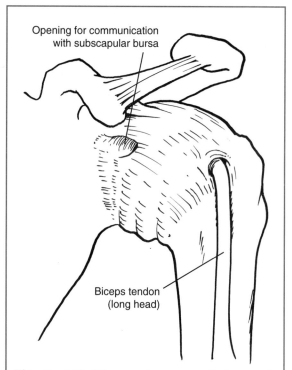

Figure 4-12. The anterior aspect of the capsule demonstrates the two constant openings of the fibrous joint capsule: the opening for the long head of the biceps and the opening for the communication with the subscapular bursa.

glenohumeral ligaments. Because these ligaments are featured primarily on the inner aspect of the anterior wall of the joint capsule, the anterior aspect of the joint capsule is noticeably thicker than the posterior part of the capsule.

The superior glenohumeral ligament (Figure 4-13) is thin and slender. It is attached to the glenoid rim immediately adjacent to the long head of the biceps tendon and travels toward the humerus paralleling the long head of the biceps, attaching to the upper aspect of the lesser tuberosity. The middle glenohumeral ligament lies just inferior to the superior glenohumeral ligament and attaches to the lesser tubercle just below the subscapularis muscle attachment.

The largest and most developed of these ligaments is the inferior glenohumeral ligament. Its breadth is such that it can be studied as three functional subparts: an anterior component (anterior-inferior glenohumeral ligament), an axillary component (axillary-inferior glenohumeral ligament), and a posterior component (posterior-inferior glenohumeral ligament).[47] The placement of this ligament on the glenoid is best described by viewing the glenoid as the face of a clock. The extent of this ligament is such that the attachments of the three components of the inferior glenohumeral ligament span an area from approximately 3 to 8 o'clock. Such an arrangement of the three components results in the ligament serving as a sling or "hammock" for the head of the humerus (see Figure 4-13). When our arm is at our side, the inferior glenohumeral ligament serves to support the head of the humerus. When our arm is abducted and externally rotated, however, the major components of the inferior glenohumeral ligament are positioned anterior to the head of the humerus and help stabilize it against anterior translation of the humeral head on the glenoid (Figure 4-14). If the applied force of abduction and external rotation exceeds the connective tissue tolerance of the inferior

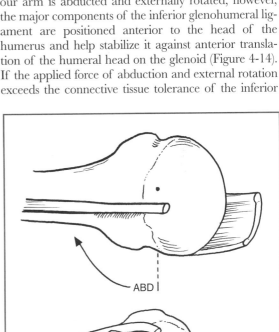

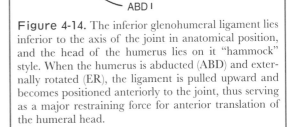

Figure 4-14. The inferior glenohumeral ligament lies inferior to the axis of the joint in anatomical position, and the head of the humerus lies on it "hammock" style. When the humerus is abducted (ABD) and externally rotated (ER), the ligament is pulled upward and becomes positioned anteriorly to the joint, thus serving as a major restraining force for anterior translation of the humeral head.

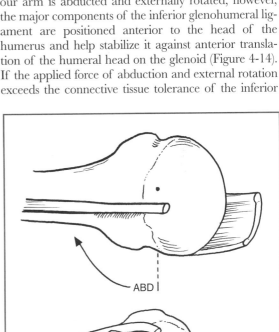

Superior glenohumeral ligament

Middle glenohumeral ligament

Posterior band of the inferior glenohumeral ligament complex

Anterior band of the inferior glenohumeral ligament complex

Figure 4-13. The superior, middle, and inferior glenohumeral ligaments reinforce the inner wall of the joint capsule. The superior glenohumeral ligament is the smallest of the three ligaments, whereas the inferior glenohumeral ligament is the largest.

glenohumeral ligament, the connective tissue fibers are torn or stretched. The lack of a restraining force to anterior translation by the inferior glenohumeral ligament potentially results in instability of the glenohumeral joint, especially when the arms are lifted away from the body.

The final capsular ligament that we discuss in this section is the coracohumeral ligament. Unlike the glenohumeral ligaments that lie on the inner wall of the shoulder joint capsule, the coracohumeral ligament lies on the external surface of the fibrous capsule. As the name implies, it extends from the coracoid process to the greater tuberosity. This ligament is located in a region of the superior joint capsule known as the *rotator interval*. The rotator interval is a space bound by the anterior border of the supraspinatus muscle and the superior border of the subscapularis muscle (Figure 4-15). Therefore, from superficial to deep, the rotator interval is occupied by the coracohumeral ligament, the joint capsule, the superior glenohumeral ligament, and the long head of the biceps tendon.

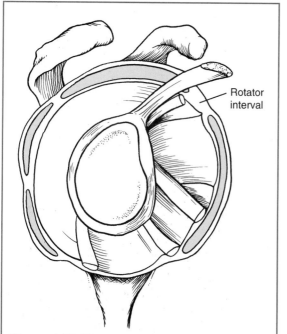

Rotator interval

Figure 4-15. The rotator interval is the portion of the capsule in which there is no reinforcement by the rotator cuff tendons. It lies between the subscapularis muscle and the supraspinatus muscle. The coracohumeral ligament supports the capsule in this space.

Pathology: Adhesive Capsulitis, or "Frozen Shoulder"

Shoulder stiffness, and the pain and disability resulting from such stiffness, can be caused by a variety of reasons. Here we discuss those elements of shoulder stiffness that appear related to changes in the joint capsule or the glenohumeral ligaments. The term *adhesive capsulitis* was first noted by Neviaser.[43] He described a clinical condition of limited shoulder movement that appeared to result from an inflammatory process, which changed the compliance of the joint capsule connective tissues. This sequence resulted in fibrosis and thickening of the capsule and ligaments. Motion limitation associated with such diffuse connective tissue changes results in all glenohumeral motions being affected rather than a limitation of motion in only one direction.

The pathogenesis of the stiff glenohumeral joint (adhesive capsulitis, or "frozen shoulder") is most likely a cascade of cellular events that begins with an inflammatory reaction. Such inflammatory events are marked by increased vascularity and the presence of inflammatory cells in the synovium.[25] The synovitis results in a fibroblastic response within the adjacent capsule. The insult initiating inflammation is typically unknown, although microtrauma and macrotrauma or autoimmune reactions associated with the cells or vasculature of the joint capsule and synovial lining may be contributing factors. The result of a chronic inflammatory process can be fibrosis, which results in thickening of the normally thin and redundant capsule with associated contractures of the collagen fibers.[44]

Cyriax proposed that inflammation of the joint capsule and a resultant limitation of motion followed a predictable pattern of limitation.[11] He called the proportional limitation of motion "the capsular pattern" and suggested that all synovial joints have a predictable proportional loss of motion when the joint capsule is the primary structure involved. The capsular pattern for the shoulder is described as a motion pattern in which the external rotation is the most limited motion, followed by glenohumeral (not total shoulder) abduction, and internal rotation as the least limited motion. The examiner will usually assess the patient for a capsular pattern when examining the shoulder using passive range-of-motion maneuvers. It is essential that the tests applied are truly passive in nature. If there is muscle guarding or the patient actively assists with the motion, a true assessment of the noncontractile tissues, such as the joint capsule, cannot occur. Although many patients with a stiff and painful shoulder may not have these exact proportions of limitations, it is quite remarkable how common it is for external rotation to be exquisitely painful and limited and a passive external rotation maneuver to quickly elicit protective muscle spasm. This is a good indication that the joint capsule is involved in the syndrome.

Asymmetric tightness of the capsule, which implies that only one region of the capsule is tight rather than the complete capsule, alters the mechanics of the humerus as it moves under the coracoacromial arch by forcing it to translate away from its central point on the glenoid.[26,38] Matsen and colleagues have used the term *obligate translation* to describe the phenomenon of the tight capsule pushing on the humerus, which shifts it off its central position on the glenoid (Figure 4-16).[38] When flexing the shoulder with a tight posterior joint capsule, the humeral head is driven up and forward into the undersurface of the anterior coracoacromial arch, compressing the soft tissues located in this region.

THE SUPRAHUMERAL-SUBACROMIAL INTERFACE

The interface between the superior aspect of the humerus and the inferior aspect of the acromion has long captured the attention of clinicians as an anatomical region from which numerous shoulder disorders may emanate. The inferior bony border of the region is the convex head of the humerus, particularly the greater tuberosity, whereas the concave undersurface of the acromion and coracoid process serve as the superior border. The complete extent of the concave arch is even more complex because it is formed by a combination of bony tissue and other specialized connective tissues. From posterior to anterior, the arch is formed by the acromion, acromion process, coracoacromial ligament, and the conjoint tendons of the short head of the biceps and coracobrachialis muscles (Figure 4-17).

The convex partner of this interface is truly unique. It consists of the head of the humerus and attached rotator cuff tendons, which are intimately blended with the glenohumeral joint capsule. The subacromial bursa lies at the interface between the

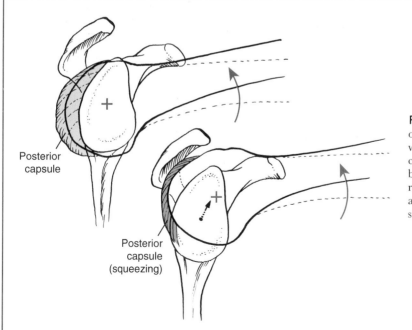

Figure 4-16. The concept of obligate translation is exhibited when tightness of the posterior capsule results in the humerus being driven superiorly and anteriorly into the coracoacromial arch, thus compressing the soft tissues in this interface.

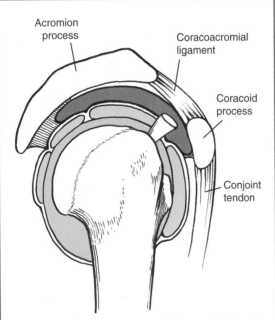

Figure 4-17. The suprahumeral-subacromial interface is shown when the concave hood is formed (from posterior to anterior) by the acromion process, coracoacromial ligament, coracoid process, and conjoint tendon of the short head of the biceps and coracobrachialis. The convex humeral head moves within this concavity, which is part bony tissue and part specialized connective tissue.

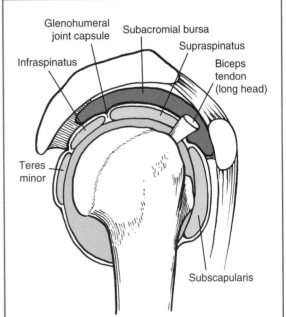

Figure 4-18. Interposed between the concave undersurface of the acromion and the convex humeral head are the rotator cuff tendons, subacromial bursa, biceps tendon (long head), joint capsule, coracohumeral ligament, and superior glenohumeral ligament.

rotator cuff tendons and the undersurface of the concave arch (Figure 4-18). The space between the convex humeral head and the arch that is formed by the acromion, coracoacromial ligament, coracoid, and conjoint tendons is approximately the thickness of the rotator cuff tendons. Attrition (thinning) of the rotator cuff tendons results in a decrease in the height of the subacromial space.

Previously we described the motion between the humerus and glenoid fossa. Note, however, that because of the attachment of the rotator cuff tendons to the head of the humerus, any movement of the humerus must result in the rotator cuff tendons themselves "gliding" under the arch in the interface formed by the acromion, coracoacromial ligament, coracoid process, and conjoint tendons (Figure 4-19, *A* and *B*). Smooth movement of this "sphere" formed by the humeral head and cuff tendons precisely within the socket created by the subacromial arch is

dependent on many factors, the most important of which are synchronized and coordinated contractions of muscles moving the humerus and scapula, the laxity of the glenohumeral joint capsule, the smoothness of the undersurface of the coracoacromial arch, and the smoothness and thickness of the rotator cuff tendons.

As a result of the arrangement of rotator cuff tendons within this space, two surfaces of the rotator cuff tendons are described: the *bursal surface* of the tendons, which refers to the superior aspect of the infraspinatus–teres minor complex, supraspinatus, and subscapularis, and the *articular surface* of the cuff tendons, which refers to the deepest part of the cuff tendons. This deep part of the cuff tendons is that portion blending in with the superficial aspect of the glenohumeral joint capsule.

This anatomical arrangement would suggest that friction might occur between the rotator cuff tendons and the undersurface of the coracoacromial arch and result in the bursal surface of the tendons, especially

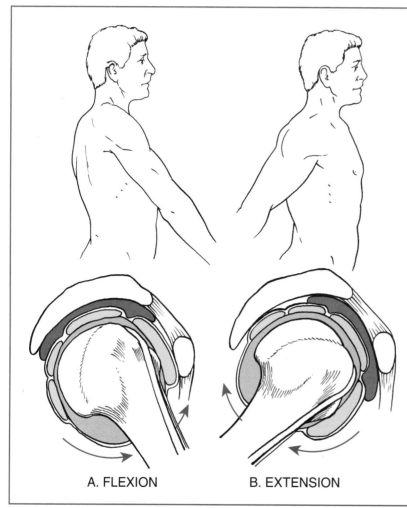

Figure 4-19. Motion of the humerus on the glenoid allows the superior aspect of the rotator cuff tendons to glide under the concave hood formed by the acromion, acromion process, coracoacromial ligament, and conjoint tendons. Note the position of the rotator cuff tendons under the hood (**A**) when the humerus is flexed and (**B**) when it is extended.

A. FLEXION   B. EXTENSION

the infraspinatus and supraspinatus, showing the earliest signs of tendon degeneration. This does not appear to be the case. Instead, the earliest signs of cuff attrition occur on the articular side of the tendon, an observation first noted by Codman in one of his classic manuscripts on the shoulder (Figure 4-20).[7,19,58]

The most distal region of the rotator cuff tendons is that portion attaching to the tuberosities of the humerus. It typically shows the first signs of rents in the tendons, cell disruption, loss of uniformity of the collagen bundles, and a loosening of the fibers from their attachment.[45] The initial point of rotator cuff

degeneration is the anterior aspect of the supraspinatus on its articular side, a region immediately adjacent to the long head of the biceps tendon. As cuff degeneration advances, it begins to involve more of the supraspinatus tendon and then typically extends into the adjacent portion of the infraspinatus tendon (Figure 4-21).[24,38]

This short discussion of the degenerative process associated with the rotator cuff is important to our understanding of the effect that cuff degeneration may have on the integrity of the suprahumeral-subacromial interface. The thickness of the cuff tendons serves as

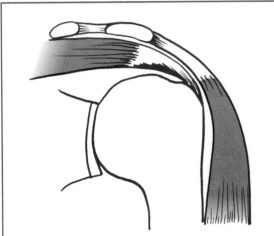

Figure 4-20. The earliest signs of rotator cuff attrition occur on the articular side of the tendon, rather than the bursal side.

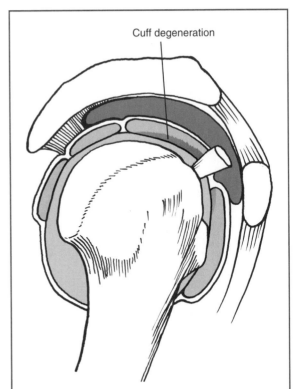

Cuff degeneration

Figure 4-21. The anterior aspect of the supraspinatus tendon near its insertion into the greater tuberosity is one of the earliest locations of cuff degeneration. This region is immediately adjacent to the long head of the biceps tendon. From this location the degenerative process can extend through the supraspinatus tendon and into the adjacent infraspinatus tendon.

the spacer that lies between the humeral head and the undersurface of the arch. This is relevant to shoulder mechanics because the pull of the deltoid results in a superior translational force of the humeral head on the glenoid (Figure 4-22). Thinning of the rotator cuff tendons can result in the humeral head riding superiorly because of deltoid contraction and more closely approximating the undersurface of the coracoacromial arch. In addition, the superior translation of the humeral head has the potential to further erode the superior lip of the glenoid labrum and the complex insertional region of the long head of the biceps tendon.

The rotator cuff plays the key role in minimizing this translation of the humerus both actively and passively when the deltoid contracts. Deficiency of the complete rotator cuff results in significant translation of the humeral head with deltoid activity.[53] The superior migration of the head of the humerus results in the head no longer being centered within the glenoid, which in further compression of the cuff tendons and bursa, affects the undersurface of the coracoacromial ligament and the biceps tendon. If, however, only the supraspinatus is markedly degenerated, the patterns of motion of the humerus on the glenoid are not significantly altered because the subscapularis and the infraspinatus are reasonably effective in maintaining the head of the humerus in the glenoid.[57]

Two pathoanatomical changes to the arch have clinical relevance. The first is the anatomical change

that occurs in the coracoacromial ligament. Note that when the head of the humerus pushes up into the undersurface of the coracoacromial ligament, the ligament is forced to deform (see Figure 4-22). Such deformation of the ligament results in a traction force at the ligament's attachments, namely, the anterior aspect of the acromion process and the posterior aspect of the coracoid process. This continuous microtrauma to the coracoacromial ligament can result in several structural changes. One is the thickening and roughening of the undersurface of the ligament. The other is a change in the shape of the acromion via resultant traction spurs that develop in the region of the attachment of the ligament to the acromion.[16,18,62] When you understand these mechanisms, it sheds a different light on the varying shapes of the acromion

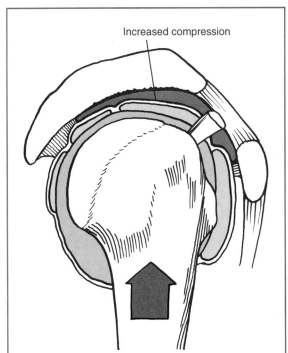

Increased compression

Figure 4-22. The pull of the deltoid results in a force that translates the humeral head superiorly. The interpositioning of the healthy, thick rotator cuff tendon acts as a spacer preventing movement of the head of the humerus superiorly. Thus the head of the humerus remains centered within the glenoid. This compression has the potential to cause deformation or thickening of the coracoacromial ligament. The trauma to the undersurface of the ligament results in degeneration of the undersurface and traction spurs at the intersection of the ligament with the acromion process.

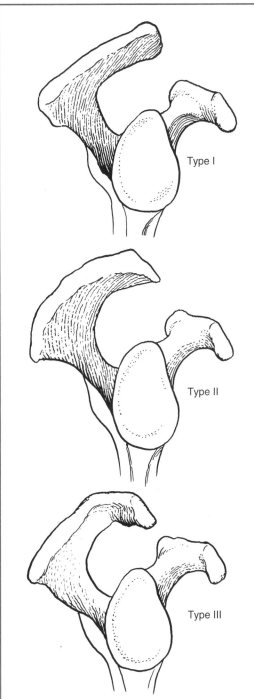

Type I

Type II

Type III

Figure 4-23. The typical shapes of the acromion include Type I, a relatively flat acromion; Type II with a more curved presentation; and Type III with a hook-shaped appearance. These different shapes may be acquired because of the force of the humeral head against the undersurface of the acromion and coracoacromial ligament.

seen on radiographic evaluation (Figure 4-23). While some of the different acromial shapes may be congenital, it appears reasonable that the shaping of the acromion process also might be an acquired phenomenon, which occurs because of the continuous and prolonged loading patterns subjected to it, especially the force of the head of the humerus on the undersurface of the coracoacromial ligament. The three acromial shapes most often described in clinical literature are Type I, which is relatively flat, Type II, which is curved in shape, and Type III, which resembles a hook.[3]

The second pathoanatomical change of note occurs in the long head of the biceps tendon. Figure 4-24 shows "flattening" of the long head of the biceps tendon with a resultant vertical crease across its substance because of its being trapped and subsequently

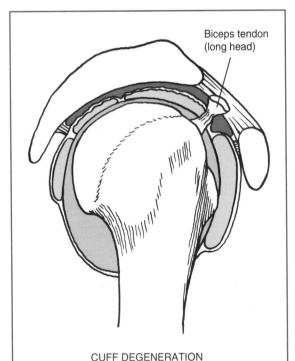

Biceps tendon
(long head)

CUFF DEGENERATION

Figure 4-24. As a result of the thinning of the rotator cuff tendons caused by cuff tendon degeneration, the long head of the biceps tendon becomes wedged between the head of the humerus and the coracoacromial arch. This results in a crease in the biceps tendon and the possibility of biceps tendonitis or a complete biceps tendon tear associated with partial or full thickness tears of the rotator cuff tendons.

Table 4-3. Compromising the Subacromial Space: Bringing the Greater Tuberosity Closer to the Coracoacromial Arch
1. Excessive superior translation of humeral head
2. Excessive anterior translation of humeral head
3. Limited external rotation of humerus
4. Decrease in scapular upward rotation
5. Altered scapular kinematics during motion

compressed between the humeral head and the coracoacromial arch.[51,60] With severe attrition of the cuff tendons, the cuff spacer effect is lost and the compressive trauma to the biceps tendon can result in loss of biceps tendon integrity with resultant rupture.

The subacromial interface is thus a socket in and of itself under which the head of the attached rotator cuff tendons must glide with any motion of the humerus. Smooth motion within this socket is dependent on the congruence of the surface of the subacromial socket with the surface of the rotator cuff tendons. Motions of the glenohumeral joint that bring the greater tuberosity in close approximation to the coracoacromial arch render the soft tissues vulnerable. These motions are noted in Table 4-3 and should be considered during evaluation of the shoulder.

The recognition of the intimate relationship between the cuff tendons and the undersurface of the coracoacromial arch has led to the development of tests used to assess for compromise of the tissues housed in this space. Although often termed *impingement tests*, it is clear that this region is much more complex and making a diagnosis by simply attempting to squeeze the cuff tendons under the arch may not always provide accurate answers. Despite limitations, impingement tests are an important part of the examination process for the patient presenting with shoulder pain because such tests begin to provide clues about the health of the tissues in this highly specialized region.

Numerous tests have been described, but those initiated by Neer and Walsh along with the application of the examination techniques were among the first.[42] The classic impingement test uses a maneuver in which passive full elevation of the arm with overpressure at endrange resulted in compression of the supraspinatus tendon under the coracoacromial arch (Figure 4-25, *A*). The forced elevation was intended to reproduce the patient's pain. If, following injection of a local anesthetic into the subacromial space, the pain was absent with the same maneuver, a cuff impingement was suspected. The Hawkins test places the humerus that is flexed to 90 degrees in full internal rotation in order to attempt to directly compress the greater tuberosity (with the attached supraspinatus tendon) against the undersurface of the coracoacromial ligament (Figure 4-25, *B*).[27] Burns and Whipple noted that the coracoacromial ligament is in contact with the supraspinatus and biceps tendons as well with varying arcs of shoulder motion (Figure 4-25, *C*).[5] Such findings have led to treatment of chronic cases of impingement via coracoacromial ligament resection in order to decrease compression to the underlying tendons.

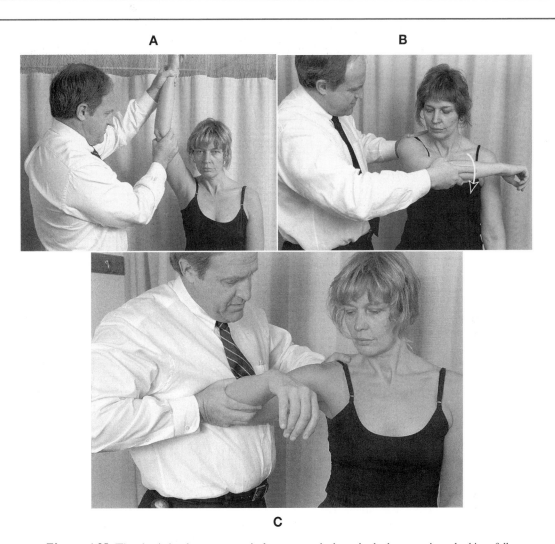

Figure 4-25. The classic impingement test is demonstrated when, **A,** the humerus is pushed into full forward elevation and overpressure is given to determine if pain is reproduced; **B,** based on the Hawkins test, the examiner brings the arm to 90 degrees and maximally to internally rotate the humerus, seeking to reproduce the patient's pain; or, **C,** as we prefer, the examiner places one hand over the top of the acromion and clavicle to fixate the scapula in downward rotation while forcibly elevating the humerus in varying arcs of motion and with varying degrees of internal and external rotation.

New anatomical studies of the various impingement tests have caused clinicans to reconsider the effect such tests might have on the articular side of the cuff tendons, which is the initial site of tendon degeneration.[59] Although this has been discussed in Chapter 3, it is worthwhile that you briefly revisit this clinical entity in the context of shoulder articulations. In these cases the deep surface of the supraspinatus tendon (articular side of the tendon) becomes compressed against the superior glenoid with all of the classic impingement positions. Whereas attrition of the bursal side of the cuff tendons is often considered to be age related, young athletes in sports requiring overhead activity, such as throwing sports, racquet sports, volleyball, swimming, and weightlifting, are often confronted with articular side lesions of the rotator cuff tendons. Compression of the deep surface of the tendon against the glenoid rim is referred to as *internal impingement*.[13] Such impingements occur between the undersurface of the tendon and the posterior-superior rim of the glenoid fossa and are secondary to repetitive microtrauma.[56] With the arm in the position of abduction, external rotation, and extension, there is markedly increased contact between the undersurface of the supraspinatus tendon and the posterior-superior border of the glenoid rim. The reader can appreciate that thousands of movement cycles in and out of this position result in increased friction and compressional loading between the tendon and rim.

Therefore the examiner must be cautious in the interpretation of pain with impingement tests since reproduction of symptoms may be due to bursal side involvement of the tendon, articular side involvement of the tendon, or both. It is important to move the humerus through various positions of potential cuff tendon stress in order to gain a better picture as to the positions and loads that reproduce the patient's symptoms.

It is clear that the discussion of impingement problems related to the suprahumeral-subacromial interface has markedly expanded beyond the simple concept of compression of the supraspinatus tendon under the coracoacromial ligament. Our expanded understanding is not simply academic: treatment interventions are based on etiological factors associated with the syndrome, and the cause of the impingement phenomenon must be identified in order to treat it most effectively. Impingement causes can include those ranging from hypomobility to hypermobility of the glenohumeral joint, loss of normal scapulothoracic kinematics, and rotator cuff weakness and fatigue. Finally, the location of the lesion can range from internal to external to full thickness.

THE ACROMIOCLAVICULAR JOINT

We discuss the acromioclavicular joint at this point in the text in order to review its mechanics and because the location of the inferior aspect of the joint is in the coracoacromial arch and may be a contributing factor in impingement syndromes. Changes in structure and function of the joint because of injury or degeneration can result in a compromise to the suprahumeral space.

The acromioclavicular joint is formed by the distal end of the clavicle and the medial aspect of the acromion. The clavicle is shaped like a "lazy S." From its attachment to the acromion, it courses posterior and then anterior to terminate on the sternum, forming the sternoclavicular joint. The clavicle serves as a source of muscle attachment (see Chapter 3) but also serves as the anterior "stabilizer" or "strut" for the scapula and glenohumeral joint. The acromioclavicular joint is unusual in that the two approximating bony ends have a variety of subtle differences in shape and joint planes, and the articulation, formed by two flat surfaces approximating each other, seems poorly designed to withstand the stresses that reach the shoulder with activities of daily living and sports.

The distal end of the clavicle typically rides higher than the acromion, which makes the palpation of the acromioclavicular joint line relatively easy on most patients (Figure 4-26). Although the joint surfaces are lined with hyaline cartilage in children and teenagers, both surfaces have fibrous cartilage by a young adult age. The joint cavity of the acromioclavicular joint also features a small meniscus or meniscoid inclusion. This meniscoid inclusion typically extends into the joint from the superior aspect of the joint capsule. Little is understood about the roles of this oddly placed meniscus, but as seen with other menisci in the body, it is assumed that the meniscus helps in the distribution of synovial fluid and in attenuation of the different forces that reach the joint. The disc degenerates during adulthood, at which time it essentially functions poorly or not at all.[48]

Because the disc is so poorly developed and the surfaces of the joint have such poor congruency, it is difficult for the acromioclavicular joint to dissipate forces in the manner seen in other joints. The weight-bearing surface area is small, and therefore forces distributed over this small area result in very large pressure (P = F/A). Large compressive and shear loads can result from simple activities in which the arm becomes weight bearing, such as leaning on our elbows or pushing a heavy object away from our body. In addition, the large pectoralis major muscle exerts significant compressive forces over the acromioclavicular joint by virtue of its attachments. Because of this peculiar

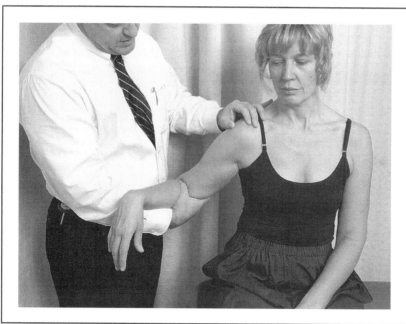

Figure 4-26. Because the clavicle typically rides a bit higher than the acromion, the joint line of the acromioclavicular joint can be easily palpated in most patients.

anatomy and associated influence on the mechanics, degenerative joint conditions of the acromioclavicular joint are very common.[15,28] Furthermore, a high incidence of coexisting pathological conditions with symptomatic acromioclavicular joint problems, such as biceps tendon pathology, full or partial thickness rotator cuff tears, and tears of the glenoid labrum, have been demonstrated.[4]

Motion of the scapula on the clavicle at the acromioclavicular joint is not as great as often suggested. The joint surface is designed to permit a small amount of sliding and rotational movement while transferring forces to the sternum through the long axis of the clavicle. In 1934 Codman noted that there was minimal motion at the acromioclavicular joint and stated that this joint "swings a little, rocks a little, twists a little, slides a little, and acts as a hinge."[7] This simple statement is still a most accurate description of this joint. Very little motion occurs separately between the clavicle and acromion, and that is the reason why the joint can be surgically fused without marked disruption of shoulder girdle mechanics. Instead, the motion of the scapula and clavicle typically occurs together and in synchrony instead of independently.[52] Approximately 20 degrees of motion of the scapula on the clavicle

occurs in the frontal and sagittal planes, which is probably more a function of the deformability of the ligamentous framework supporting the joint than the actual osteokinematics. A variety of scapular positions are thus possible, all to optimally set a scapular platform from which the glenohumeral muscles can work, including a clockwise or counterclockwise rotation of the scapula on the clavicle and a tilting of the scapula along a vertical axis, which allows the glenoid to face anteriorly or more directly laterally (Figure 4-27, *A* and *B*).

The clinician needs to recognize the mechanics of the acromioclavicular joint when designing exercises for the upper extremity in the presence of acromioclavicular joint arthritis. For example, a flat bench press (Figure 4-28, *A*) has the potential to excessively load the acromioclavicular joint not only because of the compressive load occurring as a result of pectoralis major contraction but also because of the forced retraction of the scapula and endrange loading of the acromioclavicular joint in the chest position. Several selectorized and plate-loaded resistance exercise units place significant stress on the acromioclavicular joint (Figure 4-28, *B* and *C*).

The clavicle also has the potential to rotate on its longitudinal axis. This motion primarily occurs at the

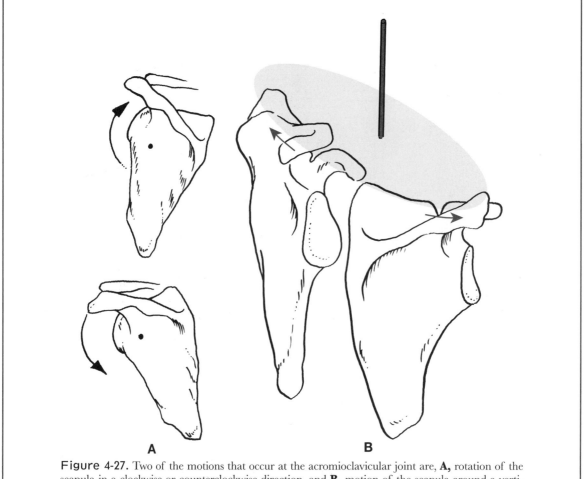

Figure 4-27. Two of the motions that occur at the acromioclavicular joint are, **A,** rotation of the scapula in a clockwise or counterclockwise direction, and **B,** motion of the scapula around a vertical axis, which allows the glenoid to have a more anterior or lateral presentation.

sternoclavicular joint, however, and as a result of scapulothoracic rotation (i.e., upward rotation of the scapula). This rotation is possible mostly because of the attachment of the coracoclavicular ligaments to the lateral undersurface of the clavicle (Figure 4-29, *A*). When the scapula moves into upward rotation (as a result of contraction of the serratus anterior and upper and lower trapezius muscles), the coracoid process moves inferiorly. Because the coracoclavicular ligaments run superiorly from the coracoid to attach to the clavicle, this movement of the scapula pulls the posterior aspect of the clavicle downward as a result of the downward movement of the coracoid process,

effectively causing a rotation of the clavicle on its longitudinal axis (Figure 4-29, *B*).

The articulation between the clavicle and acromion is inherently unstable, and because the joint has the above mentioned motion requirements, its stability is largely a result of the specialized connective tissue structures, namely the acromioclavicular ligaments and the coracoclavicular ligaments. The stronger superior acromioclavicular joint ligament and weaker inferior acromioclavicular joint ligaments surround the joint capsule. The superior and inferior acromioclavicular ligaments are not, however, the primary sources of acromioclavicular joint

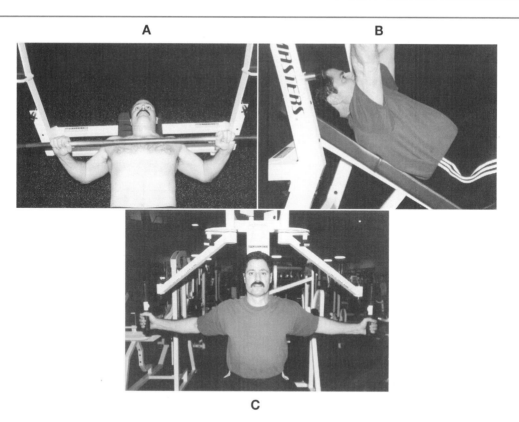

Figure 4-28. A, In the flat bench press, the acromioclavicular joint is often forced to its endrange position, which can be extremely problematic for an acromioclavicular joint with slight degenerative changes. **B,** Use of the incline bench press places less stress on the acromioclavicular joint because the scapula is not brought into such extreme retraction. **C,** Note that the bilateral pec deck exercise unit also has the potential to take the scapula into extreme endranges on the clavicle.

stability. The orientation of these ligaments is such that they help check anterior-posterior translational stress of the clavicle on the acromion, or acromion on the clavicle. The potential shifting of the clavicle posteriorly on the scapula or the scapula posteriorly on the clavicle is checked by the acromioclavicular joint ligaments.[17]

In contrast, the stability of the acromioclavicular joint, especially in regard to superior-inferior movement of the clavicle on the acromion, or the acromion on the clavicle, is largely ensured by the two portions of the coracoclavicular ligament, the conoid and trapezoid (see Figure 4-29, *A*). The two-part coracoclavicular ligament is a short, stout ligament that attaches along the apex of the convexity of the lateral

clavicle. Figure 4-30, *A*, shows the extent of the attachment of the coracoclavicular ligaments along the clavicle. The strong coracoclavicular ligament is the primary restraint against the scapula moving inferiorly on the thorax away from the clavicle. The direction of the fibers also suggests that the ligament counters or checks the strong pull of the trapezius, which is attached to the lateral clavicle. The reader can appreciate the strength of the coracoclavicular ligament by considering that the scapula and attached upper extremity literally "hang" from the clavicle via the stout coracoclavicular ligament (Figure 4-30, *B*). Disruption of this ligament markedly diminishes the vertical stability of the scapula.

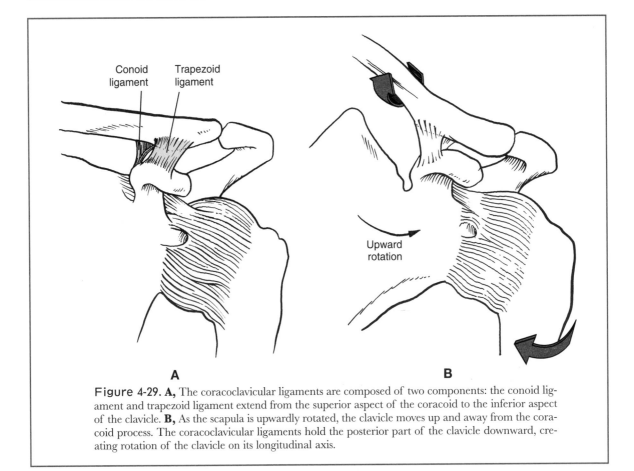

Figure 4-29. A, The coracoclavicular ligaments are composed of two components: the conoid ligament and trapezoid ligament extend from the superior aspect of the coracoid to the inferior aspect of the clavicle. **B,** As the scapula is upwardly rotated, the clavicle moves up and away from the coracoid process. The coracoclavicular ligaments hold the posterior part of the clavicle downward, creating rotation of the clavicle on its longitudinal axis.

Movement of the glenohumeral and scapulothoracic articulations ultimately terminates at the sternum via the clavicle. The acromioclavicular joint essentially acts like a stabilizing arm that has articulations at either end permitting accommodation or translatory movement. This anatomical relationship is much like a tie rod in an automobile, which functions to stabilize and direct movement from one surface to another.

Mechanical disorders of the acromioclavicular joint can be due to several factors. A fall directly on the acromion process, especially with the arm adducted into the body, violently pushes the scapula inferiorly, which potentially disrupts the acromioclavicular ligaments, joint capsule, and coracoclavicular ligaments. Acromioclavicular joint sprains are typically classified as Type I through VI injuries with an increasing level of bony, ligamentous, and muscle disruption that is more

pronounced in Types IV, V, and VI (Table 4-4). The first three classifications (Types I, II, and III) are the most common types seen in the ambulatory outpatient setting. Type I injuries feature sprain of the acromioclavicular ligaments, but since the coracoclavicular ligament is intact, there is no loss of joint stability. Type II injuries feature torn acromioclavicular ligaments but only a sprain of the coracoclavicular ligament, and therefore some joint stability is compromised. Type III injuries feature a dislocation of the clavicular and acromion joint surfaces. Type III injuries are more complex than initially meets the eye because the attachments of the deltoid and the trapezius are also disrupted depending on the direction of the dislocation. The deltoid attachment on the lateral aspect of the clavicle and the acromion is in the same insertional region as the trapezius, and since both of these muscles

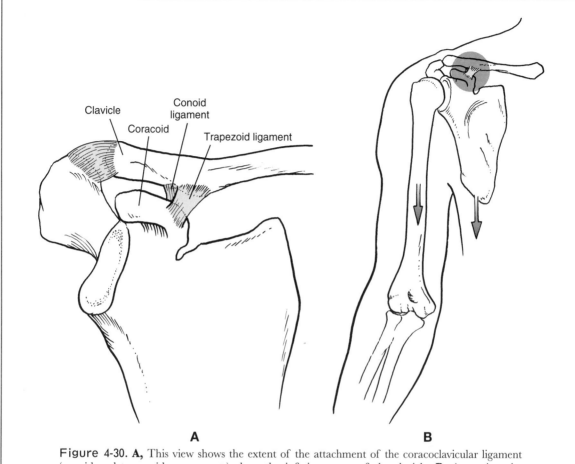

Figure 4-30. A, This view shows the extent of the attachment of the coracoclavicular ligament (conoid and trapezoid components) along the inferior aspect of the clavicle. **B,** Appreciate the strength of the coracoclavicular ligament. The scapula and upper extremity "hang" from the clavicle via the coracoclavicular ligament.

span the acromioclavicular joint, they become compromised after Type III injuries and are more grossly disrupted by an injury classified as Type IV through VI.

The acromioclavicular joint can also be symptomatic as a result of degenerative joint disease, osteoporosis, or osteolysis of the lateral aspect of the clavicle. Osteolysis is seen primarily in individuals with repeated heavy stresses to the shoulder, such as weightlifters or heavy laborers. Pain from the acromioclavicular joints is typically felt along the C3-C4 dermatomal distribution, which is localized to the superior and anterior aspects of the shoulder. Referred pain may also be felt in the anterolateral neck and trapezius-supraspinatus region.[20] It is not typical for pain from the acromioclavicular joint

to refer into the forearm or hand, and if such symptoms are present, the clinician should examine the complete upper quarter. Pain is often reproduced with palpation, and the joint can be provoked in the physical examination by maximally horizontally adducting the arm that has been elevated forward (Figure 4-31).

THE SCAPULOTHORACIC INTERFACE

Nearly all shoulder function requires movement of the scapula concurrent with movement of the humerus. Scapular motion complements glenohumeral motion,

Table 4-4. Acromioclavicular Joint Injuries

Pathology	Clinical Findings	Management
Type I Minor sprain of AC ligaments	Tender to palpation	Ice, sling 5-7 days Isometrics, ROM Return to activity after 2 weeks
Type II AC ligament rupture Distal clavicle unstable	Pain with provocation Higher riding clavicle	Ice; sling 1-3 weeks Isometrics, ROM when symptoms decreased
Coracoclavicular ligaments intact	Accessory motion increased	Return to activity after 2-4 weeks May have residual deformity
Type III AC ligament rupture Coracoclavicular ligament rupture	Marked deformity, asymmetry Distal end of clavicle unstable and palpable	Ice; sling 2-4 weeks Isometrics, ROM when tolerated
Deltoid, trapezius disruption		Consider surgical repair
Type IV AC ligament rupture Coracoclavicular ligament rupture Deltoid, trapezius disruption Clavicle lodged in trapezius	Marked deformity and disability	Surgery
Type V AC ligament rupture Coracoclavicular ligament rupture Deltoid, trapezius detachment Marked displacement of clavicle	Marked deformity and disability	Surgery
Type VI AC ligament rupture Coracoclavicular ligament rupture Deltoid, trapezius disruption Clavicle displaced behind coracoid process and conjoint tendons Rib and soft tissue injury	Marked deformity and disability	Surgery

ROM, Range of motion; *AC*, acromioclavicular joint.

and it also is essential to achieving the full range of shoulder movement possibilities. For example, reaching completely forward is the summation of scapular protraction and shoulder flexion. Likewise, reaching behind our back or attempting to scratch our own back requires the humerus to be adducted, hyperextended, and internally rotated, and the scapula must be retracted and downwardly rotated as well. These motions are complex because they involve movement of the scapula over the thorax, the scapula on the clavicle, and the clavicle on the sternum. While historically a 2:1 ratio of glenohumeral motion to scapulothoracic motion has been discussed, the scapular contribution to

elevation of the arm is much more complex in terms of the subtleties of the motion and highly variable depending on the loads the arm is lifting.[41]

Because the scapulothoracic interface is limited to the acromioclavicular joint and the glenohumeral joint in terms of bony articulations, and the scapula is only indirectly attached to the axial skeleton at the sternoclavicular joint via its linkage to the clavicle, the scapula is almost entirely dependent on the musculature for its mobility, as well as its ability to be fixated or stabilized on the thorax. The Kibler lateral scapular slide test is designed to look at the posture of the scapula as it rests on the thorax.[14,32,33] In this test the

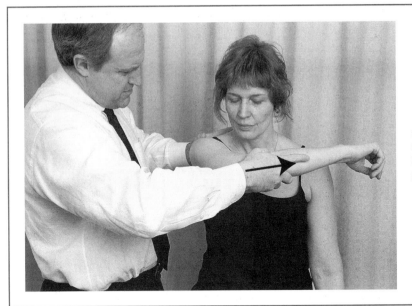

Figure 4-31. In a provocational test of the acromioclavicular joint, the arm is flexed and brought into horizontal adduction and then gentle overpressure is applied.

distance from the inferior angle of the scapula to the corresponding thoracic vertebra is measured for both scapulae. Then both sides are compared after placing the arms in three different positions: at the side, with the hands on the hips, and at 90 degrees abduction with full glenohumeral internal rotation. Differences of less than 1 cm bilaterally are considered normal, whereas differences greater than 1.5 cm are considered abnormal. Litchfield and co-workers noted further that the Kibler lateral slide test was valid for helping to identify patients with impingement.[36] In other words, patients with suspected scapular asymmetry had evidence of impingement syndrome.

Although the term *scapulothoracic interface* is used to imply motion of the scapula on the thorax, the motion interfaces are actually between the deep aspect of the serratus anterior muscle and the ribs, intercostal muscles, and serratus posterior muscles and between the deep surface of the subscapularis muscle and the superficial surface of the serratus anterior muscle. Several bursae are present at these interfaces. One large bursa is located at the superior medial corner of the scapula and lies between the serratus anterior and subscapularis muscles. Another large bursa that typically is prominent in most shoulder dissections lies between the serratus anterior muscle and the lateral wall of the chest. Therefore the scapula lies within a canopy of muscles,

and it is the muscles that must move freely among one another, as well as across the thoracic cage.

While "snapping scapula" is often thought to be a condition related to the movement across thickened bursal tissue, the causes of this syndrome are unknown. It may be caused by a variety of reasons including bony exostosis of the undersurface of the scapula or the ribs, neoplasms of the scapula, or excessive weight loss or muscle atrophy, in which the mass of the subscapularis or serratus anterior no longer provides a thick cushion in which the scapula can sit.

In addition, a change in the position of the thorax itself alters the position of the scapula at this scapulothoracic interface. For example, the forward head, rounded shoulder posture seen so often in the clinical examination is often due to a thorax that is now caudal and forward as a result of abdominal wall weakness. This collapse of the thorax forward results in the scalene muscles and sternocleidomastoid muscles passively pulling the cervical spine forward and also positions the scapula in protraction and downward rotation, which potentially compromises the tissues within the subacromial space. The relationship of the abdominal wall to the shoulder girdle muscles is detailed in Chapter 3.

Motion of the scapula occurs in numerous directions and planes simultaneously. Motions include upward and downward rotation of the scapula

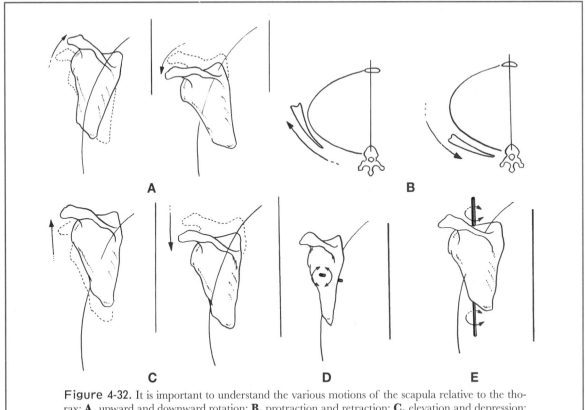

Figure 4-32. It is important to understand the various motions of the scapula relative to the thorax: **A,** upward and downward rotation; **B,** protraction and retraction; **C,** elevation and depression; **D,** tilting about a frontal axis; and **E,** tilting about a vertical axis.

(glenoid facing upward or downward, respectively), protraction and retraction (also referred to as *abduction* and *adduction,* respectively), elevation and depression, tilting about a frontal axis, and tilting about a vertical axis (Figure 4-32, *A-E*). The wide range of scapular movement is designed to provide optimal positioning of this important bone so that the muscles originating from it and moving the humerus are functioning at their optimal length-tension relationship. Scapular motion and muscle strength and endurance of the muscles directly moving the scapula are essential components of shoulder function. McQuade and colleagues noted that fatigue of the shoulder muscles has a pronounced effect on the synchrony of movement between the scapula and the humerus with a concomitant change in expected scapulohumeral rhythm.[40] This has significant implications for load distribution at the glenohumeral joint and at the

suprahumeral region for sport activities and repetitive motions associated with the work setting.

Treatment of many acute neck disorders is often best begun with passive mobilization techniques of the shoulder.[50] Because scapulothoracic motion is so essential for functional shoulder motion, mobilization of the scapula is extremely important in the treatment of many shoulder conditions, including frozen shoulder, or adhesive capsulitis syndromes, postsurgical rehabilitation for rotator cuff repair, repair of humeral fractures, and capsular repairs. Such mobilization techniques are safe and help modulate pain and maintain and restore motion of this key interface (Figure 4-33).

Several muscles move the scapula directly by virtue of their attachments. These include the serratus anterior, trapezius, rhomboid major and minor, pectoralis minor, and levator scapulae (see Chapter 3). Several

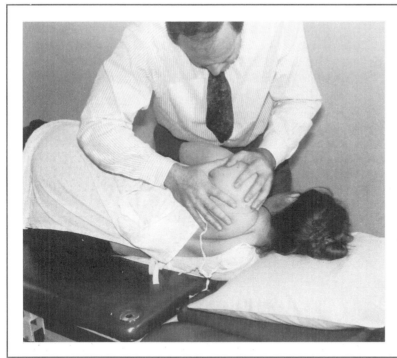

Figure 4-33. Mobilization of the scapulothoracic interface is accomplished from the side-lying position. The scapula can be easily grasped by the examiner and passively moved across the thorax for superior and inferior glides, protraction and retraction, or tilting of the scapula along a vertical axis. (From Porterfield JA, DeRosa C: *Mechanical neck pain: perspectives in functional anatomy,* Philadelphia, 1995, WB Saunders.)

other key muscles move the scapula indirectly by virtue of their attachments to the humerus. These include the latissimus dorsi (scapular depression and retraction) and pectoralis major (scapular depression and protraction). Finally, it is important to realize the synergistic activity of the thoracoscapular and scapulohumeral motions with everyday activities (Figure 4-34). For example, when you pull a heavy weight toward your body, which requires strong activity of the humeral extensor, such as the posterior deltoid and the teres major, the scapula must be fixated so that these muscles have a stable origin to pull from. In this example, the scapula retractors, such as the rhomboids and middle trapezius, must strongly fixate the scapula in order to allow the posterior deltoid and the teres major to effectively move the humerus.

THE STERNOCLAVICULAR JOINT

The sternoclavicular joint is the upper extremity's only articulation with the axial skeleton, and thus the weight of the upper extremity is continuously transferred through the clavicle to this important articulation. Disorders of the sternoclavicular joint (sprains of the joint or dislocations) are relatively rare, which implies that the articulating elements, the medial end of the clavicle and the sternum, are highly congruous and result in bony stability. This is far from the case, however, as the bony elements result, when considered alone, in the sternoclavicular joint being one of the least stable joints in the body.

Like the glenohumeral joint, the sternum and clavicle are poorly matched. Typically, less than half of the medial end of the clavicle is in contact with the concave clavicular notch of the sternum. A close look at the medial end of the clavicle reveals it to be saddle shaped, with its convex rim running vertically and its concave region running anterior to posterior (Figure 4-35, *A*). Given such poor congruency of the joint partners, the stability of the joint must come from the ligaments, namely the anterior and posterior sternoclavicular ligaments, interclavicular ligament, and the costoclavicular ligament, in addition to the articular disc that supports the sternoclavicular joint (Figure 4-35, *B*).

The articular disc of the sternoclavicular joint is unique because it attaches inferiorly at the junction of the first rib and sternum and then proceeds superiorly to attach to the superior aspect of the clavicle

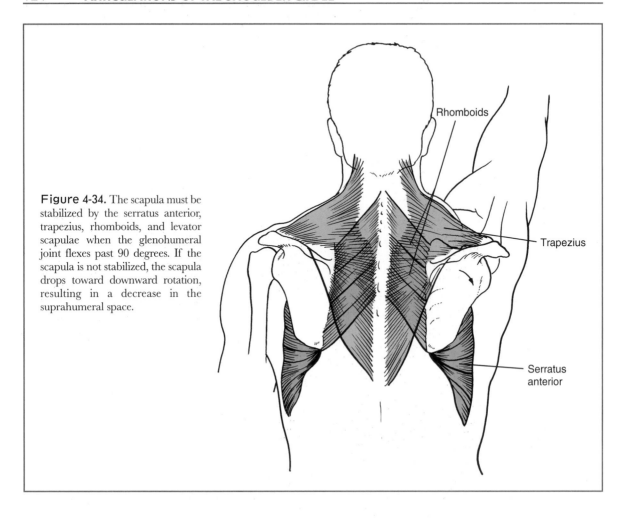

Figure 4-34. The scapula must be stabilized by the serratus anterior, trapezius, rhomboids, and levator scapulae when the glenohumeral joint flexes past 90 degrees. If the scapula is not stabilized, the scapula drops toward downward rotation, resulting in a decrease in the suprahumeral space.

(Figure 4-35, *C*). Note how the articular disc prevents superior and medial displacement of the clavicle on the sternum. Superficial to the disc is the broad costoclavicular ligament (Figure 4-35, *D*). This ligament is actually made of two parts and helps stabilize the clavicle.

Perhaps the key ligament that resists upward displacement of the clavicle away from the sternum is the capsular ligament, particularly its anterior capsule component. Just like most capsular ligaments, the anterior and posterior sternoclavicular capsular ligaments are thickenings of the joint capsule, with the anterior in this case being quite substantial. Bearn's classic work on sternoclavicular stability demonstrates that the capsular ligaments strongly resist the upward motion of the clavicle. The motion would occur simply because of the weight of the upper extremity.[2] The resting shoulder posture (point of the shoulder being held up) is in large part a result of the ligamentous structure of the sternoclavicular joint resisting upward displacement of the clavicle's sternal end (Figure 4-36, *A*).

The motion of the scapula over the scapulothoracic interface results largely from the mobility present at the sternoclavicular joint (Figure 4-36, *B*). Motion occurs in the horizontal and frontal planes, and rotation occurs around the longitudinal axis of the clavicle. This capability at the sternoclavicular joint plays a great role in allowing the shoulder girdle its extraordinary mobility.

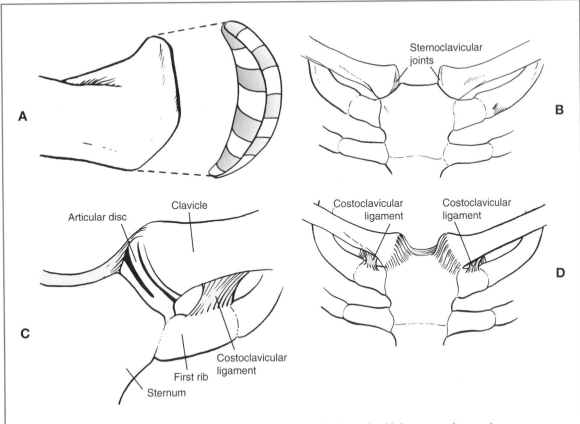

Figure 4-35. A, The medial end of the clavicle is saddle shaped, with its convex rim running vertically and its concave region running anterior to posterior. **B,** This large medial prominence (sternal end of the clavicle) is poorly matched to the clavicular notch of the sternum, as the notch is much smaller than the sternal end of the clavicle. **C,** The articular disc of the sternoclavicular joint passes superiorly from the junction of the ribs and the sternum to the superior surface of the clavicle, effectively dividing the joint into two compartments. **D,** The costoclavicular ligament originates from the junction of the first rib and the sternum and courses superiorly to attach to the inferior margin of the sternal end of the clavicle. The broadness of this ligament results in it stabilizing rotary and elevation movements of the clavicle on the sternum.

SUMMARY

We reviewed the articulations of the shoulder girdle in this chapter, including the synovial joints and key interfaces allowing shoulder motion. The study of each articulation of the shoulder girdle underscores the synchrony necessary among all moving parts and implies that dysfunction in one of the articulations or interfaces can result in overload or repetitive strain in another region. Therefore it is essential that the clinician evaluate each articulation of the shoulder girdle in order to make the most accurate diagnosis and direct a course of treatment aimed at addressing the cause of the problem instead of simply treating the symptoms associated with the disorder. The application of the clinical anatomy of any

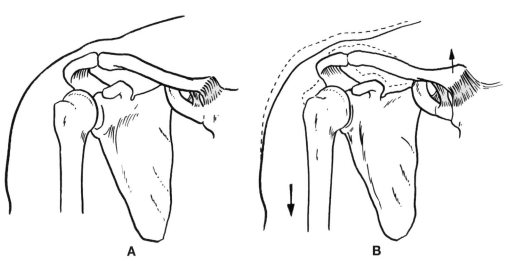

Figure 4-36. The sternoclavicular capsular ligaments and the articular disc of the joint strongly resist upward motion of the clavicle on the sternum. Note how this contributes to resting shoulder posture (**A**). The weight of the upper extremity pulls down on the lateral aspect of the clavicle through the scapula, as seen in **B**, and the medial end of the clavicle would rise from the sternal base without this ligamentous checkrein.

region of the body is best illustrated in the evaluation process for that region. In Chapter 5 we present the evaluation of the shoulder in the context of its anatomical region.

REFERENCES

1. Andrews JR, Carson WG Jr, McLeod WD: Glenoid labrum tears related to the long head of the biceps, *Am J Sport Med* 13:337, 1985.
2. Bearn JG: Direct observation of the function of the capsule of the sternoclavicular joint in clavicular support, *J Anat* 101:159, 1967.
3. Bigliani LU, Morrison D, April EW: The morphology of the acromion and its relationship to rotator cuff tears, *Orthop Trans* 10:228, 1986.
4. Brown JN, Roberts SNJ, Hayes MG, et al: Shoulder pathology associated with symptomatic acromioclavicular joint degeneration, *J Should Elbow Surg* 9:173, 2000.
5. Burns WC, Whipple TL: Anatomic relations of the shoulder impingement syndrome, *Clin Orthop* 294:96, 1993.
6. Cech D, Martin S: *Functional movement development: across the life span,* Philadelphia, 2002, WB Saunders.
7. Codman EA: *The shoulder: ruptures of the supraspinatus tendon and other lesions in or about the subacromial bursa,* Boston, 1934, Thomas Todd.
8. Conzen A, Eckstein F: Quantitative determination of articular pressure in the human shoulder joint, *J Shoulder Elbow Surg* 9:196, 2000.
9. Cooper DE, Arnoczky SP, O'Brien SJ, et al: Anatomy, histology, and vascularity of the glenoid labrum: an anatomical study, *J Bone Joint Surg Am* 74:46, 1992.
10. Crockett HC, Cook LB, Wilk KE, et al: Osseous adaptation and range of motion at the glenohumeral joint in professional baseball players, *Am J Sport Med* 30:20, 1992.
11. Cyriax J: *Textbook of orthopaedic medicine,* vol 1, London, 1978, Bailliere Tindall.
12. D'Alessandro DF, Fleischli JE, Connor PM: Superior labral lesions: diagnosis and management, *J Athletic Training* 35(3):286, 2000.
13. Davidson PA, Elattrache NS, Jobe CM, et al: Rotator cuff and posterior-superior glenoid labrum injury associated with increased glenohumeral motion: a new site of impingement, *J Shoulder Elbow Surg* 4:384, 1995.
14. Davies GJ, Hoffman SD: Neuromuscular testing and rehabilitation of the shoulder complex, *J Orthop Sports Phys Ther* 18:449, 1993.
15. Edelson JG: Patterns of degenerative change in the acromioclavicular joint, *J Bone Joint Surg Br* 78B:242, 1996.

16. Flatow EL, Soslowsky LJ, Ticker JB, et al: Excursion of the rotator cuff under the acromion: patterns of subacromial contact, *Am J Sports Med* 22:779, 1994.

17. Fukuda K, Craig EV, An K, et al: Biomechanical study of the ligamentous system of the acromioclavicular joint, *J Bone Joint Surg (Am)* 68A:434, 1986.

18. Fukuda H, Hamada K, Nakajima T, et al: Pathology and pathogenesis of the intratendinous tearing of the rotator cuff viewed from en bloc histologic sections, *Clin Orthop* 304:60, 1994.

19. Fukuda H, Hamada K, Yamanaka K: Pathology and pathogenesis of bursal side rotator cuff tears viewed from en bloc histologic sections, *Clin Orthop* 254:75, 1990.

20. Gerber C, Galantay RV, Hersche O: The pattern of pain produced by irritation of the acromioclavicular joint and the subacromial space, *J Shoulder Elbow Surg* 7:352, 1998.

21. Graichen H, Stammberger T, Bonel H, et al: Glenohumeral translation during active and passive elevation of the shoulder girdle—a 3-D open-MRI study, *J Biomech* 33:609, 2000.

22. Green MR, Christensen KP: Arthroscopic Bankart procedure: two- to five-year follow-up with clinical correlation to severity of glenoid labral lesion, *Am J Sports Med* 23:276, 1995.

23. Guidi EC, Zuckerman JD: Glenoid labral lesions. In Wilk KE, Andrews JR, editors: *The athlete's shoulder*, New York, 1994, Churchill Livingstone.

24. Hadler A, Zobitz ME, Schultz F, et al: Mechanical properties of the posterior rotator cuff, *Clin Biomech* 15:456, 2000.

25. Hannafin JA, DiCarlo ED, Wickiewicz TL, et al: Adhesive capsulitis: capsular fibroplasias of the glenohumeral joint, *J Shoulder Elbow Surg* 3S:5, 1994.

26. Harryman DT II, Sidles JA, Matsen FA III: Laxity of the normal glenohumeral joint: a quantitative in vivo assessment, *J Shoulder Elbow Surg* 1:66, 1992.

27. Hawkins RJ, Kennedy JC: Impingement syndrome in athletes, *Am J Sports Med* 8:151, 1980.

28. Henry MH, Liu SH, Loffredo AJ: Arthroscopic management of the acromioclavicular disorder: a review, *Clin Orthop* 316:276, 1995.

29. Howell SM, Galinat BJ: The glenoid-labral socket: a constrained articular surface, *Clin Orthop* 243:122, 1989.

30. Howell SM, Galinat BJ, Renzi AG, et al: Normal and abnormal mechanics of the glenohumeral joint in the horizontal plane, *J Bone Joint Surg Am* 70A:227, 1988.

31. Kelkar R, Flatow EL, Bigliani LU, et al: A stereophotogrammetric method to determine the kinematics of the glenohumeral joint, *Adv Bioeng* 19:143, 1992.

32. Kibler WB: Role of the scapula in the overhand throwing motion, *Contemp Orthop* 22:525, 1991.

33. Kibler WB, Livingston BR: Current concepts in shoulder rehabilitation, *Adv Oper Orthop* 3:249, 1995.

34. Kronberg M, Brostrom LA, Soderlund V: Retroversion of the humeral head in the normal shoulder and its relationship to the normal range of motion, *Clin Orthop* 253:113, 1990.

35. Lippitt SB, Vanderhooft JE, Harris SL, et al: Glenohumeral stability from concavity-compression: a quantitative analysis, *J Shoulder Elbow Surg* 2:27, 1993.

36. Litchfield R, Hawkins R, Dillman CJ, et al: Rehabilitation of the overhead athlete, *J Orthop Sports Phys Ther* 18:433, 1993.

37. Ludewig PM, Cook TM: Alterations in shoulder kinematics and associated muscle activity in people with symptoms of shoulder impingement, *Phys Ther* 80:276, 2000.

38. Matsen FA III, Lippitt SB, Sidles JA, et al: *Practical evaluation and management of the shoulder*, Philadelphia, 1994, WB Saunders.

39. McMahon P, Debski R, Thomson W, et al: Shoulder muscle forces and tendon excursions during glenohumeral abduction in the scapular plane, *J Shoulder Elbow Surg* 4:199, 1995.

40. McQuade KJ, Dawson J, Smidt GL: Scapulothoracic muscle fatigue associated with alterations in scapulohumeral rhythm kinematics during maximum resistive shoulder elevation, *J Orthop Sports Phys Ther* 28:74, 1998.

41. McQuade KJ, Smidt GL: Dynamic scapulohumeral rhythm: the effects of external resistance during elevation of the arm in the scapular plane, *J Orthop Sports Phys Ther* 27:125, 1998.

42. Neer CS, Welsh RP: The shoulder in sports, *Orthop Clin North Am* 8:583, 1977.

43. Neviaser JS: Adhesive capsulitis of the shoulder, *J Bone Joint Surg* 27:211, 1945.

44. Neviaser JS: Adhesive capsulitis and the stiff and painful shoulder, *Orthop Clin North Am* 11:327, 1980.

45. Nixon JE, DiStefano V: Ruptures of the rotator cuff, *Orthop Clin North Am* 6:423, 1975.

46. Norris TR, Fischer J, Bigliani LU: The unfused acromial epiphysis and its relationship to impingement syndrome, *Orthop Trans* 7:505, 1983.

47. O'Brien SJ, Neves MC, Arnocsky SP, et al: The anatomy and histology of the inferior glenohumeral ligament complex of the shoulder, *Am J Sports Med* 18:449, 1990.

48. Petersson CJ: Degeneration of the acromioclavicular joint: a morphological study, *Acta Orthop Scand* 54:434, 1983.

49. Poppen NK, Walker PS: Normal and abnormal motion of the shoulder, *J Bone Joint Surg (Am)* 58:195, 1976.

50. Porterfield JA, DeRosa C: *Mechanical neck pain: perspectives in functional anatomy*, Philadelphia, 1995, WB Saunders.

51. Refior HJ, Sowa D: Long tendon of the biceps brachii: sites of predilection for degenerative lesions, *J Shoulder Elbow Surg* 4:436, 1995.

52. Rockwood CA Jr: Dislocations about the shoulder. In Rockwood CA Jr., Green DP, editors: *Fractures*, vol I, Philadelphia, 1975, JB Lippincott.

53. Sharkey NA, Marder RA, Hanson PB: The entire rotator cuff contributes to elevation of the arm, *J Orthopaedic Res* 12:699, 1994.

54. Snyder SJ, Banas MP, Karzel RP: An analysis of 140 injuries to the superior glenoid labrum, *J Shoulder Elbow Surg* 4:243, 1995.

55. Snyder SJ, Larzel RP, Del Pizzo W, et al: SLAP lesions of the shoulder, *Arthroscopy* 6:274, 1990.

56. Sonnery-Cottet B, Edwards TB, Noel E, et al: Results of arthroscopic treatment of posterosuperior glenoid impingement in tennis players, *Am J Sports Med* 30:227, 2002.

57. Thompson WO, Debaki RE, Boardman ND, et al: A biomechanical analysis of rotator cuff deficiency in a cadaveric model, *Am J Sports Med* 24:286, 1996.

58. Uhthoff HK, Loehr J, Sakar K: The pathogenesis of rotator cuff tears. In *Proceedings of the Third International Conference on Surgery of the Shoulder*, Fukuora, Japan, 1986.

59. Valadie AL, Jobe CM, Pink MM, et al: Anatomy of provocative tests for impingement syndrome of the shoulder, *J Shoulder Elbow Surg* 9:36, 2000.
60. Walch G: Posterosuperior glenoid impingement. In Burkhead WZ Jr, editor: *Rotator cuff disorders,* Media, Pa, 1996, Williams & Wilkins.
61. Williams PL, Warwick R, Dyson M, et al: *Gray's anatomy,* New York, 1989, Churchill Livingstone.
62. Yuzici M, Kapuz C, Gulman B: Morphological variants of the acromion in neonatal cadavers, *J Pediatric Orthop* 15:644, 1995.

CHAPTER **5**

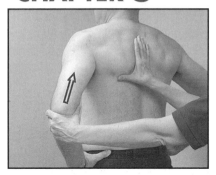

FUNCTIONAL ASSESSMENT OF THE SHOULDER GIRDLE COMPLEX

GENERAL CONCEPTS

Pathomechanical Versus Pathoanatomical Diagnosis

There are many tissues within the shoulder girdle complex that are potential sources of pain. In addition, the cervical spine, visceral structures such as cardiac and pulmonary tissues, and select abdominal viscera, all have the capacity to refer pain to the shoulder region. Once referred pain from visceral structures has been ruled out, the clinician must identify the precise anatomical tissue causing the painful syndrome within the shoulder complex or determine those movements and combinations of applied stresses that reproduce familiar signs or symptoms. The shoulder complex can be assessed from either a pathoanatomical or pathomechanical perspective. This may, however, present a dilemma in the development of an active treatment program or an exercise prescription. For example, does the clinician prescribe exercise in order to minimize stress to a suspected lesion of the long head of the biceps because he surmises that is the painful tissue? Or does he prescribe exercises around the nociceptive mechanics evaluated, designing an exercise program around the motions and forces that clearly reproduce the patient's signs and symptoms? The pathoanatomical approach to examination seeks to discover the tissue that might be at fault, whereas the pathomechanical approach seeks to identify those

motions, postural positions, stresses, or combinations of stresses that are contributing to the painful syndrome.

The first and most basic question to ask is: What is the precise anatomical lesion causing pain in most shoulder conditions? Even a well-understood condition such as impingement syndrome presents great difficulty in identifying the exact tissue that might be at fault. The anatomy described in Chapters 3 and 4 illustrates that in addition to mechanical linkages and anatomical connections among the various tissues, the structures lie in very close proximity to each other. Is it possible, for example, to definitively conclude that pain resulting from an impingement test is actually from the anterior aspect of the supraspinatus tendon rather than the posterior portion of the long head of the biceps tendon, since they are so closely placed? Likewise, with the intimate blending of the anterior aspect of the infraspinatus tendon to the posterior aspect of the supraspinatus tendon, is it possible to identify the specific symptomatic tendon? Shoulder instability provides another example. Classic shoulder instability is relatively easy to identify based on information gained from the patient history and several passive motion maneuvers. It is not as easy to identify the exact anatomical tissue that is the nociceptive generator because so many tissues are typically compromised when the glenohumeral joint is unstable. Chapter 4 reviewed the possible joint structures that might be implicated with instability, along with the potential for secondary compromise to surrounding tissues such as the rotator cuff tendons and long head of the biceps.

Certainly the increased use of imaging and arthroscopic techniques optimizes the chances of identifying the tissues that appear to have been injured or are in the varying stages of degeneration. In some clinical conditions the tissue at fault can in fact be identified. For example, the history of an abrupt loss of the ability to lift the arm following shoulder trauma, coupled with a positive drop-arm test (described later in detail) and diagnostic arthroscopy revealing a full thickness tear of the supraspinatus tendon, allows us to appropriately conclude which tissue is at fault.

In many shoulder syndromes the history, signs, and symptoms are less clear. It is important to recognize that the similarities and differences between normal age-related changes and pathology have not been clearly elucidated. It is difficult to be certain that the nociceptive generator in someone complaining of shoulder pain is due to pathology of the cuff tendons rather than surrounding tissues because rotator cuff tendons begin to show age-related changes as early as the second and third decades and yet can be asymptomatic.

Another example relates to glenoid labrum damage. We previously mentioned that the superior aspect of the glenoid labrum is less firmly attached to the glenoid rim than the inferior aspect (see Chapter 4). Short of an obvious tear in the superior aspect of the labrum, when should the superior labrum be considered pathological because it is identified as "too loose" and hence diagnosed as a SLAP lesion (see Chapter 4) as opposed to simply being the normal loose attachment for that particular patient? Consideration of the questions these clinical examples raise is fundamentally important because ultimately the conclusions that the examiner reaches after taking the history and conducting the physical examination direct the course of treatment, whether it is surgical or nonsurgical.

The Concept of Applied Physical Stresses

Perhaps the most compelling reason for the thorough discussion of the shoulder anatomy in the previous chapters is that it provides the clinician with an appreciation of the anatomy in three dimensions. Combining a comprehensive understanding of the anatomy and biomechanics of the articulations comprising the shoulder complex with knowledge about fiber direction, connective tissue linkages, and spatial relationships of the muscles allows the examiner to resolve every force the patient applies during the physical examination into component vectors. For example, what might look like a simple anterior-to-posterior shear of the head of the humerus on the glenoid by the examiner with the patient in the supine position may in fact have the following concurrent stresses applied to associated tissues:

1. Compression of all soft tissue (skin, anterior deltoid, vasculature, neural tissue, subscapularis, long head of biceps tendon, joint capsule, coracohumeral ligament, glenohumeral ligaments) between the skin and the head of the humerus
2. Compression of the head of the humerus into the posterior part of the labrum and glenoid if the application of the anterior-posterior shear stress is not applied parallel to the glenoid surface
3. Stretch of the posterior joint capsule and the cuff muscles reinforcing the posterior aspect of the capsule by movement of the humeral head against the inner capsule wall

We suggest that in the nonsurgical management of many musculoskeletal conditions, it is not as critical to determine the anatomical tissue that is at fault but rather to find out what abnormal or excessive stresses or combinations of stresses are reproducing familiar pain by stimulating the nociceptive system. Nociceptive stimulation occurs as a result of the tissue's inability to attenuate such stresses, typically because of injury as a result of age-related tissue changes.

Therefore the examination methods discussed in this chapter largely describe efforts to reproduce familiar symptoms through the application of three primary stresses: compression, tension, and shear. Whether the examination procedure involves active motion, passive motion, resisted motion, palpation, or the use of shoulder-specific special tests, the unifying feature of these tests is that they are typically assessing the shoulder tissues' ability to attenuate compression, tension, or shear. Such an approach provides clinical utility for several reasons:[30]

- It allows the clinician to use the results of the examination as the basis for designing an exercise program around these nociceptive mechanics.
- It correlates the patient's vulnerable and invulnerable positions and movements to his work and activities of daily living.

- It provides information to the patients in understandable and practical terms.

Thinking in terms of applied physical stresses also provides meaningful information regarding the irritability of the tissues. The examiner needs to be able to correlate the magnitude of their applied stress to the ease or difficulty in evoking a painful response. The goal is to identify the intensity and direction of the forces used in the physical examination in order to determine the relationship of the applied stresses to the painful syndrome. After this information has been gained, an appropriate active treatment plan can be established, which minimizes further tissue damage and promotes connective tissue and muscle growth while simultaneously decreasing sensitivity to pain.

INFORMATION GAINED FROM THE EXAMINATION

Perhaps no area of the musculoskeletal system besides the shoulder complex has such a broad array of special tests available to help with assessment. Numerous tests have been described for the biceps tendon, thoracic outlet syndrome, and shoulder instability, to name just a few. Indeed, there are enough special tests for specific tissues of the shoulder to warrant their own complete chapters in textbooks.

This presents a challenge for the examiner. How can a comprehensive clinical examination of the shoulder be conducted while maintaining a balance between thoroughness and efficiency? What are the best tests to use? It is not enough to have a particular sequence of examination in mind. The clinician must also use the patient history in a manner that dictates the essential pieces necessary to the physical examination so that he can conduct it in a manner that avoids unnecessary redundancy while simultaneously substantiating what has already been discovered up to that point in the examination process.

Regardless of the examination scheme chosen, there are a few essential pieces of information that must be gleaned on completion of the history and physical examination. Recognizing such end points allows the examiner to conduct an effective and efficient examination. The minimal essential pieces are threefold and fall under the categories of *pathomechanics*, *syndrome classification*, and presence or absence of *stability*.

Pathomechanics

During the physical examination the clinician guides the patient through a series of systematic motions and then applies various stresses and combinations of stresses to and through the tissues. As implied in the previous section, the examiner ultimately concludes which series of motions and combinations of stresses reproduce familiar pain. The application of overpressure to these motions results in increased tension, compression, or shear to the structures. The clinician seeks the specific combination of stresses that exacerbates the condition or provokes familiar pain. The pathomechanics that reproduce familiar pain or are recognized to yield atypical responses such as abnormal motion, muscle or motion guarding, or apprehension are acknowledged by the examiner and then substantiated by applying similar stresses in other positions. Applying similar stresses with the shoulder in dependent and nondependent positions, for example, and from different starting points in the range of motion, allows the examiner to correlate these responses and determine their relationship to the painful syndrome.

Syndrome Classification

The second piece of necessary information relates to the syndrome presentation itself. Is the patient presenting with an acute shoulder problem, an exacerbation of a previous problem, or a syndrome exhibiting chronic pain behaviors? The great majority of shoulder joint disorders fall into one of the first two categories. It is only when there is evidence of little or no direct relationship between the physical stimulus applied in the examination and the pain response from the patient, combined with the complaint of persistent pain well beyond expected healing time, that the clinician begins to consider the presence of *chronic pain syndrome*.

Acute injuries are those in which the response of the patient to various stresses is proportional to the time since the onset of the painful syndrome and the pathomechanics of injury. Because of the predictability of the healing times for many of the specialized connective tissues and based on work that has been done with spinal disorders, acute injuries are generally considered to be those that are less than 7 weeks old.

Because acute injuries are typically accompanied by swelling and the associated alteration of the chemical milieu of the tissues, morning stiffness and discomfort are positive indicators of swelling and the acuteness of the injury. When an injured tissue is placed at rest and very little movement occurs, fluid stasis chemically activates the nociceptive system (see Chapter 6). The remaining category of syndrome classification is the *exacerbation of previous injury* patient presentation. Within this group patients typically describe previous injuries, past symptoms, or an antecedent event from which a pattern of pain develops over the course of time, with varying levels of pain intensity and varying intervals of time between episodes. The pain pattern described gives the examiner a sense of the limited capacity of the injured tissues to attenuate compression, tensile, and shear loads. This syndrome is related to tissues that have been previously subjected to macrotrauma and those tissues affected by the age-related, degenerative processes. In both cases the optimal loading capacity or limit of the tissue's tolerance to compression, tension, or shear is being exceeded (see Chapter 1). Patients in this category describe similar episodes of their unique problem, which typically worsen over time.

Presence or Absence of Stability

The third piece of information that must be determined from the examination concerns the stability of the key articulations of the shoulder complex. Stability of the articulations within the musculoskeletal system is primarily due to two reasons: the integrity of the connective tissues associated with the articulations and the status of the neuromuscular control over these articulations.[16] This is especially true for the glenohumeral joint. As seen in many other areas of the musculoskeletal system, the body type, connective tissue integrity, and neuromuscular health of the region determine how the forces of weight bearing and movement converge on the region and are attenuated. Do these forces result in aberrational motion between the articulating structures, and is this abnormal motion excessively loading support tissues and resulting in stimulation of the nociceptive receptors associated with the articulations? This is a key question that the examiner needs to ask while administering tests during the examination process.

In Chapter 1 the concept of the optimal loading zone of tissues was explained. In Chapter 3 the role of the muscular system over the articulations was discussed in detail. Chapter 4 focused on the specialized connective tissues associated with the shoulder. The important point to be gleaned from these chapters is that the precision and interplay of neuromusculoconnective tissues are vital for joint stability and subtle changes in any of these tissues have the potential to contribute to joint instability. Therefore the patient history and physical examination for mechanical disorders of the shoulder have to be designed to ultimately confirm the presence or absence of stability, which then guides the examiner in determining the causative factors if instability is suspected.

In the remaining sections of this chapter, we will provide the reader with a pattern of examination for activity related disorders of the shoulder complex. Using a consistent pattern of examination is important because it helps ensure thoroughness and allows physical findings to be compared among patients. The examiner must understand the potential relevance of key elements in the history and be able to administer important provocative tests to tissues, palpate key structures, and identify those factors that may be contributing to the pain pattern or dysfunction at the shoulder. The composite of this information provides the examiner with information regarding the pathomechanics, the syndrome classification, and the presence or absence of stability.

COMPONENTS OF THE PATIENT HISTORY

Initial Considerations

The patient history often dictates the direction that the remaining portion of the musculoskeletal examination will take. During questioning, pay close attention to patient affect, posturing, and willingness to give information. Be a focused listener, and think in terms of joints or soft tissues under the area of complaint that might be causing the problem and any anatomical region that might refer pain to the shoulder and associated regions of the upper quarter. Frame questions in such a way that you and the patient can reach a common understanding of the problem. This is the first step in helping the patient recognize how important his role will be in the management of his problem. During the history, the therapeutic relationship between clinician and patient begins, as well as the patient's educational process.

And as mentioned earlier, it is important to be complete but also succinct. Table 5-1 lists key questions

Table 5-1. Questionnaire for Patient History: Shoulder

1. How old are you? What is your occupation?
2. In your words, what is the problem?
3. How long have you had shoulder pain? How would you describe it?
4. Show me where you have pain. (Consider using a body chart.) Do you ever have pain, numbness, or tingling in any other areas? Do you notice any numbness or tingling in the arm or hand? Does your pain extend toward elbow or wrist? Does it stay localized to the shoulder?
5. What position were you in when you were initially hurt?
6. Is it difficult to perform activities that require reaching above shoulder level?
7. Describe previous episodes of shoulder pain. How long did these episodes last?
8. What positions or activities increase your pain? What activities are limited by this problem? Are you able to lie on that shoulder at night? Does the shoulder pain awaken you at night?
9. Do you have any neck pain, or do neck movements increase your shoulder pain?
10. Is your pain worse in the morning on awakening, or is it worse toward the end of the day? Are you more stiff or sore in the morning as compared with the end of the day?
11. How would you rate your level of activity? What activities are limited and why?
12. How would you rate your level of pain?
13. Are you currently taking any medications?
14. Have you had any surgeries in the past?
15. What do you think is the cause of your shoulder pain?
16. What goals do you have for treatment results?

Special Questions Related to General Health

1. Have you had any recent weight loss? Do any other joints in your body have this same type of pain?
2. Does your pain prevent you from sleeping? Is it worse at night?

than during activity, visceral pathology referring pain to the shoulder must be considered and appropriate medical referral made for additional diagnostic workup. Visceral pathology such as vascular disturbances leading to avascular necrosis and the presence of heart disease, lung tumors, and gallbladder disease has a propensity to refer pain to the shoulder. If the patient has similar complaints at other joints, for example, bilateral shoulder pain or bilateral wrist pain, then rheumatoid disease or one of the rheumatoid variants must be ruled out. Likewise, a past history of cancer such as lung cancer, breast cancer, or any other metastatic tumor should alert the clinician that the current pain complaints might not be associated with the musculoskeletal tissues of the shoulder girdle. Therefore the examiner should always be aware that other disorders might be the source of pain when the pain pattern, aggravating factors, and easing factors do not follow recognized musculoskeletal patterns. The clinician should be suspicious when the patient cannot find any position that eases discomfort, has night pain that far exceeds pain during the day or during his activities, or is complaining of a pain pattern that does not follow the typical referral zones for musculoskeletal tissues of the neck or shoulder. Chapter 2 thoroughly detailed the referral pattern for pain from the cervical joints and nerve roots.

Even before beginning the physical examination, answers given by the patient to some of the questions noted in Table 5-1 cue the clinician to a potential cause or causes of the problem and allow him to prioritize which special tests might be indicated. In addition, a thorough history directs him to properly plan the examination of the joints and soft tissues that are under the area of complaint and the tissues that have the capacity to refer pain to the region.[17]

that the examiner needs to ask a patient who is complaining of pain or change in function in the shoulder girdle. These questions help the clinician begin to discern if the pain is of mechanical origin.

Screening for Medical Conditions That Might Present as Shoulder Pain

Musculoskeletal tissues react and respond predictably. When signs and symptoms begin to fall out of expected patterns, such as the inability to reproduce familiar pain with motions or postures, continuous and unrelenting pain, or pain that is greater at rest

Predisposing Factors

Examples of questions that lead the clinician to consider predisposing factors include *"How old are you?" "What is your occupation?"* and *"What sports or activities are you involved in?"* Answers to these questions help him focus on the tests and measures that need to be included during the physical examination.

It is important to know how old a patient is because common shoulder conditions such as instability and rotator cuff pathology are often associated with age. For example, instability would be less likely in a patient under the age of 30 than in a patient of 65.

By comparison, frank pathology of the rotator cuff is more common in patients over 40, whereas the earlier stages of rotator cuff disorders such as tendonitis are more common in the 25 to 40-age-group.[24] The Neer classification scheme for shoulder impingement illustrates the cascade of age-related degenerative changes of the rotator cuff that progress from edema and hemorrhage of the tendon through tendon fibrosis and ultimately tendon rupture (Table 5-2). Understanding these stages and correlating them with the age of the patient provide more clues.

Another example of shoulder pathology influenced by age is nontraumatic primary "frozen shoulder," or adhesive capsulitis.[7,12] This phenomenon is poorly understood and most often is seen in women from 45 to 60 years of age. It is characterized by three stages, any of which might be the first point of contact with the clinician. The first stage is the initial *freezing stage* in which the abrupt loss of motion and excessive pain begin. This is followed by the *frozen stage* in which pain decreases but the motion is markedly restricted, and then a final stage of *thawing* during which slow, spontaneous recovery occurs, often over a period of 1 to 3 years.[22]

Finally, it is essential to conduct a careful analysis of the patient's activities of daily living and sport activities, especially those related to overhead activities or repetitive motions of the upper extremity. The requirements of the shoulder complex are typically sport and job specific, so the examiner's suspicions based on this information regarding which movements and stresses will be painful in the physical examination and tissues that are most likely compromised are usually accurate. For example:

- Swimming is associated with a high incidence of impingement problems, especially in a swim stroke such as the butterfly and during training with the use of swim paddles and elastic bands.[8] Internal rotation during the stroke increases the compression of tissues in the suprahumeral space.

- Throwing sports can place a significant stress to the anterior aspect of the glenohumeral joint complex, especially during the late cocking and acceleration phase of throwing.[11,29] Pain during these phases is usually felt anteriorly or superiorly as a result of anterior subluxation of the humerus and impingement of the rotator cuff as the humeral head migrates superiorly. Throwers also have increased stresses to the rotator cuff muscles in the cocking, acceleration, and follow-through phases of throwing. Pain in the acceleration phase of throwing can be due to strain on the posterior cuff tendons, whereas the deceleration phase of throwing can result in pain due to humeral head translation further increasing rotator cuff strain as a result of eccentric workload and long head of the biceps tendon strain. Table 5-3 lists the phases of throwing and selected biomechanics related to clinical problems often noted in the shoulder. Contact sports including football may result in glenohumeral subluxation, tensile injuries to the brachial plexus, or acromioclavicular joint injuries. When the patient describes contact injuries, the examiner must also prepare to assess cervical nerve root and brachial plexus function.

- Tennis may lead to cumulative microtrauma in the posterior rotator cuff tendons and the long head of the biceps since the athlete must eccentrically control the lever, now lengthened because of the racquet, during the deceleration phase of the stroke. The result is excessive tension to these tissues. The overhead activity that occurs during the cocking and acceleration phases also results in the tissues of the suprahumeral space being compromised via compression and renders the articular surface of the tendons susceptible to internal impingement.

- Weight lifting practiced with poor technique and weak scapulothoracic muscles places the tissues of the suprahumeral space in a compromised position while performing upper extremity elevation

Table 5-2. The Neer Classification Scheme for Shoulder Impingement

Stage	Age	Clinical Course	Treatment
I: Edema and hemorrhage	<25	Reversible	Conservative
II: Fibrosis and tendonitis	25-40	Recurrent pain with activity	Consider subacromial decompression
III: Bone spurs and tendon rupture	>40	Progressive disability	Subacromial decompression and cuff repair

From Neer CS II: Impingement lesions, *Clin Orthop* 173:70, 1983.

Table 5-3. Biomechanics of Throwing

Phase	Features	Pain
I. Windup and cocking phase	Abduction, extension, and external rotation of the humerus • Strong *deltoid* action in this phase • Tension placed on the anterior joint structures • *Supraspinatus* provides a stabilizing force through its action in compressing the humeral head in the glenoid • *Infraspinatus* and *teres minor* maintain humeral head in fossa through inferior directed forces and also provide concentric contraction • *Subscapularis*, aided by the *pectoralis major*, restricts the terminal external rotation of this first phase through eccentric control and helps stabilize head of humerus in glenoid	Pain in the later part of the cocking phase is usually felt anteriorly or superiorly because of anterior subluxation of the humerus and impingement of the rotator cuff, and the humeral head moves superiorly.
II. Acceleration phase	Complete reversal of above motion that begins with internal rotation • Internal rotators, notably the *subscapularis* and *pectoralis major*, provide the force • Eccentric contraction of *posterior cuff* muscles • *Latissimus dorsi, serratus anterior,* and *triceps* provide additional force through concentric activity • Very strong contraction of the serratus anterior, trapezius, rhomboids, and levator scapulae, implying that scapular stabilization is essential during this phase • Large valgus stress at the elbow	Pain in the acceleration phase is often caused by strain on the posterior cuff tendons. Pain in the elbow is caused by valgus stress.
III. Deceleration and follow-through phase	Strong activity of the rotator cuff to slow the arm down as motion is completed • *Subscapularis* continues to rotate internally • *Posterior cuff* works to decelerate the arm and maintain the humeral head within the glenoid; the posterior cuff muscles are the key stabilizing force resisting glenohumeral distraction and anterior subluxation forces • *Supraspinatus* works to keep head of humerus compressed to glenoid • *Biceps* acts eccentrically to control the rate of elbow extension; *supinator* acts to eccentrically control the rapidly pronating forearm	Pain in the deceleration phase may be caused by humeral head translation, rotator cuff strain, and long head of the biceps tendon strain.

exercises. Movements such as overhead presses or shoulder raises that maintain the humeral head in the internally rotated position potentially increase compression under the coracoacromial arch and shear at the glenohumeral and acromioclavicular joints. Poor control of heavy weights during bench press maneuvers stresses the acromioclavicular joint and the anterior and posterior capsular tissues.

• Work-related movements in an industrial setting may jeopardize arms and shoulders during their work tasks. Often, poorly designed workstations contribute to overuse syndromes not only of the shoulder but also of the cervical spine and scapulothoracic complex. Perhaps even more importantly, the gradual loss of range of motion in the lower cervical and upper thoracic spine, coupled with loss of glenohumeral motion, as occurs with age, contributes to the inability to position the arms completely overhead or in the necessary work position. Full extension of these regions of the spine is necessary for full shoulder girdle range of motion. This is one of the primary reasons that the forward head, rounded shoulder position of the upper quarter, which is often accompanied by a slouched, kyphotic posture, is a contributing factor to the development of impingement syndromes. When these types of postural changes are coupled with weakness and fatigue of scapular muscles such as the serratus anterior and trapezius in conjunction with weakness of the abdominal wall, tissues in the suprahumeral space have an even greater potential for compromise (see Chapters 3 and 6).

Mechanism of Injury

Answers to questions such as *"What position were you in when you were initially hurt?"* and responses to statements such as *"Describe previous episodes of your shoulder pain and tell me how long the episodes have lasted"* allow the examiner to begin analyzing whether increased compression, tension, or shear stresses may have occurred or are recurring. Does the patient describe either a fall on the point of the shoulder that results in damage to the coracoclavicular ligaments and acromioclavicular joint separation, or a fall on the outstretched hand (a FOOSH injury) (Figure 5-1)? Either can cause a potential fracture to the humerus, scapula, or clavicle or result in significant trauma to the soft tissues of the shoulder. Falls also may result in subluxations of either the acromioclavicular joint or the glenohumeral joint. Landing on the point of the shoulder can completely disrupt the coracoclavicular ligaments (conoid and trapezoid), which are the key support ligaments of the acromioclavicular

joint, or result in significant trauma to the rotator cuff tendons over the greater tuberosity, which may cause tendon rupture. Likewise, falling on the elbow may violently drive the humerus superiorly into the suprahumeral space and result in mechanical trauma to the glenohumeral joint capsule, rotator cuff tendons, and subacromial bursa.

Was there excessive motion that put the shoulder into an extreme range of motion? Does the patient now feel a "giving away" sensation with movement? Did the patient feel the shoulder "come out"? One of the most common mechanisms of injury resulting in anterior instability of the shoulder is forced abduction and external rotation of the glenohumeral joint, which stresses the joint capsule, the labrum, and the inferior glenohumeral ligaments (Figure 5-2).

Pain Location and Associated Symptoms

Statements such as *"Show me where you have pain"* and questions such as *"Do you notice any numbness or tingling in the arm or hand?"* *"Does your pain extend toward the elbow or wrist?"* *"Does your pain stay localized to the shoulder?"* *"Do you have any neck pain or does neck pain reproduce your shoulder discomfort?"* and *"Do you feel your shoulder 'gives out'?"* all provide key information that ultimately directs the level of scrutiny of the physical examination. For example, instability of the glenohumeral joint can also compromise the brachial plexus as it courses through

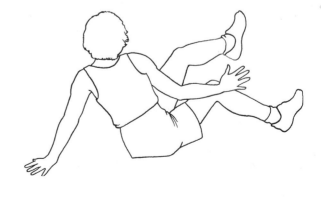

Figure 5-1. Shoulder injury can occur via a fall on the point of the shoulder that results in damage to the coracoclavicular ligaments and acromioclavicular joint separation, or a fall on the outstretched hand (FOOSH injury), as illustrated here, that results in fracture about the glenohumeral joint.

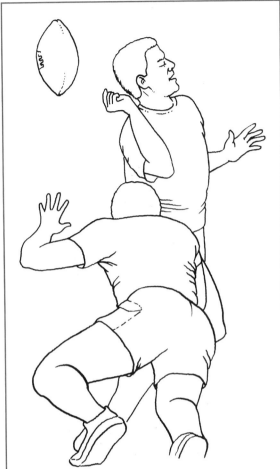

Figure 5-2. Forced external rotation in an abducted position can damage the anterior aspect of the glenohumeral joint capsule and the inferior glenohumeral ligament complex. Such injury can occur during an afternoon touch football match.

glenohumeral joint. For example, the axillary nerve, which courses around the neck of the humerus with the posterior humeral circumflex artery, can be injured with a glenohumeral dislocation. Injury to the axillary nerve may result in paralysis or weakness of the deltoid and teres minor muscles. Other terminal branches of the brachial plexus, such as the musculocutaneous and radial nerves, potentially may be compromised by the inferior position of the head of the humerus, which can occur with dislocation (see Chapter 2). Therefore when there is a history of dislocation, the examiner is prepared to clinically assess the muscles supplied by the terminal branches of the brachial plexus.

When instability is suspected, the clinician will clarify whether or not there was a traumatic event, the positions and motions in which symptoms are reproduced or the shoulder feels "unstable," and whether or not the patient can voluntarily sublux or dislocate his glenohumeral joint. A wide range of shoulder instabilities exist, from the TUBS type (traumatic onset in a unilateral direction, often causing a Bankart lesion and optimally treated with surgery) to the AMBRI type (atraumatic etiology with multidirectional instability pattern bilaterally, often responsive to rehabilitation, and if surgery is indicated, an inferior capsular shift procedure is commonly used). If the history leads the examiner to suspect glenohumeral joint instability, he performs several tests in the course of the physical examination.

The examiner needs to carefully determine the area of pain. It is one of the most important pieces of information to be ascertained. The location of pain may indicate that the structures have been injured and alert him to stresses that might be poorly tolerated during the physical examination (Figure 5-3, A and B). For example, pain felt at the region of the deltoid insertion (an area within the C5 dermatome) is often a referred pain pattern from lesions of the rotator cuff tendons. Problems of the glenohumeral joint termed *capsulitis* refer pain along the C5 and C6 dermatomes, which include the area of skin over the deltoid insertion and the lateral border of the arm and forearm. Note that since many of the tissues of the shoulder are derived from the fifth and sixth cervical cord segments, referral of pain to the arm and forearm is common, whereas referral to the hand from lesions of the shoulder is less common. Acromioclavicular joint problems typically remain localized to the top of the shoulder region because the acromioclavicular joint is derived from the third and fourth cervical cord segments.

the axilla. This results in a patient's complaints of transient numbness in the arm or hand, a "dead" feeling in the arm with certain movements, or paresthesia. The examiner needs to visualize how the head of the humerus could compromise the brachial plexus if it assumes a more anterior and inferior position with different postures or movements or how the brachial plexus might have been compromised during the trauma of the injury.

Clinicians must recognize the potential for peripheral nerve injury secondary to dislocation of the

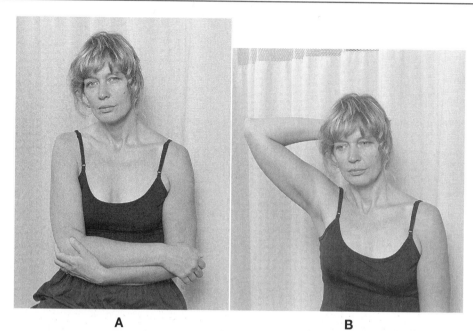

Figure 5-3. A and **B,** Patients with cervical nerve root problems often need to support the shoulder girdle in some way in order to minimize tensile stresses through the brachial plexus and cervical nerve root complex.

Patients with multidirectional instabilities of the humerus on the glenoid typically complain of diffuse shoulder pain with global muscle soreness about the shoulder girdle. This is in contrast to unidirectional instabilities that characteristically result in complaints of pain on the opposite side of the instability. For example, the patient with anterior instability will often describe soreness and aching of the shoulder posteriorly, as well as being tender to palpation over the region of the anterior glenoid.

Aggravating Factors

Questions that assess the nociceptive mechanics include *"Is it difficult to perform activities that require reaching above the shoulder level?" "What positions or activities increase your pain?" "What activities are limited by this problem?"* and *"Are you able to lie on that shoulder at night?"* When answering these questions, the patient has an opportunity to describe those positions, movements, or activities that reproduce familiar pain in the shoulder complex. Based on an in-depth understanding of the clinical anatomy of the region, the examiner can begin to visualize how compression, tension, and shear stresses potentially compromise the musculoskeletal tissues in the positions or movements the patient describes.

Many patients with shoulder disorders complain about an increase in pain when they attempt to sleep on the side of the shoulder disorder. This is especially common in late stage adhesive capsulitis disorders and rotator cuff problems. In both cases, the tissues are markedly irritable, and the combination of no movement, which promotes stasis, and pressure from lying on the shoulder increases pain and results in increasing the referred pain pattern along the lateral aspect of the arm.

Pain Behavior and Intensity

Questions such as *"On a scale of 0 to 10 with 10 being the most discomfort you have had with this particular problem, what level of pain are you currently experiencing?"* and *"Is your pain greater in the morning than in the evening?"* provide the clinician with the patient's own interpretation of his pain. Mechanical disorders of the musculoskeletal system typically feature pain patterns that are aggravated with increased compression, tension, and shear stresses to the injured tissues (mechanical stimulation of the nociceptive system) or continued activation of the nociceptive system by chemical irritation (i.e., a change in the chemical milieu as a result of tissue injury). For example, pain felt in the morning when the patient awakens that eases as the day progresses is typical for injured tissues that have an associated inflammatory process (Figure 5-4). With rest and sleep in the recumbent position, there is no muscle pumping action to decrease fluid stasis and therefore the chemical environment associated with stasis results in chemical activation or depolarization of the nociceptive system. When we get up and begin to move, muscle contraction around the injured tissues creates pressures that restore microcirculation and lymph drainage. This results in a change in the chemical environment of the injured region. The Blazina classification of pain, presented in Table 5-4, offers a way to assess the severity of the complaint.

Assessment of Functional Limitations

Patients seek help for their musculoskeletal problems for one of two reasons: pain or a problem that is now compromising desired function. Questions such as *"What activities are limited because of this problem?"* or *"On a scale of 0 to 10 with 0 being no limitation to activity and 10 representing all activity that you normally do, what level of activity are you at because of this problem?"* begin to provide the clinician with information regarding the patient's perception of his problem and how this problem is affecting his life. Answers to these types of questions need to be correlated with self-reports of pain because a reasonable relationship between pain intensity and compromise to function will exist.

Several tools designed to provide a convenient way to systematically document shoulder function are available. We refer the reader to two different shoulder questionnaires that are reliable and are more sensitive to change in patients with shoulder pain than a generic questionnaire.[2] The tools are the Simple Shoulder Test (SST) and the Shoulder Pain and Disability Index (SPADI).

The SST is a self-report questionnaire that takes approximately 5 to 10 minutes to complete and consists of 12 *yes or no* questions that assess functional limitations caused by shoulder pathology.[18] The questions focus on an individual's ability to tolerate or perform multiple activities of daily living.

The second outcome tool is the SPADI.[10,31] This is a self-report questionnaire that consists of two subscales identifying pain and projecting disability. The

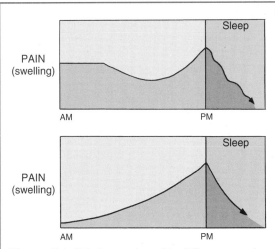

Figure 5-4. Pain is experienced in different ways during the AM and PM time periods as shown in this graphical representation of pain behavior. Pain that is greater in the morning but decreases as we move the injured region is suggestive of inflammatory conditions and swelling of the injured tissues. Such a reaction indicates a chemical cycle of pain (top graph). Pain that is greater toward the end of the day suggests muscular fatigue and a resultant loss of neuromuscular control of the affected regions that cause mechanical overload in the connective tissue elements. Such reaction indicates a mechanoreceptor cycle of pain (bottom graph).

Table 5-4. The Blazina Classification of Pain
Grade I: Pain with activity
Grade II: Pain during and after activity, but not disabling
Grade III: Pain during and after activity and disabling
Grade IV: Pain with activities of daily living

Data from Blazina ME et al: Jumper's knee, *Orthop Clin North Am* 4(3):665, 1973.

pain dimension is measured based on the severity of an individual's pain, whereas the disability dimension is measured based on the degree of difficulty an individual has with various activities of daily living that require upper extremity use. The time needed to complete this 13-item index is also 5 to 10 minutes. Both tools can easily be used to assess a patient's own perception of the pain and functional limitations he now has because of his shoulder condition.

The Patient's Description of the Problem

Ask the patient, *"What do you think is the cause of the pain?"* or *"What goals do you have as a result of treatment?"* His analysis of the cause of his pain provides you with additional information regarding nociceptive mechanics. For example, patients often talk about "pressure," "grinding" or "slipping," or a fear of different positions. If the patient states that he does not know what the problem is, encourage him to describe his own shoulder in *his* terms. The intent is to further your understanding of how the patient views his problem. This information is used to more tightly focus the physical examination.

Asking the patient to articulate his goals for treatment establishes his role in the total rehabilitation process. In addition, it allows the clinician to begin determining whether these goals are realistic when compared with the results of the examination. Injured connective tissues are repaired rather than regenerated. Injured tissues and those tissues with age-related degenerative changes have newly imposed mechanical stress limits that imply what activities of daily living and sport may need to be modified (see Chapters 1 and 6).

To review, three essential pieces of information need to be gained from the questions asked. They are the pathomechanics, the pain syndrome that is being presented, and the presence or absence of stability. Whatever the format of the questions, each question needs to be asked within a logical order so that the patient can follow the sequence of this history. When the patient is following the line of questioning, he can better relate one question to the other. Furthermore, a logical line of questioning gives the clinician opportunities to show the patient how one piece of information begins to correlate with another. Thus the teaching process for self-management of the condition has already begun.

Physical Examination

Carry out the physical examination in a manner that does not require the patient to change positions continuously. Organize it in logical fashion so that subsequent portions of the physical examination build on the results of tests immediately completed and the patient history. The challenge is to be thorough yet avoid unnecessary redundancy. If the examiner is able to conclude from the history the pathomechanics, syndrome classification, and presence or absence of stability, the essential tests needed in the active, passive, resisted, and palpation sequences of the examination, coupled with observation of static and dynamic postures, become more obvious. We will review and discuss each part of the sequence of the physical examination that we typically use here.

Observation and Inspection

The physical examination begins with the patient in the standing position (Table 5-5). Observation of the patient presenting with shoulder complaints includes the head, neck, shoulder girdle, thoracic spine, and abdominal wall. Key aspects of the observation portion of the physical examination are noted in Table 5-6. Inspecting the posture in the sagittal plane is the best way to assess for the presence of the forward head, rounded shoulder posture, which provides an excellent indication of the function of the abdominal wall musculature.

Frontal plane postural assessment often reveals asymmetry associated with handedness patterns. Typically the dominant side shows slightly greater hypertrophy and a lower riding scapula on the rib cage. Noting the levels of the iliac crests, posterior superior iliac spines, and the lumbar waist angle also provides information regarding the overall frontal plane posture.

Clarify bruises or scars and clearly understand past surgeries to any region of the upper quarter. Compare

---

Table 5-5. Sequence of Physical Examination: Standing Position

1. Have patient place hands on hips.
2. Observe static upper quarter and trunk posture.
3. Manipulate active physiological motions with overpressure if indicated.

Table 5-6. Observation and Inspection: Key Points

1. Check sagittal and frontal plane postural relationships of head, neck, shoulder girdle, thorax, and abdominal wall.
2. Observe posture of arm and shoulder girdle and position of scapula on rib cage.
3. Check symmetry.
4. Check the relationship of clavicle to acromion process.
5. Observe arm swing.
6. Check for evidence of atrophy.
7. Check for scars and bruises.
8. Observe contour: does the patient tend to support arm or hold arm close to chest?
9. Always compare bilaterally.

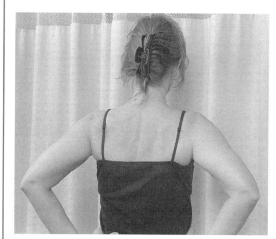

Figure 5-5. The hands on hips position makes it easier to detect the various shoulder asymmetries, such as those affecting the scapular position or muscle atrophy.

the contour of the shoulders bilaterally, giving special attention to the humeral heads on both sides of the body, the acromioclavicular joints, and the muscle girth in the infraspinatus fossa. The humeral head inspection is especially important because even a slight inferior displacement of a subluxed humeral head and the resultant sulcus sign over the suprahumeral space can be detected in lean individuals. We prefer to look at the resting posture of the shoulder girdle with the patient placing his hands on his hips. Scapula positions and the detection of shoulder girdle muscle atrophy especially over the infraspinatus fossa are much easier to compare bilaterally from this position (Figure 5-5).

Finally, how the individual is holding the upper extremity is instructive. Note how the individual protects or supports the upper extremity and the manner in which he carries his upper quarter. This can reveal how fearful he might be during further aspects of the examination. For example, shoulder-hand syndromes are extremely complex disorders accompanied by vasomotor changes in the upper quarter and extreme guarding and fear of movement of the complete upper extremity. Be cognizant of the potential for such syndromes with any type of trauma or surgery associated with the upper extremity.

Active Motion

The best way to begin the provocation portion of the physical examination is to start with active motions. We prefer to carry out the active motions with the patient in the standing position (Table 5-7). Active motions provide information regarding the patient's ability and willingness to move. During the active motion examination

of the shoulder girdle, look at the glenohumeral motion, the scapulothoracic motion, and the motion of the cervical and thoracic spine. As mentioned throughout Chapter 4, the ability to elevate the arm completely overhead is dependent on full mobility and strength for all shoulder girdle articulations, as well as for cervical spine and upper thoracic spine extension. During any motion, clarify if familiar pain is reproduced and the location of that particular pain.

The sequence of active motions is noted in Table 5-7. A quick screen of the cervical spine begins active motion assessment. The patient is asked to move the head and neck into the forward (Figure 5-6, *A*) and

Table 5-7. Assessment of Active Motion

1. Clearing of cervical spine
2. Glenohumeral assessment: consider having the patient start by simultaneously moving both arms
   Flexion, extension
   Abduction, adduction
   Internal and external rotation
   Horizontal adduction
   "Scaption," or movement with arm in internal and external rotation
3. Scapula: Elevation, depression, protraction, retraction

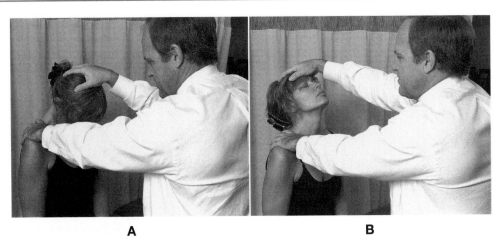

Figure 5-6. Ask the patient to move the cervical spine in the forward bending and backward bending quadrants. In **A,** apply overpressure to the forward bending quadrant, and in **B,** apply overpressure to the backward bending quadrant.

backward (Figure 5-6, *B*) bending quadrants, and the examiner can overpressure these motions to see if shoulder pain is reproduced. If the examiner suspects that the upper quarter pain is from cervical spine involvement, then a complete cervical spine examination is indicated.

Now active movement of the shoulder girdle can be assessed. *Elevation* is the terminology typically used for any movement of the arm overhead and includes the contributions for all articulations of the shoulder complex. Such motion can occur in the sagittal (pure flexion motion) or frontal (pure abduction) cardinal planes, but from a functional standpoint, elevation of the arm typically occurs in an arc that lies somewhere between the frontal and sagittal planes. We typically have the patient elevate the arm overhead several times and in varying positions between the sagittal and frontal planes. The patient is asked to raise his arms forward as high as he can several times in different portions of the arc between the sagittal plane and frontal plane. The plane midway between the sagittal and frontal planes is referred to as the *scaption plane* and is the approximate plane of the scapula as it sits on the thorax. We then ask the patient to place his shoulders in varying degrees of internal and external rotation as he elevates the arm in order to assess how symptoms might be affected (Figure 5-7, *A-E*). Note any apprehension to motion and points in the range of motion

that reproduce familiar pain. We do not hesitate to apply gentle overpressure at the patient's limits of active arm elevation because we now have the ability to clarify the effects of increased compression, tension, or shear to the motion with simple adjustments of hand position or direction of force application. The ranges of motion can then be recorded, with 175 to 180 degrees of motion being the normal ranges of overhead motion.

Acromioclavicular joint pain is typically increased at the extremes of shoulder range of motion, so overpressure to arm elevation at 170 to 180 degrees may provoke this joint. Likewise, horizontally adducting the glenohumeral joint fully eventually begins to force the scapula into protraction, and further overpressure of this maneuver increases stress to the acromioclavicular joint and increases compression of the soft tissues between the humerus and coracoid process. Therefore the examiner needs to apply overpressure to active motions using several different lines of force, all the time visualizing the tissues that are simultaneously being compressed or that are subject to shear and tension with such maneuvers.

During active elevation of the arm overhead the presence of a painful arc may be revealed. Although not as valuable a sign with an acutely painful shoulder, a painful arc has been defined as an arc of motion in which there is a beginning range without

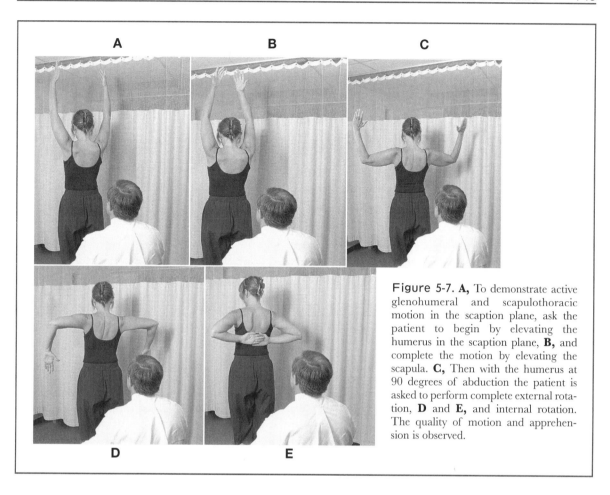

Figure 5-7. A, To demonstrate active glenohumeral and scapulothoracic motion in the scaption plane, ask the patient to begin by elevating the humerus in the scaption plane, **B,** and complete the motion by elevating the scapula. **C,** Then with the humerus at 90 degrees of abduction the patient is asked to perform complete external rotation, **D** and **E,** and internal rotation. The quality of motion and apprehension is observed.

pain (Figure 5-8, *A*), followed by a portion of the arc with pain (Figure 5-8, *B*), whereas the last part of the arc is without pain (Figure 5-8, *C*).[4,23,25] *No pain–pain–no pain* constitutes the classic painful arc as the arm moves from a position at the side of the body to complete elevation and has been attributed to irritation of tissues in the suprahumeral space, which are maximally stressed in compression during the middle range of elevation as the tuberosity of the humerus engages with the undersurface of the coracoacromial arch. The structures potentially irritated include the supraspinatus, the infraspinatus, the long head of the biceps tendon, the subacromial bursa, and the superior aspect of the glenohumeral joint capsule.

Notice the difference between a painful arc due to impingement and loss of the arc of motion because of suspected capsular restriction. In a capsular restriction pain and motion limitation would begin at some point

in the arc and progressively become more problematic without an easing of pain toward the end of the motion. The pattern of the capsular restriction is thus *no pain followed by increasing pain,* as compared with a painful arc where we see pain toward the middle of the arc of motion.

All motions of lifting the arm overhead include scapulothoracic motion that is smooth and relatively symmetrical without winging from the rib cage. The pattern of scapular motion is actually quite unpredictable as it moves in varying amounts of upward rotation and protraction depending where in the arc between the sagittal and frontal plane the arm is elevating. The clinician also needs to realize that the majority of scapular motion occurs after humeral elevation exceeds approximately 90 degrees and it is only in coronal plane motion that the scapula begins its rotation at lower degrees of elevation.[5]

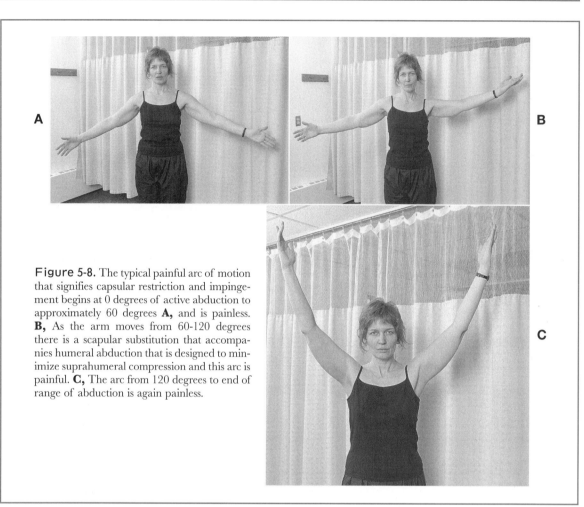

Figure 5-8. The typical painful arc of motion that signifies capsular restriction and impingement begins at 0 degrees of active abduction to approximately 60 degrees **A,** and is painless. **B,** As the arm moves from 60-120 degrees there is a scapular substitution that accompanies humeral abduction that is designed to minimize suprahumeral compression and this arc is painful. **C,** The arc from 120 degrees to end of range of abduction is again painless.

The range of motion for active internal rotation is normally 70 degrees, whereas that of active external rotation is approximately 90 degrees. Although it often is suggested that having the patient reach behind his low back and attempt to bring his hand up the spine is an excellent way to assess internal rotation, such a motion results in so much scapular movement on the thorax that the value of assessing internal rotation in this way is questionable. It is much easier, and perhaps has greater functional implications, to assess active rotation in these two ways:

1. With the arm at the side and elbow flexed to 90 degrees and then observing active internal and external rotation
2. With the humerus abducted in the coronal plane to

approximately 90 degrees and then asking the patient to internally and externally rotate his shoulders. From this position it is very easy to see how early the scapula comes into play during external rotation and whether or not there is a significant difference in the scapulothoracic and glenohumeral motions when comparing the two sides (Figure 5-9, *A-C*).

If overpressure is applied to the rotations of the glenohumeral joint at this point, special attention needs to be paid to potential subluxations. The patient may feel especially vulnerable with overpressure in external rotation, so do not attempt to push through any muscle guarding that may be present. Consider

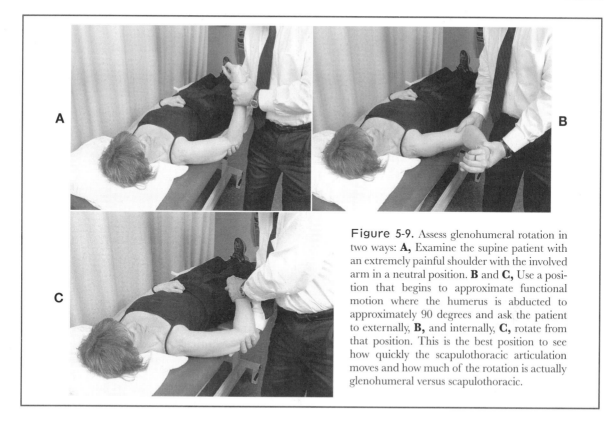

Figure 5-9. Assess glenohumeral rotation in two ways: **A,** Examine the supine patient with an extremely painful shoulder with the involved arm in a neutral position. **B** and **C,** Use a position that begins to approximate functional motion where the humerus is abducted to approximately 90 degrees and ask the patient to externally, **B,** and internally, **C,** rotate from that position. This is the best position to see how quickly the scapulothoracic articulation moves and how much of the rotation is actually glenohumeral versus scapulothoracic.

stabilizing the anterior aspect of the humerus and glenoid if overpressure in external rotation is applied at this point in the examination. Subtly removing and reapplying this stabilization force over the anterior aspect of the glenohumeral joint offers significant clues regarding the presence or absence of joint stability.

During all requested movements, it is essential to view scapular motion and humeral motion simultaneously. Assess whether the overhead motion attempted by the patient is primarily scapulothoracic motion that might occur with adhesive capsulitis or rotator cuff problems. With these two clinical problems, very little humeral motion occurs on the glenoid, and instead, the arm moves upward or out to the side primarily by motion of the scapula on the thorax. The scapulothoracic articulation is quite mobile in all planes, and the clinician can be misled into thinking that more glenohumeral motion is present than is actually available. The final portion of the active motion tests look at isolated scapular motion, such as elevation, retraction, depression, and protraction, and the effect these motions may have on the familiar pain.

On completion of the assessment of the active motions of the shoulder girdle, we have a good idea of the pain location, where throughout the ranges the patient has the most difficulty (due to pain, weakness, motion limitation, or feeling of instability), and the ease in which the symptoms can be provoked. We have the patient repeat these active motions numerous times because the self-report of any difficulties experienced during active ranges needs to be consistent and reproducible to be of value. Subsequent portions of the examination use the information already gleaned to place selected stresses into the various tissues in order to provide further clarification of the painful syndrome.

Passive Motion Assessment and Passive Provocational Tests

At this point we ask the patient to be seated. Typically we conduct several of the passive tests described in this section from the seated position (Table 5-8) and then conduct the remaining passive tests from the supine position. If necessary, the side-lying or prone positions can also be used to further substantiate findings from the seated or supine positions.

The passive tests are designed primarily to provoke familiar pain through carefully applied compression, tensile, or shear stresses to the glenohumeral structures. Most passive tests for the musculoskeletal system take advantage of an understanding of the three dimensional relationships of anatomical structures, and thus many of the tissues can be passively prepositioned so that the examiner can apply a passive force and assess the response. Thus passive tests are not limited to assessing the connective tissues, such as the joint capsule and ligaments, but can also be used in physical examination of the shoulder to assess muscle-tendon tissues.

We feel that the passive tests are the most important part of the physical examination for mechanical shoulder pain. Although there are many different passive tests for physical examination of the shoulder, two key items are important to consider regardless of the test used:

1. Recognize *exactly* where the forces you apply ultimately converge in the region and what movements of the articulation might occur with the application of such forces. It is essential to have the ability to visualize the anatomy and understand exactly which force or combinations of forces are being applied to tissues of the region.
2. Apply overpressure carefully during the test and note the end feel (e.g., the feeling imparted to the examiner's hands during the passive test) and the relationship of that end feel to the patient's response. Does pain occur before, during, or after your hands meet resistance? This information is important for examination purposes and when considering and planning the treatment process.

Table 5-8. Sequence of Physical Examination: Seated Position

Sulcus test
Load and shift test
Drawer tests
Palpation
Neuromuscular resisted tests
Impingement tests
Assessing generalized connective tissue laxity

The examiner has most likely decided whether or not stability is a question from the information obtained in the patient history and the active tests. Further corroboration can be gained using a series of passive tests from the seated position.

The first test we prefer to conduct is the *sulcus test*, which assesses inferior glenohumeral joint instability (Figure 5-10). In this test the patient is seated with the arm comfortably at the side. The examiner palpates the suprahumeral space with one finger, and the opposite hand applies an inferiorly directed force through the long axis of the humerus. A positive sulcus test results in a "gaping" at the suprahumeral space because of excessive inferior translation of the head of the humerus.[6,19]

After repeating the sulcus test, and thus developing the ability to visualize the anatomical relationships of the patient's scapulohumeral interface, we perform the *load and shift test* (Figure 5-11, *A-C*).[9] In this test the patient is seated with his hand resting on his thigh. The examiner grasps the humeral head and compresses it into the glenoid fossa, thus seating the head of the humerus within the glenoid. This is considered the "load" portion of the load and shift test. From this point the examiner attempts to translate the head of the humerus anteriorly and posteriorly, noting humeral motion, and ascertains whether the humeral head is clicking over the glenoid rim. Because of the loading portion of the examination, less movement would be expected in this test than the next test that we perform: the *drawer test*.

Drawer tests also assess translation of the humeral head. Normally translation is equal anteriorly and posteriorly and is best assessed with the arm toward 90 degrees abduction and neutral rotation (Figure 5-11, *D-E*). Carefully assess motion and whether the humeral head, if unstable, clicks over the glenoid rim during the test. Again, it is important to compare the first with the opposite shoulder. If it is difficult to hold the arm and apply the translatory stresses, or if excessive muscle guarding develops as the arm is passively brought out to the start position, the test can easily be done when the patient is moved to the supine position.

Palpation

Although some clinicians prefer to wait until the end of the examination to conduct a palpation sequence, the examination process has already revealed a significant amount of information from the history, the active tests, and the beginning battery of

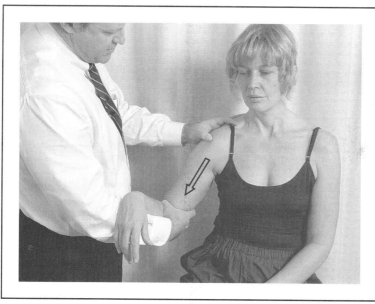

Figure 5-10. Perform the *sulcus test* to assess inferior glenohumeral joint instability with the patient seated with the arm comfortably at the side. Palpate the suprahumeral space with one finger, and use the opposite hand to apply an inferiorly directed force through the long axis of the humerus. A positive result on the sulcus test is marked by a "gaping" at the suprahumeral space because of excessive inferior translation of the head of the humerus.

stability tests. Thus the information that can be gained from conducting a palpation examination at this point is valuable because it confirms findings that have already been arrived at and helps provide the focus for the remaining portion of the physical examination.

Palpation is usually performed to detect tenderness in underlying musculoskeletal structures but also needs to be performed to assess for the presence of muscle spasm, nodules, temperature and swelling, and changes in contour when the two sides are compared. We prefer to start away from the area of pain and then move toward the existing complaint. Table 5-9 lists the essential areas for palpation in the shoulder examination. The examiner cradles the humerus and the arm as it is moved to varying positions in order to palpate and repalpate the shoulder. We pay particular attention to the region over the anterior glenoid, the complete surfaces of the tuberosities, the suprahumeral space, and the acromioclavicular joint. We typically use the following sequence when palpating the shoulder:

Anterior

Key palpations on the anterior aspect of the shoulder include the acromioclavicular joint and along the length of the clavicle. The clavicle usually rides slightly higher than the acromion and can be checked to reveal whether or not a subluxation or dislocation of the acromioclavicular joint is present. Old fractures of the clavicle may have formed a large, bony callus, which can mechanically compromise the neurovascular bundle as it travels between the clavicle and first rib. Acromioclavicular joint arthritis can manifest as pain with palpation over the joint line. At this point in the examination, the clavicle also can be gently moved inferiorly or posteriorly to assess the response of the acromioclavicular joint to accessory movement. The undersurface of the acromioclavicular joint is often associated with compromise to the rotator cuff tendons, contributing to impingement syndrome. The sternoclavicular joint region can be palpated as well, although its involvement in shoulder joint pathologies is significantly less likely than involvement of the acromioclavicular joint.

The anterior aspect of the glenoid labrum is another important structure to palpate (Figure 5-12, *A* and *B*). The glenoid labrum is often tender to palpation in patients with subluxation or instability problems of the glenohumeral joint. From this point in the palpation, the examiner can move to the region of the lesser tuberosity, which serves as the insertion for the subscapularis muscle, and then just laterally to the bicipital groove. The examination of the anterior structures is usually concluded with the soft tissues of the anterior axillary fold and the supraclavicular tissues.

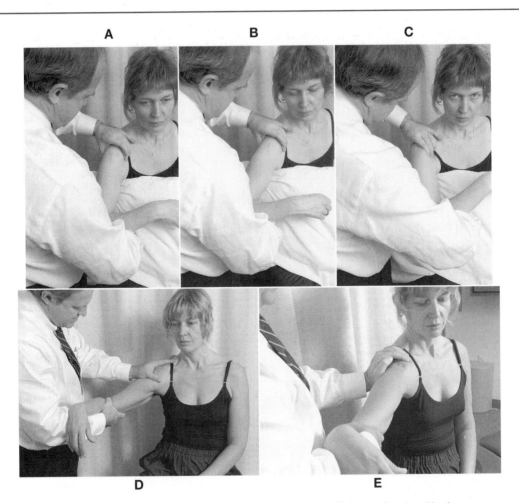

Figure 5-11. In the load and shift test, **A,** first the examiner uses his bottom hand and body to exert a superior and medial force along the humerus to increase compression at or "seat" the gleno-humeral joint. **B,** The opposite hand cups the humeral head, and then the thumb and middle finger create a transitional force that moves the head of the humerus anteriorly, **C,** and posteriorly. The drawer test examines passive mobility or stability of the glenohumeral joint. A positive finding allows the examiner to feel the humeral head rise up on the glenoid labrum, often producing an audible click. This can be interpreted as one or a combination of capsular instability, a labral tear, or detachment of the glenoid labrum. Other techniques, **D** and **E,** can be used to assess the integrity of the glenoid labrum. Such techniques use the humerus and the base of the hand to specifically direct the desired force to the head of the humerus.

magnetic resonance imaging, or CT arthrography is often necessary to make the definitive diagnosis.

Lateral and Posterior

One of the key areas for palpation is the suprahumeral space. Several key tissues, notably the glenohumeral joint capsule, the supraspinatus and infraspinatus tendons, the long head of the biceps tendon, and the subacromial bursa, lie in this region. The examiner needs to carefully palpate the region immediately under the acromion and continue the palpation inferiorly over the complete greater tuberosity. We prefer to place the humerus in various degrees of external and internal rotation and then palpate the greater tuberosity as increasing areas of the cuff and bursa become exposed with this technique.

Many tests have been described for assessing labral defects, and several are illustrated here that are useful in identifying labral problems, including the "clunk test"[1] (Figure 5-13, *A* and *B*), the Kibler test[15] (Figure 5-14), and the O'Brien test,[28] or active compression test (Figure 5-15, *A* and *B*). Further examination via arthroscopy,

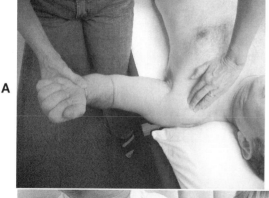

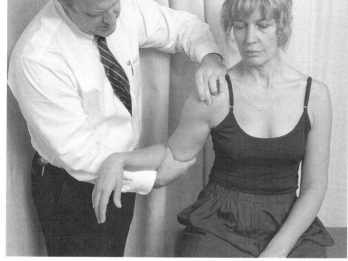

Figure 5-12. Palpation of the anterior aspect of the glenoid labrum can be done with, **A,** the patient in a supine position, or **B,** the patient seated. This is an important palpation because tenderness in this region is common in patients with subluxation or instability problems of the glenohumeral joint. Tenderness also may indicate anterior labral lesions.

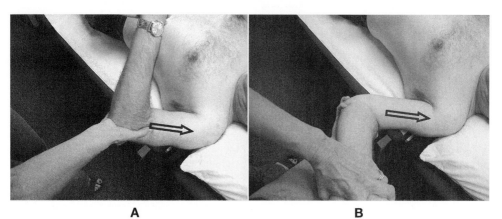

A   **B**

Figure 5-13. The "Clunk test" is performed by positioning a supine patient's shoulder in 0 degrees abduction and 90 degrees elbow flexion and then slowly **A,** internally and **B,** externally rotating the humerus while maintaining strong joint compression through the long axis of the humerus. A "catching or clunking" of the humerus during the rotation is considered to be a positive sign.

The supraspinatus and infraspinatus muscles can then be palpated in their respective fossae. We conclude the examination of the posterior structures by assessing the soft tissues of the posterior axillary fold and the paraspinal muscles. Tenderness over the superomedial corner of the scapula is often found in patients with rotator cuff tendonitis. One potential reason for this is the mechanical linkage between the supraspinatus and levator scapulae muscles at the medial aspect of the supraspinous fossa (see Chapter 3).

Muscle-Tendon and Neuromuscular Examination via Resisted Tests

Once the information from the patient history is confirmed via palpation and stability tests and with the patient still seated, we proceed with tests that are intended to answer two questions:

1. Do contractions of the muscles associated with the shoulder girdle reproduce familiar pain?
2. Are there any neural conduction problems?

Resisted tests were first described by Cyriax as a means to discern muscle-tendon lesions from lesions of the inert tissues.[4] While instructive for reviewing the functional anatomy of the shoulder, it is probably not possible to completely isolate the muscle-tendon units from the connective tissue structures. As noted in

Chapter 3, the attachments of the rotator cuff muscles are not simply connected to the tuberosities of the humerus, but rather via a blending with the glenohumeral joint capsule. Likewise, the muscle tissues are intimately related to the fascial networks of the

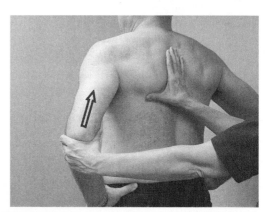

Figure 5-14. In the Kibler test, the standing patient has his hands on his hips, with his thumbs draped over the posterior aspect of the iliac crest. Stabilize the shoulder girdle with one hand and push strongly through the elbow along the long axis of the humerus while the patient pushes back in the opposite direction. Pain, popping, or clicking in the shoulder is considered a positive sign.

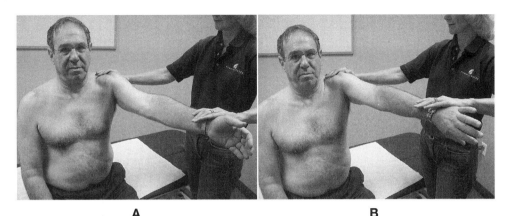

A   **B**

Figure 5-15. Perform the O'Brien or active compression test by having the patient bring the shoulder to 90 degrees flexion and 15 degrees adduction. **A,** With the humerus externally rotated (thumb up), resist further shoulder elevation, and **B,** Repeat the same maneuver with thumb down position. The thumb down position exhibits increased loading of the labrum-biceps tendon complex. Consider the test positive if the thumb up position relieves pain compared to the results in thumb down position.

shoulder, and contraction of the muscle exerts tensile stresses to the fascia and ligaments via direct pull and through the broadening effects of the muscle within its fascial envelope, such as the compartmentalized infraspinatus muscle.

Despite the limitation of not being able to completely isolate the muscle-tendon unit, screening the shoulder muscles is essential because of the possibility of provoking pain and detecting weakness. If weakness is detected, the examiner needs to comprehensively test the muscles of the shoulder girdle. The motions that should be tested as part of the routine shoulder examination are listed in Table 5-10. We pay particular attention to those tests that can potentially detect strength or weakness of the cuff tendons and whether contraction of the muscles reproduces familiar pain because a large proportion of shoulder pathologies are related to involvement of the rotator cuff.

We do the initial portion of resisted testing with the patient's arm at the side and without any movement allowed between the humerus and the scapula. The intent of such an isometric test is to minimize forces on surrounding capsule or ligamentous structures. We request that the patient "hold" the position while the testing force is being applied rather than encouraging him to "push against us." Using the former command instead of the latter one ensures that the examiner is in complete control of the test and allows for specific gradations of resistance force to be applied. Figure 5-16, *A-F,* demonstrates selected tests for the resisted tests portion of the shoulder examination.

Since rotator cuff pathology is so common, special attention usually is given to assessment of the muscles that make up this important complex. The supraspinatus

Table 5-10. Resisted Tests of the Shoulder

Assess for weakness and reproducibility of symptoms using:
   Forward flexion in neutral
   Forward flexion with arm forward (Speed's test)
   Shoulder extension
   Shoulder abduction in neutral
   Shoulder abduction in impingement position
   Shoulder adduction
   Internal rotation
   External rotation
   Elbow flexion
   Elbow extension

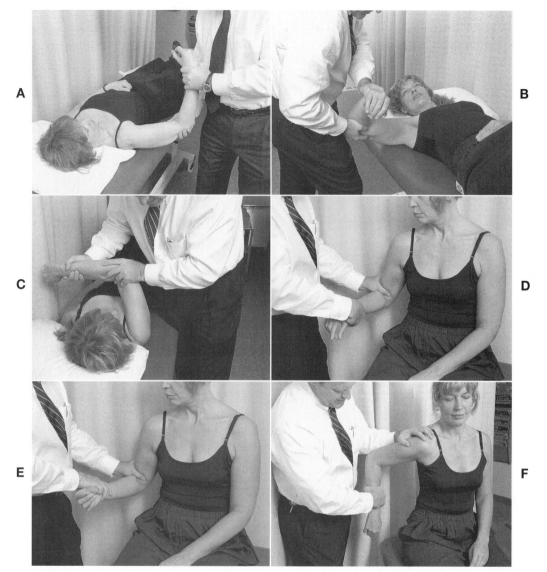

Figure 5-16. There are a number of resisted tests for examination of the shoulder. Examples include: **A,** Resisted external rotation from neutral position. **B,** Resisted external rotation with the arm pre-positioned in internal rotation. Note that this position stretches the infraspinatus and teres minor, and then asks the muscle to contract strongly from the stretched position. Generally, if more passive pre-stretch is needed to provoke pain with muscle contraction, the lesion is considered to be less severe. **C,** Impingement test position with the arm forward flexed and internally rotated. The patient is asked to "hold," and pain with contraction usually incriminates the supraspinatus muscle. **D,** Speed's test is an excellent tool to assess the biceps tendon, specifically for the SLAP lesion. The examiner resists shoulder flexion while the arm is first supinated, and then with it pronated **E,** while the elbow remains extended. An even better assessment that uses Speed's test actively resists an eccentric movement of the arm into extension. This puts increased tension onto the biceps tendon and moves the bone under the tendon. **F,** Position the shoulder to place maximal stress to the biceps tendon by creating a posterior to anterior force to the humeral head with the left hand while the right hand resists shoulder and elbow flexion. This uses the head of the humerus as a fulcrum, which increases the tensile stress of the biceps tendon. Resisted pronation and supination further stress the tendon and its attachment.

muscle is often tested using the "empty can" test, in which the patient's arm is abducted to approximately 90 degrees without any rotation of the humerus.[13] A resistance force to abduction is applied, and the arm is brought forward into the scaption plane while the humerus is internally rotated (thumb toward the floor as if emptying a can), with resistance to abduction being applied once again. Weakness or pain is indicative of supraspinatus involvement.

A variation of the empty can test is used to detect complete tears of the rotator cuff tendons and is known as the "drop-arm" test.[21] Here the examiner passively lifts the shoulder to the abducted position and asks the patient to hold the position and begin to slowly lower the arm to the side. The test is considered positive when the patient cannot hold the position or lower the arm slowly and the arm falls back to the patient's side.

In our experience simple resisted flexion of the elbow as described by Cyriax rarely elicits pain from involvement of the long head of the biceps tendon. This is because lesions of the long head of the biceps tendon are primarily of two types: the SLAP (superior labral anterior to posterior) lesion, which is a partial avulsion of the long head of the biceps and superior glenoid labrum from the glenoid, and tendonitis or tenosynovitis as a result of friction of the tendon in the bicipital groove of the humerus. SLAP lesions are among the most complex because they can be subdivided into four different classifications based on the extent of the labral and biceps tendon detachment.[33] One of the best tests to assess the long head of the biceps is to pre-position the shoulder in forward flexion and apply resistance to forward flexion in a manner that makes the test an eccentric contraction of the shoulder flexors (Speed's test). In other words, the examiner carefully pushes the patient's shoulder back toward extension, gently overcoming the resistance of the shoulder flexors. Further tension can be placed through the long head of the biceps by simultaneously resisting forearm supination during the flexion movement, or by passively pre-positioning the forearm in full pronation for the test. The examiner needs to be careful during this test because an abrupt force, or one that is too great, can cause further injury to the long head of the biceps tendon and the glenoid labrum.

Performing these tests places a strong tensile stress to the long head of the biceps tendon and moves the humerus under the tendon. The examiner needs to realize that sometimes it is this movement rather than the resistance that reproduces shoulder pain; movement of the humerus under the tendon creates a frictional force between the tendon and the bicipital groove. The biceps tendon does not slide in the bicipital groove, but rather the bony groove slides under the tendon. Understanding this subtle difference between these mechanics becomes important in developing an exercise program. Patients with a suspected tenosynovitis problem must learn that decreasing motion of the affected arm from flexion to extension (such as in rowing exercises, work, or sport) is the best way to rest the injured long head of the biceps tendon, rather than simply decreasing the movements of elbow flexion and extension.

Finally, muscle tests can be performed to confirm or rule out any neural conduction problem (see Tables 2-1 and 2-2).

Impingement Tests

The patient history, along with results of palpation and resisted tests, provides the examiner with important information about the tissues under the coracoacromial arch. Next, we typically conduct the various impingement tests with the patient in the seated position. As mentioned in Chapter 4, the examiner's frame of reference must include both external and internal impingement. We simplify the examinations for these two conditions by considering external impingement to be primarily related to the bursal side of the cuff tendon and the intimate association that this side of the tendon has with the coracoacromial arch and internal impingement to be more closely related to the articular side of the tendon and the relationship that this region of the tendon has with the glenoid labrum.

External impingement is recognized as a component of cuff disorders and frequently, and perhaps even more commonly, a secondary phenomenon associated with activities or adaptive changes in the connective tissues of the glenohumeral joint capsule. Overuse and fatigue related to eccentric overload of the rotator cuff muscles resulting in intrinsic fiber failure of the cuff and biceps tendon constitutes the primary etiology in the active, young population (throwers, lifters, workers). The initial failure of the fibers may lead to secondary impingement as external forces, such as those with throwing, pull the cuff superiorly. Patients with anterior instability are also at risk for impingement because of the architecture of the subacromial region. Those with loose shoulders or multidirectional instabilities may develop cuff tendonitis because of overwork and overstretching of the gleno-humeral joint capsule.

There are several special passive tests for external impingement (Figure 5-17, *A-D*). Pain on forced forward flexion in which the greater tuberosity is forced up against the acromion is often referred to as the *Neer impingement test*.[26] This test may be varied through an attempt to provoke pain with forced internal rotation of the 90-degree forward flexed arm. We use a combination of these tests in which the humerus is forced up against the acromion with the humerus initially in maximal external rotation. After the humerus is lowered away from the arch, it is internally rotated and then again forced up against the arch. This is repeated several times with the arm internally rotated slightly

more each time until it reaches full internal rotation. Testing in this manner presents a significant portion of the greater tuberosity and the bicipital groove to the undersurface of the coracoacromial arch.

Internal impingement is a phenomenon most often found in shoulders that exhibit laxity, whether that laxity is congenital or, more commonly, a result of acquired laxity seen in overhead athletes. An abduction and external rotation motion with a lax shoulder results in the humerus subluxing anteriorly. When this subluxation occurs, the greater tuberosity impinges on the posterior-superior aspect of the glenoid rim. The deep surface of the rotator cuff may be pinched between these two structures and under repetitive loading can lead to partial thickness tears of the

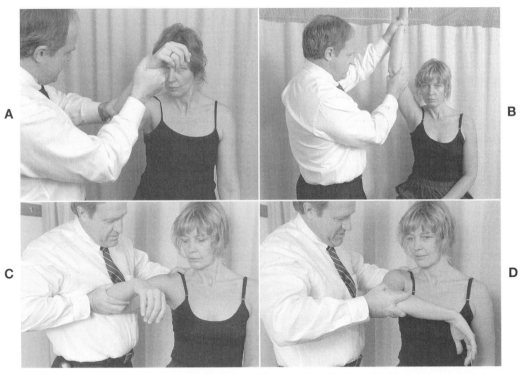

Figure 5-17. Passive tests for impingement are illustrated in **A-D. A** and **B,** Passive forward elevation is used in which the greater tuberosity approximates the under surface of the acromion, often referred to as the Neer test. The movement impinges on the suprahumeral tissues between the bony surfaces. **C** and **D,** Another passive test for impingement abducts the humerus to 90 degrees and a force is generated by the examiner's right hand along the humerus. This position and force increases the compression load or impinges these tissues and directs increased loads to the acromioclavicular joint. A patient with swelling in her suprahumeral tissues or at the AC joint will experience pain as compression increases.

tendon's undersurface. Continuous compressive loading of the tuberosity on the labrum can also result in the labrum loosening or becoming detached, thus compounding the instability problem. We typically use a noninvasive test for internal impingement. We position the shoulder toward abduction and external rotation and then subtly use controlled and careful glides of the humeral head while noting whether posterior shoulder joint pain results with the position or gentle translations.

Assessing Generalized Connective Tissue Laxity

Before we move the patient from the seated position to the supine position, we conduct an assessment of generalized ligamentous laxity. Body type influences the mobility of the joints because of the inherent elasticity of the connective tissues. The examiner needs to check quickly how much thumb hyperabduction, index finger metacarpophalangeal (MCP) joint hyperextension, and elbow hyperextension is present to get a sense of the patient's connective tissue makeup. When the examiner does this at this stage, he can conduct the remaining mobility and stability tests with the patient in the supine position with more accurate interpretation.

Physiological Motion Testing

At this point, we move the patient to the supine position (Table 5-11). Tests that have been performed from standing and sitting positions may be repeated in order to confirm the patient's previous responses to the compressive, tensile, and shear stresses of the examination. Confirmation of the patient's responses also occurs with variations of the previously administered tests and additional tests that are best conducted from the supine position.

The passive physiological motion tests are the first that we typically perform from the supine position. We take the patient's arm through passive flexion-extension, abduction-adduction, internal-external rotation, and horizontal adduction. Note that a significant amount of shoulder joint motion in the cardinal planes is from the contribution of the scapulothoracic articulation. Therefore when the patient is lying supine with the scapula compressed against the table, the endrange of passive glenohumeral motion is reached much earlier than when the scapula is free to move. Be sure to assess carefully

Table 5-11. Sequence of Physical Examination: Supine Position
Passive physiological motions
Joint play to glenohumeral joint
Stability tests (relocation tests)
Apprehension tests
Joint play to acromioclavicular and sternoclavicular joints

what is actually true glenohumeral motion, rather than total shoulder motion, with passive tests. More clinical skill is needed with assessment of true glenohumeral motion from the supine position than typically meets the eye.

Rather than limiting the assessment to the cardinal planes only, the examiner needs to move the humerus in arcs of motion throughout the quadrant between the sagittal and frontal planes, noting available range, where in the range pain is felt, and the end feel that limits the passive motion. Rotations are assessed from varying positions in the different quadrants. It is important to passively rotate the glenohumeral joint in varying degrees of abduction, scaption, and flexion in order to stress all parts of the glenohumeral joint capsule and intrinsic ligaments.

Horizontal adduction is included in the passive physiological tests for its assessment of the joint capsule and the effect of increased tensile stress to the posterior cuff muscles and a means to assess the endrange capabilities of the acromioclavicular joint and the ability of the tissues under the coracoacromial arch and over the coracoid process to tolerate compression.

The capsular pattern of the glenohumeral joint as described by Cyriax is a passive pattern of motion that reveals a marked limitation of glenohumeral external rotation and an accompanying limitation of glenohumeral abduction and internal rotation.[4] The most typical "pattern" is one in which the external rotation limitation is the most significant motion loss and glenohumeral abduction is the second most significant loss. The usual explanation for the pattern of motion loss is the loss of elasticity of the anterior pleats of the glenohumeral joint capsule (limiting external rotation) and a loss of the elasticity of the inferior pleats of the capsule (limiting abduction).

Although this explanation helps us begin to understand the relationship of the anatomy of the joint capsule to movement, the syndrome adhesive capsulitis is much more complex because physiological changes are mostly at the cellular level (see Chapter 4). Typically the inflammatory process and tissue fibrosis are centered in the subsynovial layer of the joint capsule and the joint capsule may be adhered to the humeral head itself.[27] Tissue fibrosis also may occur in other regions of the joint capsule, leading to differing patterns of movement. For example, a "reverse" capsular pattern for impingement problems of the shoulder has been described in which there are more limitations in glenohumeral internal rotation than in glenohumeral abduction and external rotation.[34] Additionally, it is important to realize that patients with diabetes have a much higher incidence of shoulder joint capsule problems than those without the disease.[3,20,32] Therefore the pathogenesis of capsulitis is probably multifactorial and not simply a disuse phenomenon. We noted earlier that there are three phases of "frozen shoulder," or adhesive capsulitis. Although a pattern may be present, it is perhaps more important to concentrate on the end feel when passive tests are used in the physical examination because it is the end feel, coupled with the patient's response to pain when the end feel is reached, that ultimately identifies the phase of the syndrome present and directs the treatment process.

Joint Play and Stability Tests

We focus the next part of the examination on the quality of and the patient's reponse to glenohumeral joint play. Joint play refers to the accessory motions of the glenohumeral joint, as well as those incorporated via specific tests to determine the possible presence of glenohumeral instability. Three of the more important signs that we look for include conditions in which the humerus has less-than-normal movement with translatory motion of the humerus on the glenoid (capsule hypomobility), movements that either increase pain or result in apprehension by the patient, or excessive mobility of the humerus on the glenoid with or without pain (capsule hypermobility). Be aware that if there is any muscle guarding or muscle spasm while the passive tests are performed, mobility of the humerus on the glenoid cannot be accurately assessed.

Simple anterior, posterior, and inferior glides of the head of the humerus on the glenoid with the patient in the side-lying position and the shoulder joint in the "loose packed" position (55 degrees abduction, 30 degrees forward flexion, neutral rotation) are an excellent way to begin this portion of the examination (Figure 5-18, *A* and *B*).[14] The examiner needs to apply the anterior and posterior forces in the scaption plane

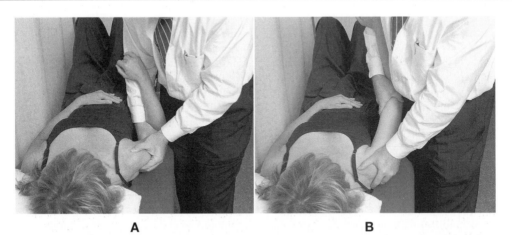

A   **B**

Figure 5-18. Examination of anterior and posterior translations of the head of the humerus on the glenoid with the patient in the supine position with the shoulder in the "loose-packed" position (55 degrees abduction, 30 degrees forward flexion, neutral rotation). We secure the head of the humerus with one hand and grasp the distal humerus with the other hand. A simple anterior (**A**) and posterior (**B**) glide is used with the force being applied in the plane of the scapula (scaption plane) rather than the force being applied in the cardinal sagittal plane. Varying degrees of traction can be applied to the humerus with the right hand.

rather than the sagittal plane and determine the patient's response to the motion or the presence of increased or decreased mobility in comparison with the opposite side. Although abnormal anterior laxity of the glenohumeral joint is the most common type of instability, posterior and multidirectional instabilities are increasingly recognized.

Numerous classification mechanisms for instability can be used, including *frequency and chronology, direction and degree of instability, etiology, and presence or absence of voluntary control:*

1. Acute, recurrent, or chronic conditions may be described with regard to temporal background of the patient's complaints.
2. Instability may occur anteriorly, posteriorly, or inferiorly, or it may be multidirectional.
3. Articular surfaces may be completely separated (dislocation), or symptoms may result from abnormal translation without complete separation (subluxation).
4. Episodes of macrotrauma are common. Microtrauma associated with repetitive use is very common, especially in throwers, swimmers, and workers with continual overhead demands.

Apprehension tests and *relocation tests* are often used to examine the shoulder for instability. The simplest apprehension test is one in which the patient's shoulder is moved toward abduction and external rotation. Typically, the patient with a history of subluxations or dislocation has markedly increased muscle guarding or voices fear *(apprehension)* of the shoulder "popping out" as external rotation is increased. We perform a *relocation test* by placing one hand over the anterior shoulder of the supine patient (Figure 5-19, *A-C*). A posteriorly directed force is applied with the hand to prevent anterior translation of the head. Then the shoulder is abducted and externally rotated in the same manner used with the anterior apprehension test. A positive result is obtained when this pressure used to stabilize the head of the humerus and prevent it from subluxing anteriorly allows increased external rotation and diminished associated pain and apprehension.

Finally, the joint play of the acromioclavicular and sternoclavicular joints can be assessed from the supine

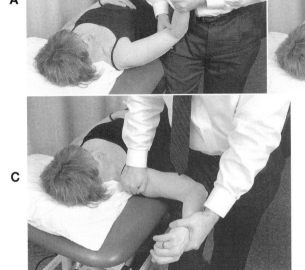

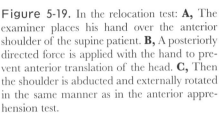

Figure 5-19. In the relocation test: **A,** The examiner places his hand over the anterior shoulder of the supine patient. **B,** A posteriorly directed force is applied with the hand to prevent anterior translation of the head. **C,** Then the shoulder is abducted and externally rotated in the same manner as in the anterior apprehension test.

position. Simple anterior-posterior pressures on the lateral aspect of the clavicle just adjacent to the acromioclavicular joint assess this joint's tolerance to shear loads. The same anterior-posterior pressures at the medial end of the clavicle just adjacent to the sternum assess the sternoclavicular joint's responses to shear.

Special Tests

Special tests including radiographic assessment, arthograms of the glenohumeral joint, magnetic resonance imaging of the shoulder, or diagnostic arthroscopy are important adjuncts to the patient history and physical examination (Table 5-12). Neural tension and thoracic outlet tests are controversial in both their application and interpretation. The relevant anatomy for such tests and clinical considerations have already been described in Chapter 2.

SUMMARY

We have provided a template from which to conduct the patient history and physical examination for problems related to the shoulder girdle as a basis for evaluation. Although there are numerous special tests available for the analysis of the shoulder, many are redundant. We encourage the reader to learn and understand the clinical anatomy and choose provocational tests that make good clinical sense and can be reproduced from patient to patient. We have offered an examination sequence that moves the patient infrequently and allows the information gained to be applied continuously to the next portion of the physical examination. It is important to recognize that a diagnosis for shoulder problems is rarely made using a singular test but instead relies on correlating the information gained from the history and results of the physical examination.

In Chapter 6 we will look at specific problems related to the shoulder and make suggestions regarding the organization of various interventions in order to optimize treatment outcomes. The examination described here typically provides the information from which a treatment plan can be developed and perhaps more importantly results in gaining information, which allows the patient to assume responsibility for important aspects of the management process.

REFERENCES

1. Andrews JR, Gillogly S: Physical examination of the shoulder in throwing athletes. In Zarins B, Andrews J, Carson W, editors: *Injuries to the throwing arm*, Philadelphia, 1985, WB Saunders.
2. Beaton D, Richards RR: Assessing the reliability and responsiveness of five shoulder questionnaires, *J Shoulder Hand Surg* 7:565, 1998.
3. Bridgman JF: Periarthritis of the shoulder and diabetes mellitus, *Ann Rheum Dis* 31:69, 1972.
4. Cyriax J, Cyriax P: Diagnosis of soft tissue lesions. In Cyriax J: *Textbook of orthopedic medicine*, ed 6, Baltimore, 1970, Williams and Wilkins.
5. Fung MF, Kato S, Barrance PJ, et al: Scapular and clavicular kinematics during humeral elevation: a study with cadavers, *J Bone Elbow Surg* 10:278, 2001.
6. Gerber C, Ganz G: Clinical assessment of instability of the shoulder, *J Bone Joint Surg Br* 66:551, 1984.
7. Hawkins RJ, Kennedy JC: Impingement syndrome in the athletic shoulder, *Am J Sports Med* 8(3):151, 1980.
8. Hawkins RJ, Mohtadi NG: Clinical evaluation of shoulder instability, *Clin J Sports Med* 1:59, 1991.
9. Hazleman BL: Why is a frozen shoulder frozen? *Br J Rheumatology* 29:130, 1990.
10. Heald SL, Riddle DL, Lamb RL: The shoulder pain and disability index: the construct validity and responsiveness of a region-specific disability measure, *Phys Ther* 77(10):1079, 1997.
11. Howell SM, Galinat BJ, Renzi AJ, et al: Normal and abnormal biomechanics of the glenohumeral joint in the horizontal plane, *J Bone Joint Surg* 70A:227, 1988.
12. Hulstyn MJ, Weiss AP: Adhesive capsulitis of the shoulder, *Orthop Rev* 22:425, 1993.
13. Jobe FW, Moynes DR: Delineation of diagnostic criteria and rehabilitation program for rotator cuff injuries, *Am J Sports Med* 10:336, 1982.
14. Kaltenborn FM: *Mobilisation of the extremity joints: examination and basic treatment techniques*, Oslo, 1980, Olaf Bokhandel.
15. Kibler WB: Specificity and sensitivity of the anterior slide test in throwing athletes with superior glenoid labral tears, *Arthroscopy* 11:296, 1995.
16. Levine WN, Flatow EL: The pathophysiology of shoulder instability, *Am J Sports Med* 28(6):910, 2000.
17. Maitland GD, Hengeveld E, Banks K: *Maitland's vertebral manipulation*, ed 6, London, 2000, Butterworth-Heinemann.

Table 5-12. Special Tests for Examination of the Shoulder

Imaging studies of the shoulder complex
Arthrograms
Angiography
Diagnostic arthroscopy
Tests for thoracic outlet
Upper limb neural tension tests

18. Matsen FA, Lippitt SB, Sidles JA, et al: *Practical evaluation and management of the shoulder*, Philadelphia, 1994, WB Saunders.

19. Matsen FA, Thomas SC, Rockwood CA: Glenohumeral instability. In Rockwood CA, Matsen FA, editors: *The shoulder*, Philadelphia, 1990, WB Saunders.

20. Moren-Hybbinette I, Moritz V, Shersten B: The clinical picture of the painful diabetic shoulder—natural history, social consequences and analysis of concomitant hand syndrome, *Acta Med Scand* 221:73, 1987.

21. Mosely HF: Disorders of the shoulder, *Clin Symp* 12:1, 1960.

22. Murnaghan JP: Adhesive capsulitis of the shoulder: current concepts and treatment, *Orthopedics* 11:153, 1988.

23. Neer CS II: Anterior acromioplasty for the chronic impingement syndrome in the shoulder: a preliminary report, *J Bone Joint Surg Am* 54A:41, 1972.

24. Neer CS II: Impingement lesions, *Clin Orthop* 173:70, 1983.

25. Neer CS II: *Shoulder reconstruction*, Philadelphia, 1990, WB Saunders.

26. Neer CS II, Welsh RP: The shoulder in sports, *Orthop Clin North Am* 8:583, 1977.

27. Neviaser RJ, Neviaser TJ: The frozen shoulder: diagnosis and management, *Clin Orthop* 223:59, 1987.

28. O'Brien SJ, Pagnani MJ, Fealy S, et al: The active compression test: a new and effective testfor diagnosing labral tears and acromioclavicular joint abnormality, *Am J Sports Med* 26:610, 1998.

29. Perry J: Anatomy and biomechanics of the shoulder in throwing, swimming, gymnastics, and tennis, *Clin Sports Med* 2(2):247, 1983.

30. Porterfield JA, DeRosa C: *Mechanical low back pain: perspectives in functional anatomy*, Philadelphia, 1998, WB Saunders.

31. Roach KE, Buhiman-Mak E, Songsiridej N, et al: Development of a shoulder pain and disability index, *Arthritis Care Res* 4(4):143, 1991.

32. Sherry DD, Rothstein RRL, Petty RE: Joint contractures preceding insulin-dependent diabetes mellitus, *Arthritis Rheum* 25:1362, 1982.

33. Snyder SJ, Karzel RP, Del Pizzo W, et al: SLAP lesions of the shoulder, *Arthroscopy* 6:274, 1990.

34. Wilk KE, Arrigo CA: Current concepts in the rehabilitation of the athletic shoulder, *J Orthop Sports Phys Ther* 18:365, 1993.

CHAPTER **6**

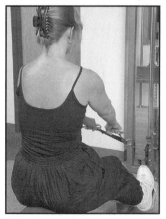

TREATMENT OF MECHANICAL SHOULDER DISORDERS

INTRODUCTION

In this text we have emphasized that a detailed understanding of the anatomy, especially the relationships of individual tissues and structures to one other, is requisite to effective application and interpretation of various aspects of the physical examination and to implementation of appropriate treatment interventions. References to video clips have been placed at key points throughout Chapters 2, 3, and 4 to enhance this understanding, highlight its clinical relevance, and provide the reader with a three-dimensional appreciation of the pertinent anatomy. On gaining a thorough understanding of the region, it becomes easier to visualize the mechanisms by which different structures related to the shoulder girdle are stretched and compressed and move in relation to one another during exercise or as a result of the application of any manual techniques. We encourage the reader to use the accompanying anatomical DVD often during this discussion of rehabilitation for the shoulder, especially when considering exercises. Visualizing the anatomy in this way will augment the reader's ability to scientifically analyze the potential effects of every aspect of treatment and allow appropriate modification of exercises or movement patterns based on examination findings.

The basic tissues of primary concern in the treatment of mechanical disorders of the shoulder are the connective, muscle, and nerve tissues. Examples of the most commonly seen medical diagnoses of the shoulder, with reference to the tissues of primary concern, include:

- Shoulder instability (connective tissues)
- Rotator cuff tears and surgical repairs (muscle and connective tissues)
- Calcific tendonitis (connective tissues)
- Complex regional pain syndrome (nerve tissue)
- Repetitive strain syndrome (muscle tissue)
- Glenoid labral lesions (connective tissues)
- Neurovascular compression syndromes (nerve tissue)
- Acromioclavicular joint disorders (connective tissues)
- Fractures and total joint arthroplasty (connective tissues)

When working from this tissue construct, the principles of treatment are very similar to those for the extremities and the spine. In this chapter we will suggest that by coupling the four objectives of treatment (patient education, pain modulation, movement promotion through strategically applied forces, and neuromuscular efficiency enhancement) with an understanding of the response of tissues to aging and injury, a logical and effective plan of care can be established.

Disorders of the shoulder are a particular challenge because of the inherent instability of the various articulations and the limited understanding of the complex yet highly coordinated roles the neuromuscular system plays over these same articulations. The enormously wide range of surgical and nonsurgical interventions (for example, thermal capsular shrinkage, exercise, acromial resection, rotator cuff repair, capsular shifts, bone and tendon translocations, subacromial debridement, rest, prolotherapy) not only reinforces that science has a surprisingly limited understanding of the shoulder complex but also suggests that no one formula exists for shoulder treatment.

Trying to determine the best treatment for shoulder disorders is extremely difficult owing to the realities of clinical practice. Since it is problematic to select a homogenous group of patients with precisely the same anatomical lesion responsible for the shoulder disorder, it is very difficult for outcome studies to compare and contrast the results of treatment interventions between patient populations. Diagnostic labels must be valid and reliable if treatment results are to be compared. Yet it is not simply the difficulty in establishing a meaningful diagnostic label that renders analysis of a homogenous group of patients with mechanical shoulder disorders difficult but also such factors as the patient's work requirements, social roles, myriad insurance and legal influences, and the unique and individualized responses that each individual has to pain stimuli and disability.

Despite such limitations, treatment can be based on the known sciences related to tissue aging, injury, healing, and repair. In addition, the effect of exercise on the promotion of general health, physical well-being, and enhancement of tissue strength and function is well accepted and understood. It is on these strong foundational principles that this chapter is based.

GENERAL CONCEPTS

For the most part musculoskeletal tissues heal predictably. This is an important point to recognize in planning the treatment process for mechanical disorders of the shoulder. The literature is replete with information regarding the healing potential of bone,[4,5] tendon,[16,19,25] ligament,[2,8] muscle,[14] nerve,[3,20] and cartilage.[6,17,18] Therefore rehabilitation for any musculoskeletal disorder should by definition follow foundational guidelines that have been established for these tissues.

The uniqueness of any rehabilitation program, however, becomes dependent on the functional demands of that region. Therefore while the foundational rehabilitation principles regarding tissue repair might be similar for rehabilitation of the shoulder, low back, or knee, the *uniqueness* of the rehabilitation prescriptions is dependent on the functional demands that the region is currently being subjected to and is expected to be subjected to in the future.

This is the primary reason that the concept of force attenuation was introduced in Chapter 1 and then continuously reiterated in subsequent chapters, culminating in Chapter 5, with this paradigm being the essential focus of the examination process. The relationship of the loading response from functional demands to treatment of mechanical shoulder disorders is extremely important. Management strategies will need to be tailored to and implemented for conditions as varied as those seen in the throwing athlete, the older adult patient with full thickness tear of the rotator cuff, the swimmer, the overhead worker, the gymnast, the tennis player, the patient with neurovascular compromise to a component of the brachial plexus, or an individual who insidiously loses glenohumeral capsular resiliency within a few days.

Accurate mechanical diagnosis and the implementation of appropriate interventions are thus intimately related. Being able to predict the outcome of the treatment dosage based on the interpretation of the findings of the history and physical examination, along with meaningful and practical patient education, is closely related to quality patient care. In the shoulder, particularly with the dominant side, the key to any treatment approach is to minimize, and in the best of circumstances, prevent the overload to the injured tissue while staying active. The assessment process suggested in Chapter 5 helps the clinician determine the "barrier," the position of the extremity or the loading response of the tissues that just begins to stimulate the nociceptive system or reproduces signs or symptoms similar to the original problem for which the patient has sought help. Once such a barrier is determined, the clinician must decide whether rehabilitation should work *through* that barrier, mechanically stressing the repairing tissues, or be designed to work *away* from the barrier, recognizing that the force attenuation capabilities of the tissues have been irrevocably lost. Such a decision becomes part of the guiding philosophy behind designing the plan of care and is scientifically grounded when the loading responses of tissues, the effects of age and injury on tissues, and recognition of the three major influences on the painful response (chemoreceptor activation of the nociceptive system, mechanoreceptor activation of the nociceptive system, and the influence of psychosocial factors on the pain response) are understood.

In order for any rehabilitation program to be effective, the patient must also take "ownership" of his problem. It is therefore important for the patient to see and understand the similarities of the positions and forces mentioned above in his activities of daily living or the requirements of his work or sport. In order for collagenous structures to repair, a balance between tissue loading and controlled rest must be struck. This becomes one of the primary dilemmas with rehabilitation of the shoulder, especially in regard to work and sport requirements. The successful clinician helps the patient analyze movement and the relationship of movement to healing and potential reinjury. The patient must then pay particular attention to those activities that are more reflexive or subconscious in nature, such as arising from his chair, opening and closing heavy glass doors, reaching overhead for cups and dinner plates, lying on his shoulder when falling asleep, or abruptly lifting heavy objects, among a wide array of movements, and be able to relate these to his shoulder impairment or functional loss. The successful patient will make the temporary changes in physical behavior that minimize the overload, while remaining active. At the risk of being redundant, it is important to remember that this is the primarily purpose of the evaluation system as outlined in Chapter 5: to provide the clinician and the patient with a knowledge base that allows for the implementation of practical solutions to balance activity and rest.

We have already seen that the neurology of the upper quarter is complex and intricate. Also, it must always be considered in the design of treatment programs. In many ways, the upper quarter neurology is more complex than that of the lower extremities because of the density of sensory receptors and muscle spindles present here. Unlike other areas of the body, pain anywhere in the upper quarter has the potential to exacerbate symptoms within the entire region. Several examples illustrate this:

- The source of pain may be in the neck, but the patient also complains of his entire arm aching, as well as ringing in the ears.
- The patient with a degenerative segment in his cervical spine feels pain "right between my shoulder blades" when he extends his neck and laterally flexes toward one side.
- The patient complains of pain along the back of the arm, scapular regions, and neck after injuring himself while performing a pull-up.
- The patient with the frequently dislocated shoulder complains of headaches and pain at the superior medial border of the scapula.
- The patient with a trivial injury to the wrist and hand develops edema, pain, and discoloration of the complete arm and forearm and is unable to tolerate any sensory stimulus to the upper quarter.
- The patient presents with carpal tunnel syndrome but on close examination also has shoulder pain and evidence of cervical nerve root involvement.
- The patient attempts a new exercise on a selectorized exercise machine at his local exercise facility and feels an immediate discomfort in the shoulder, which then results in neck stiffness and diffuse arm pain the following day.

These examples demonstrate that it is not only the anatomical linkages of tissues that have been described in this text that are important to recognize but also the neurology of the region. Both must be taken into consideration when examining any patient with upper quarter pain.

Finally, we must mention the importance of movement in the early phases of rehabilitation. With most injuries, the sooner the injured region can be moved into and through a painful range of motion with an intensity, frequency, and duration that does not exacerbate the condition, the more rapid the recovery. Moving through the painful range at the appropriate rate and amplitude requires guidance by the clinician and is an essential factor in facilitating functional healing and ultimately the determination of future functional limitations.

INTENT OF TREATMENT

The intent of treatment has four basic components:[26]

1. Optimize the healing environment.
2. Restore anatomical relationships between the injured and noninjured tissues.
3. Maintain the normal function of the noninjured tissues.
4. Prevent excessive stress or strain to the injured tissues.

Optimize the Healing Environment

Healing of collagenous structures can be described in three phases: reaction, regeneration, and remodeling.[26] The reaction phase calls on specific cells to create the cellular and chemical environment required for tissue repair. Mast cells, granulocytes, leukocytes, fibroblasts, and myofibroblasts respond and reach the injured and surrounding regions quickly. This barrage of cells, when coupled with the inflammatory exudate that results, creates a "biological soup."[28] This is an excellent analogy because it provides a strong visual image of the thickened fluid–like nature of the environment and the tissue stasis that result. This soup becomes the basis for increased tissue pressure, which retards lymph drainage and microcirculation, rendering the area hypoxic and acidic. The depolarization threshold of the nociceptive free nerve endings lessens as the pH decreases, resulting in axonal depolarization and increased afferent input into the central nervous system. The resultant pain can begin a cascade of events, including muscle spasm, decreased blood flow, and increased fluid congestion.

The goal with treatment is to maximize the healing environment through restoration of the microcirculation environment and is often best accomplished through graded and controlled movement. This is best introduced by the clinician in the form of passive, active assistive manual techniques, active movements, or controlled muscle contractions over the area.

Time frames need to be considered with this treatment intent and are dependent on the circulation present in the region and the age of the patient. In an adolescent a well-vascularized area may require as little as 6 to 8 weeks for reasonable repair of connective tissues, whereas a young adult may require 8 to 12 weeks. At the other end of the spectrum, the older adult patient with an injury in an area with less optimal vascularization, such as the rotator cuff tendons, may require 6 to 9 months for reasonable repair, if repair is even possible. In all cases, repair of collagenous tissues ultimately results in some loss of function.[10,22,29]

Restore Anatomical Relationships Between the Injured and Noninjured Tissues

This second intent of treatment refers to the introduction of movement designed to stress the injured tissues in a way that stimulates functional healing and allows the tissues to begin assuming their role of load attenuation in concert with the surrounding tissues. Restoration of the strength, length, and motion capabilities of the injured tissue relative to the surrounding region is important if loads are to be effectively distributed via multiple tissues in the region. Tissues must be able to glide over, compress onto, and exert tension to the attached tissues. This ultimately results in functional healing.

Maintain the Normal Function of the Noninjured Tissues

The third intent of treatment is designed to introduce the right dosage of movement and tissue loading in order to simultaneously maintain tissue health and reduce disuse atrophy. The dosage is important, and clinicians always must keep in mind that symptom reduction in and of itself is not the best indicator of tissue repair. For example, the degenerated and painful rotator cuff may become asymptomatic, but its ability to tolerate loads may not have appreciably changed. Excessive load to the degenerated asymptomatic rotator cuff tendon can result in a partial thickness tear increasing to a full thickness tear. A fine line always exists between too much and too little activity. A direct relationship exists between the restoration of microcirculation, the required healing times for injured or surgically repaired tissues, and the introduction of movement for healing.

Prevent Excessive Stress or Strain on the Injured Tissues

The final intent of treatment requires an understanding of the mechanics of the articulations related to the shoulder girdle and the requirements of muscle activity during functional activities. Clinicians can design exercise programs or apply manual techniques safely and without compromise to the injured region only when those interventions are based on a complete understanding of the anatomy and biomechanics of the region. For example, when any exercise is being performed, the clinician should be able to clearly visualize:

- When the acromioclavicular joint is placed at its endrange
- When the supraspinatus tendon is simultaneously loaded in compression and tension

- What position of the glenohumeral joint places the greatest tension to the anterior-inferior glenohumeral ligament
- What motions of the upper extremity place the greatest stress to the long head of the biceps tendon
- What position of the shoulder puts the greatest stress to a subacromial region that has recently been surgically debrided
- What exercises place the greatest degree of frictional loading on a recently repaired anterior glenoid labrum
- What sleeping postures stress an inflamed and irritated glenohumeral joint capsule

These types of joint and tissue specific analyses continually guide the clinician's treatment approach, especially regarding development of the exercise prescription. While it is important to guide the patient through a painful range of motion without further exacerbation of symptoms, it cannot be done at the expense of placing excessive stress on the injured tissues.

PRIMARY INFLUENCES ON THE PAIN RESPONSE

When considering the wide range of clinical presentations possible in patients with shoulder girdle disorders, two theoretical questions should be considered in order to better appreciate the complexity of the pain response:

1. Can pain exist without inflammation?
2. Can inflammation exist without pain?

Theoretically, both scenarios have the potential to exist. Pain without inflammation might best be interpreted as mechanical pain, that is, stimulation of the mechanoreceptor nerve endings when endranges of motion result in tissue distortion great enough to result in depolarization of the afferent nerve endings without tissue damage. When the excessive force or motion is removed, the discomfort decreases or is diminished.

It is reasonable to assume that the answer to the second question is also "yes" because, again, we must take into account the depolarization threshold of the nociceptive system, this time chemically instead of mechanically. High depolarization threshold refers to the necessity of a larger stimulus being required for axonal discharge, while a low threshold requires less or little stimulus for axonal depolarization. The threshold is reached because of sufficient

chemical activation of the nociceptive system. In many patients with shoulder disorders, one often hears of a "pre-pain continuum" during the history, which begins with stiffness and movement complaints, after which an appreciation of pain occurs at a later time.

Pain is also influenced by emotions and the individual's behavioral responses to his surrounding environment. Factors such as family stress and job stress and emotional states including fear and depression all contribute to the complexity and uniqueness of the perception of pain, the pain response, and the ultimate response to treatment. Therefore in planning the treatment of mechanical disorders of the musculoskeletal system, the clinician should first consider these three influences on pain:

- Chemoreceptor or biochemical cycle
- Mechanoreceptor cycle
- Emotional or behavioral cycle

The clinician also needs to be cognizant of the various behavioral and physiological responses that occur as a result of these three stimuli. Figure 6-1 illustrates this via the use of a clockwise spin of three cycles: chemoreceptor, mechanoreceptor, and emotional/behavioral. Each cycle includes the associated physiological or behavioral changes that occur. Pain perception is typically due to a contribution from each cycle, and during the assessment and reassessment processes, the clinician is always attempting to ascertain which three cycles are "spinning" to the greatest degree. In other words, what is the primary stimulus contributing to the disorder?

Determining which of the three cycles predominates ultimately influences what interventions will be applied. For example, pain syndromes that are thought to be primarily influenced via the chemoreceptor cycle are best treated with carefully controlled motion and appropriate rest. Working through the barrier would most likely exacerbate the condition, as might the initiation of resistance exercises. Pain that is primarily caused by the mechanoreceptor cycle has less inflammation and tissue damage associated with the disorder and can tolerate more loading to the tissues. Thus it can be treated with more active approaches such as incorporating resistance exercises and more aggressive joint mobilization and stretching activities. Such conditions can often be treated into and through the barrier. When the emotional/behavioral cycle is the major influence, patient education becomes the

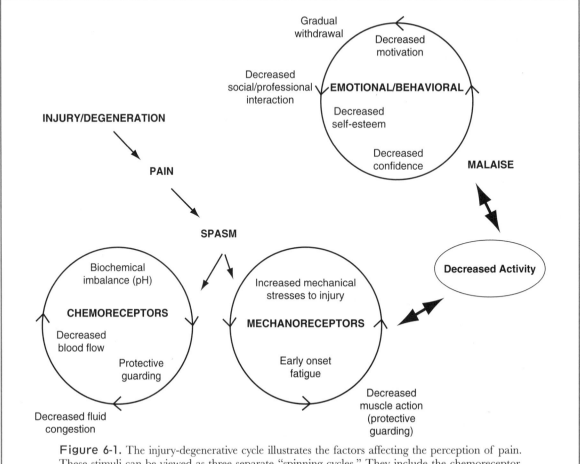

Figure 6-1. The injury-degenerative cycle illustrates the factors affecting the perception of pain. These stimuli can be viewed as three separate "spinning cycles." They include the chemoreceptor, mechanoreceptor, and emotional-behavioral cycles. Pain can be related to each individual cycle or to a combination of the three. *Chemoreceptor cycle:* The nociceptive effects of fluid stasis and altered biochemistry of the injured region, often noted as morning stiffness by the patient. *Mechanoreceptor cycle:* The effects of early onset fatigue and decreased activity, often noted as pain at the end of the day by the patient. *Emotional-behavioral cycle:* Shows the influence of psychosocial stressors on the patient. When viewing these three components as spinning cycles, the clinician attempts to determine which of the cycles is dominant or the most responsible for the pain perception and therefore should take precedence in establishing the treatment process. (From Porterfield JA, DeRosa C: *Mechanical low back pain: perspectives in functional anatomy,* ed 2, Philadelphia, 1998, WB Saunders.)

primary treatment approach. Less hands-on intervention is used because the pain generator has minimal mechanical or chemical basis. While all three cycles contribute to the painful syndrome, the clinician is attempting to determine the hierarchy of each cycle's influence and then use the appropriate treatment techniques indicated to match each cycle with such a hierarchy.

OBJECTIVES OF TREATMENT

While there are anatomical differences and unique functional demands for each region of the musculoskeletal system, four basic objectives of treatment for orthopedic mechanical disorders exist that should be considered regardless of the region. These objectives are:

1. Patient education and biomechanical counseling
2. Modulation of pain and the promotion of analgesia
3. Application of controlled forces to promote patient activity
4. Enhancement of neuromuscular health and performance

We will consider each of these objectives in relation to the development and implementation of treatment interventions for painful disorders of the shoulder complex.

Patient Education and Biomechanical Counseling

Appropriately directing the responsibility of recovery to the patient via education is the key to any successful rehabilitation program. It is important to realize that if a patient is treated in a clinical environment 3 days a week for 1 hour at each visit, the clinician is interacting with the patient only for a very small percentage of the time that the patient is awake and active. What the patient is doing away from the clinical environment becomes critical to care management. In order to obtain the best results from a rehabilitation program, the patient must understand his injury and what his own contribution must be to the rehabilitation process. Establishing reachable, realistic, short- and long-term goals becomes a very important aspect of this process since it underscores the significance of the patient's involvement in the treatment process.

Patient education needs to include an explanation of anatomical and biomechanical aspects of the injury or condition, the rationale for the suggested treatment program, and the expected outcomes. One very important aspect of the initial stages of the treatment process is to assist the patient in understanding the relationships between the intervention and the expected outcome. In most cases, the initial outcome is a decrease in pain and an increase in function, after which there are more complex outcomes such as the development of specific neuromotoric skills that can be set as goals. The latter are especially important in dealing with the painful shoulder of the patient returning to sport or industry.

When treating the patient with an acute injury, the optimal reassessment of the patient has to take place within the most immediate time period following treatment. Often the constraints of authorized visits

and insurance limitations influence this, but optimal care is achieved when the results of treatment for the acute injury are promptly assessed. A daily reassessment, for example, permits the clinician to substantiate his findings and understanding of the extent of the injury. Following an initial treatment, the clinician might predict such changes as the extent of pain relief that the patient should experience, a change in the referral zone of pain, how easy or difficult it will be for the patient to sleep that night as a result of treatment, and the amount of stiffness that the patient might experience the following morning upon awakening. When the patient returns to the clinic on a subsequent visit, the predictions are revisited by both clinician and patient and revised decisions regarding further interventions are made. Outcome prediction following the subsequent treatment is repeated again, with the result being that the clinician ultimately can confidently predict the extent of the injury and the short- and long-term course of the rehabilitation program. If the clinician has gained the essential information from the patient history, clearly understands the ease in which painful responses can be elicited, and knows how the shoulder girdle will be used in work and activities of daily living, such predictions often can be made with a high degree of accuracy.

Biomechanical counseling establishes those positions, movements, and forces that have the potential to compromise the patient's shoulder injury in activities of daily living, work, and sport throughout each phase of the recovery process. Making correct judgments and providing clear explanation about the demands of various activities of daily living on his injury is an important clinical skill. Decisions regarding the patient's gradual progression of activity during rehabilitation and the demands associated with return to work or reactivation into sport must be based on observation, accurate prediction, and effective planning. The shoulder complex is involved in almost all activities of daily living and sport, and therefore keeping the loads under the injury threshold throughout rehabilitation is important.

In most mechanical shoulder disorders, it is unusual to progress completely through the rehabilitation process without some form of exacerbation of the condition. It could be successfully argued that a mild increase in symptoms along the rehabilitation continuum is helpful in determining the upper limit of tissue tolerance as the patient progresses from one stage of activity to the next. The dialogue established between patient and clinician is one of the main factors in the successful return to painless activity.

There are numerous examples of patient education and biomechanical counseling that are used to help the patient manage his shoulder disorder. Many can be surmised from the mechanics of injury discussed in Chapters 2, 3, and 4, and additional examples are included in the case studies in the final section of this chapter. Several practical examples to share with patients are listed here in order to relate this objective of treatment to selected shoulder impairments and functional limitations:

- Avoid carrying heavy purses or backpacks over one shoulder when symptoms of brachial plexus involvement or neural entrapment are present.
- Avoid excessive scapular retraction in the presence of symptomatic degenerative joint disease of the acromioclavicular joint.
- Modify rowing exercises in the presence of long head of the biceps tenosynovitis.
- Avoid any shoulder elevation exercises that leave the glenohumeral joint in a relatively internally rotated position.
- Realize the importance of trunk rotation (when throwing) during the acceleration and deceleration phases.
- Make sure enough body roll is occurring during the recovery phase of swimming in order to avoid abnormal glenohumeral joint motion.
- Realize increased thoracic extension and scapular retraction occur when carrying out tasks in the overhead position for extended periods of time.

These examples use the biomechanical knowledge of shoulder girdle function to provide specific and individualized advice to a patient regarding protection of his injury.

Modulation of Pain and the Promotion of Analgesia

Shoulder pain often is poorly tolerated. Pain tolerance is lessened by the inability to assume a comfortable position for sleep, the inability to move the shoulder in activities of daily living without provoking pain, or the presence of sharp episodes of pain on simple shoulder movements. Because pain is also a part of the healing process, it serves as a warning signal that assists us in making the correct decisions regarding motions and tissue loading patterns.

Pain modulation interventions are important in order to begin to reintroduce functional activities at the earliest possible opportunity. Several different strategies are available that meet this objective of treatment. Controlling exuberant inflammation and hence pain is the primary reason for using medication as a strategy to meet this objective. This includes nonsteroidal antiinflammatory drugs (NSAIDs), steroidal medications, and corticosteroid injections. In several disorders of the shoulder, the rapid control of inflammation brought about by corticosteroid injections is the best management strategy, as in the case of the rapid onset subacromial bursitis. Although such a problem might also be treated with ice and antiinflammatory medication, an injection of corticosteroid and analgesic into the region provides rapid relief and more importantly does not allow the glenohumeral joint to remain immobilized as a result of pain for an extended period of time. Analgesics used alone in the treatment of mechanical shoulder disorders are primarily used for pain modulation without antiinflammatory qualities.

The most difficult question here is determining the length of time to use such a medication and how to couple its use with the active rehabilitation process. Monitoring the changing level of pain represents one of the best guides in directing the progression toward recovery. Oftentimes medication is used until the patient can comfortably sleep through the night.

Avoid muscle relaxants during the active rehabilitation process. They are primarily used to enhance the patient's ability to sleep and often may make the patient groggy. The appropriate resting state of muscle activity helps to control the loads that need to be attenuated for injured tissues during even the simplest of movements and postures. Therefore, depending on the problem, decreasing muscle activity is not always in the patient's best interest.

Proper hydration is essential while taking medications. Fatigue, one of the more common indicators of dehydration, is most often seen as a side effect when patients are taking medication and needs to be monitored by the clinician.

Thermal and electrical modalities administered to the injured region of the shoulder in the most comfortable position can often be coupled with manual techniques to stimulate fluid dynamics and help decrease pain as a result of alteration of the chemical environment associated with the injured tissue. Ice applied to the shoulder in the form of ice massage, coupled with soft tissue and joint mobilization techniques, also produces advantageous results.

Application of Controlled Forces to Promote Patient Activity

The objective of applying controlled forces refers to the clinician's ability to introduce motions in such a way that active movements by the patient are subsequently encouraged. There are numerous ways in which controlled forces can be effectively used in the management of mechanical disorders of the shoulder. Table 6-1 lists active, manual, and mechanical treatment techniques that are often used in this objective of treatment. Although many different explanations have been made regarding the effects of these techniques, we believe that the physiological outcomes of all of the techniques are remarkably similar and can be distilled to a combination of the following:

- *Stimulation of fluid dynamics.* As previously mentioned, stasis results in an altered biochemical environment associated with the region of injury and this chemical environment activates the nociceptive system. Active motion and some of the passive motion techniques help move tissue fluid along a gradient, thus altering the chemical milieu associated with injured tissue.
- *Increasing afferent input into the central nervous system.* Many of the manual and active techniques provide mechanoreceptor input into the central nervous system, which has a twofold reflexive effect.
- *Enhanced modulation of pain.* Many of the joint and soft tissue techniques have sufficient mechanoreceptor stimulation to help modulate the afferent pain impulse emanating from the injured region at the central nervous system level; this is especially important when dealing with the exquisitely painful glenohumeral joint capsule.
- *Modulation of the resting state of muscle contraction.* Many of these techniques are effective in decreasing muscle spasm and guarding through the reflex connections associated with mechanoreceptor input.
- *Modification of connective tissue.* This is especially important when considering rehabilitation following surgery; recently injured or surgically repaired connective tissues respond to applied forces by stimulation of new fibroblast formation and realignment of collagen fibril orientation.

The total endrange time or time that the joint is held at the end of its available range becomes an important consideration because it is this parameter that has the most significant effect on the modulation of connective tissue length.[7,15]

Soft tissue techniques (Figure 6-2) and joint mobilization techniques (Figure 6-3) are often used to manage pain and inflammation and can be obstacles to active movement. As noted in Chapter 4, various accessory joint mobilizations are designed to improve general joint mobility. Do not think of them as increasing one particular physiological motion over another. The longer the time frame of the injury, however, or the more the healing scar proliferates, the greater the cross linking of the collagen fibrils. Thus at some point there is a reduced ability to actually modify connective tissues through any mobilization or stretching techniques.

Oftentimes manual treatment of the upper quarter has physiological effects on the surrounding area as well, most likely because of the increased afferent input afforded by the stimulation of the joint, muscle, tendon, and skin mechanoreceptors. Therefore treatment often is directed to the primary region of

Table 6-1. Application of Controlled Forces to Promote Patient Activity		
Passive Manual Techniques	**Mechanical Interventions**	**Active Techniques**
Glenohumeral joint mobilization	Shoulder slings	Active range of motion
Scapulothoracic mobilization	Shoulder taping	Muscle energy techniques
Acromioclavicular and sternoclavicular joint mobilization	Shoulder abduction splints	Proprioceptive neuromuscular facilitation
Soft tissue mobilization		Isometric stabilization
Physiological joint and muscle stretching		
Cross friction massage		
Effleurage		
Acupressure		

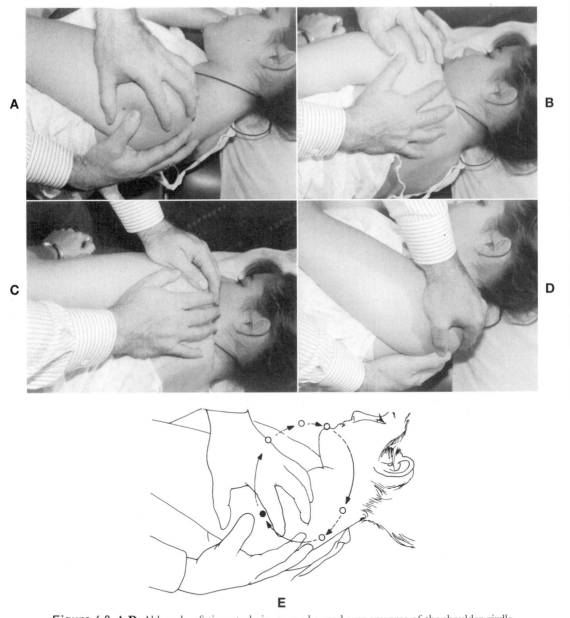

Figure 6-2. A-D, Although soft tissue techniques can be used over any area of the shoulder girdle, the tissue techniques are primarily used over the scapulothoracic articulation. In these examples the scapula is passively moved by the examiner along all available planes of motion. **E,** The sequence moves clockwise. (From Porterfield JA, DeRosa C: *Mechanical neck pain: perspectives in functional anatomy,* Philadelphia, 1995, WB Saunders.)

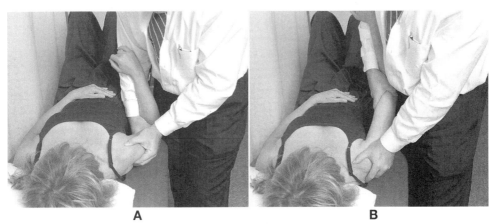

Figure 6-3. General mobility of the glenohumeral joint can be encouraged with the use of passive physiological motion in conjunction with various translations of the humeral head on the glenoid. Shown in this example are anterior, **A,** and posterior glides, **B,** of the humerus on the glenoid, useful as a supplemental technique to help restore or improve general joint mobility. During these accessory motion techniques, one must be cognizant of the joint plane and then be certain that movement of the two bones relative to one another remains parallel to this joint plane.

involvement, as well as associated regions. For example, internal derangement within the glenohumeral joint, such as seen in a torn glenoid labrum, may initiate protective guarding (spasm) and pain throughout the upper quarter. This, in turn, results in cervical spine discomfort, scapulothoracic complaints, and headaches, perhaps as the result of abnormal and excessive spine and scapula muscle activity.

Finally, splints and taping of the various shoulder articulations often are used in an attempt to control how forces reach the region and therefore such interventions also fall under this objective of treatment. Abduction splints are especially important in some surgical repairs because the positioning of the arm with such splints minimizes the chances that adhesive capsulitis will develop. Taping of the anterior aspect of the glenohumeral joint in the case of chronic anterior subluxation is another such intervention.

The following examples illustrate how this objective of treatment is used in selected shoulder disorders:

- Passive stretching to increase glenohumeral external rotation in order to allow the patient to avoid subacromial compression when raising the arm overhead
- Small and controlled translations of the humeral head on the glenoid using very specific handholds to

treat the patient with a humeral shaft fracture in order to help maintain some degree of capsular mobility and avoid secondary adhesive capsulitis
- Use of a sling to support the upper extremity in order to counter the gravitation pull to the scapula on the clavicle in the recently injured acromioclavicular joint
- Cross friction to the infraspinatus tendon to help mobilize the connective tissue and also induce a hyperemic response in the mildly involved case of infraspinatus tendonitis
- Glenohumeral joint mobilization using an inferior glide translation "stretch" to help decompress the subacromial space and allow for active overhead movement to be initiated
- Use of rhythmic internal and external rotation oscillations in order to treat the acutely painful capsulitis
- Manual stretching of the pectoralis major and minor to decrease the shoulder protraction position and minimize subacromial compression
- Use of a shoulder wand or L bar to introduce active assistive motion in the shoulder that has been recently surgically repaired
- Codman's exercises to apply passive range-of-motion techniques to the glenohumeral joint, which allows gravity to decompress the loading between the humeral head and the glenoid

Enhancement of Neuromuscular Health and Performance

The rehabilitation process shifts toward resisted exercise once motion has been restored, the patient is sleeping through the night and waking up without excessive stiffness or soreness (one of the best indicators of an inflammatory condition), the time of pain relief from treatment is lengthening, and the intensity of pain has been lessened. Injuries to the connective tissues associated with the articulations of the shoulder girdle result in a loss of stability. Because connective tissues repair rather than regenerate, restoration of stability will not come from the connective tissue contribution but instead from enhanced neuromuscular control. Therefore this objective is very important.

Several definitions are important to understand. An operating definition of *strength* indicates that the recruitment of motor units allows the muscle to generate sufficient tension to overcome a given load or resistance. *Power* refers to the amount of force that can be generated over a unit of time, whereas *endurance* is the ability of the neuromuscular system to sustain a given force or repeated contractions. *Coordination*, the most complex of motor functions, is the integration of cortical, subcortical, and spinal cord levels of control with the receptor system associated with the joints and soft tissues. Coordination also includes the motor planning that actually precedes the activity. Exercise programs designed around the enhancement of neuromuscular health and performance need to include these parameters.

Use of poor exercise technique can result in further injury, oftentimes compounding the original injury. It is very important then that the clinician is able to assess the biomechanics of each exercise, especially as resistance or repetitions are increased, and successfully match these mechanics to the positions and movements that have been altered as a result of the injury or degeneration. The successful clinician visualizes the anatomy of the shoulder girdle, spine, and trunk in three dimensions during movement and then assesses the structural and load-bearing changes imparted to the joint structures and related tissues. This knowledge permits the clinician to customize the strengthening program to meet the needs of each patient. The goal is to develop resisted movement patterns that appropriately load each tissue within the shoulder complex without injury. Such treatments are based on the following concepts:

- Movement enhances healing.
- Movement against resistance can enhance connective tissue strength and muscle strength.
- Greater overload applied causes greater tension generating demands of the muscle and thus the potential for muscle hypertrophy.
- Resistance coupled with repetition leads to neuromotoric changes and motor learning.

The challenge is to effectively teach the patient how to exercise against resistance using proper biomechanics until a change in the quality of the motion occurs and proper form is lost. The patient must develop the ability to move the humerus irrespective of the scapula, scapula irrespective of the humerus, and both in concert with the trunk. Fatigue of any one aspect of the shoulder girdle mechanism can result in movement substitution and thus the loss of the targeted training stimulus. Strict form is essential, and the clinician must continually monitor trunk, cervicothoracic, scapulothoracic, and upper extremity move-ments and positioning until the patient gains the necessary awareness of the proper mechanics for the exercise.

The goal of weight training is to increase and improve all aspects of the neuromuscular system, including strength, power, and endurance without injury. The challenge to both clinician and patient is to learn proper technique in order that controlled, noninjurious, resisted movement can be consistently carried out. To accomplish these goals, a process must be developed and adhered to at the beginning of exercise. We recommend the following training process:

1. Establish the range of motion. Start with a small range of motion and gradually increase the range of motion to points just short of compromising tissue stress.
2. Establish the speed of motion. The emphasis is to learn to move in a smooth, rhythmical, and controlled fashion without excessive pauses at either end of the range of motion or ballistic quick starts to the motion.
3. Complete the motion. Include as many of the articulations of the shoulder girdle and trunk as possible while maintaining control of the loads as they pass into and through the injury. For example, in the seated row exercise, the motion can begin with simple humeral movement, progress to include scapular protraction and retraction, and then continue to include the entire coordinated motion of the trunk and shoulder girdle, which

adds spinal flexion and resisted spinal extension to the complete exercise. Starting with a simple humeral extension and ending with compound trunk and shoulder girdle motion is most desirable. Note how the most comprehensive approach to training the shoulder girdle involves monitoring the activity of the muscles of the abdominal wall and extensors of the trunk.

4. Monitor substitution of motion. Once range of motion is established, the speed is constant, and compound movements have been integrated, the next step is to recognize the subtle signs of fatigue or what is referred to as "repetitions to substitution." Fatigue can be defined as performing consistent movement patterns against resistance until change in speed and/or range of motion is realized. Fatigue can take place in any represented part of the motion and over any articulation of the shoulder girdle. For example, during one exercise session, the first muscle group to fatigue may be the scapular retractors and those muscles responsible for controlling the scapula. The patient recognizes the gradual changes in the position of his scapula as it completes its excursion over the thorax. In a subsequent exercise session the fatigue may not be in the scapula retractors but instead in prime movers associated with glenohumeral motion. "Clinical" fatigue is a change of speed or change in motion that alters the loading patterns of each involved tissue. Again, the role of the abdominal wall cannot be overemphasized.

Once the patient is appropriately instructed and involved in strengthening in this manner, the coordination or control of weight bearing will be accomplished, and each repetition and set of resisted exercises will appropriately stimulate the tissues. We feel that in a therapeutic condition, it is a mistake to develop the exercise prescription that states "do 3 sets of 10 repetitions." One day 10 repetitions might be excessive for the tissue, resulting in injury, whereas the next day 10 repetitions may be more easily tolerated and the training effect not even realized. This is especially important in the rehabilitation of the shoulder because it is very easy to overstress the rotator cuff tendons.

Once the patient comprehends this four-step process, the chances of reinjury decrease markedly. The exercise prescription is then further developed to meet specific training needs. The question becomes, "To what sport or activity of daily living is the patient attempting to return?" Understanding the goal is obviously a major component in determining the intensity, frequency, and duration of the rehabilitation process. Designing the rehabilitation to fit the task is ultimately the goal that we need to progress toward, closely replicating the movements and forces that mimic the activity to which the patient expects to return. Effective strength training will result in neural and musculofascial changes.[13,23]

THE EXERCISE SECTION

A unique aspect of this text is marked by the inclusion of a comprehensive series of exercises that can be selected for many of the mechanical shoulder conditions that we have discussed. The sequence of exercises also includes clinical commentary regarding essential considerations for positioning, in addition to positions or movements that have the potential to compromise a particular tissue or structure. This "set" of exercises is meant to serve as a "palette" from which the clinician can make selections based on desired outcome.

The exercise section provides an array of exercises designed to improve the strength, power, and endurance of the global and local muscles associated with the shoulder girdle. The reader is encouraged to revisit Chapter 3 to understand where different muscle fiber crossing relationships occur because these often represent foci for resistance exercises. Such crossing relationships exist between the following:

- Latissimus dorsi and serratus anterior
- Latissimus dorsi and gluteus maximus
- Serratus anterior and abdominal wall bilaterally
- Trapezius and rhomboids
- Pectoralis major bilaterally
- Long head of the triceps and the teres major and infraspinatus
- Coracobrachialis or short head of the biceps brachii and the subscapularis

These regions of muscle crossing, with each other or as a result of the muscle fiber direction when the muscles are considered bilaterally, are a focus for strengthening exercises. This type of training complements and enhances specific, localized strengthening, such as isolated rotator cuff strengthening. Isolated strengthening is an excellent point at which to introduce resistance exercises, but it is necessary for each of the shoulder girdle articulations to work in concert with the trunk and spine in order to optimize upper quarter function. Therefore the exercise section that follows illustrates therapeutic exercises essential for scapulothoracic, trunk, and spinal stability or motion, as well as those that cross the glenohumeral joint. Appropriately strengthening the tissues at the apex of these relationships enhances the ability to stabilize the trunk and neuromuscularly "link" the extremities.

Closely examine the starting, midrange, and finishing positions for each of the exercises presented. Whereas one clinician may look at a particular exercise and recognize its utility for a specific clinical problem, another may see the same exercise and consider it useful for a markedly different problem. Many times exercises are categorized according to muscle groups (e.g., exercises for the anterior deltoid, exercises for the pectoralis major, exercises for the rhomboids). The reader will appreciate after reviewing Chapters 2, 3, and 4 that no muscle group works in isolation regardless of the exercise. Trunk, spine, scapula, and humeral muscles are all required to serve as stabilizers or prime movers or contribute muscle forces, which cancel the unwanted motions that the prime mover would introduce to the desired movement pattern as a result of its muscle fiber orientation.

We have organized this section to serve the clinician seeking strengthening strategies for his patients and to illustrate exercises considered essential for general conditioning of the upper quarter. The exercises appear in the following order:

- *Exercises 1 through 7*. An excellent group of exercises that the clinician incorporates for the patient in the prone position to strengthen the scapular retractors and those muscles of the glenohumeral joint associated with pushing, pulling, and moving the arm overhead.
- *Exercises 8 through 11*. Seated resistance exercises for the prime movers and scapular and trunk stabilizers involved with arm elevation.
- *Exercises 12 through 15*. Rowing exercises from different positions are some of the most useful exercises for strengthening the shoulder extensors, scapular retractors, and spine extensors.
- *Exercises 16 through 18*. The pull-downs and assisted pull-ups are powerful exercises for the latissimus dorsi, teres major, and the downward rotators of the scapula, such as the rhomboids.
- *Exercises 19 through 35*. Functional strengthening exercises include the variations of the standing row and pulling exercises. These exercises combine the stimulus of stabilization via the lower extremities with trunk and shoulder girdle movement. Depending on the instructions given by the clinician, these exercises can exert a training effect to the spinal extensors, abdominal muscles, and scapulothoracic and glenohumeral muscles.
- *Exercise 36*. The classic dumbbell curl.
- *Exercises 37 through 45*. Pushing exercises are essential for training the muscles of the anterior chest wall, the shoulder protractors, the abdominal muscles, and, with the arms beginning in the overhead position, the glenohumeral extensors.
- *Exercises 46 through 48*. Exercises emphasizing sensorimotor integration, quickness, and speed of movement.

Exercise 1—Prone Lying Scapular Retraction

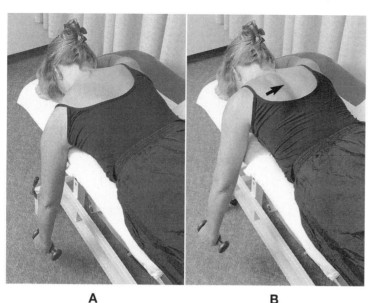

Beginning Position: Lie in a comfortable prone position with a light weight in hand. The table height permits complete scapular protraction without weight touching the floor. Retract scapula while the arm remains straight.

Focus: Isolated and complete scapular retraction.

Sequence: A, B, A, B, A.

A

B

Exercise 2—Prone Lying Humeral Extension and Scapular Retraction With Elbow Flexion

Beginning Position: Lie in a comfortable prone position with a light weight in hand. The table height permits complete scapular protraction without weight touching the floor. Extend humerus while flexing elbow and then retract the scapula. Perform one or more scapular retractions before returning to the starting position.

Focus: Complete scapular retraction.

Sequence: A, B, C, B, C, B, A.

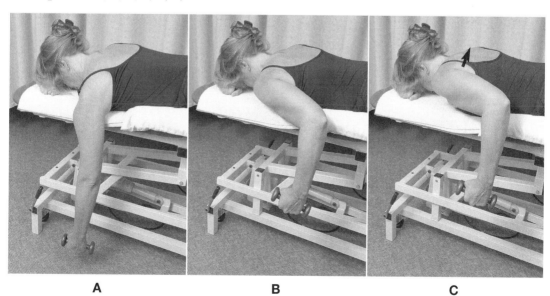

A

B

C

Exercise 3—Prone Lying Humeral Abduction

Beginning Position: Lie in a comfortable prone position with a light weight in hand. The table height permits complete scapular protraction without weight touching the floor. Abduct and externally rotate the humerus to horizontal position and then retract the scapula. Perform one or more scapular retractions before returning to the starting position.

Focus: Complete scapular retraction and external rotation of the humerus.

Sequence: A, B, C, D, C, D, C, B, A.

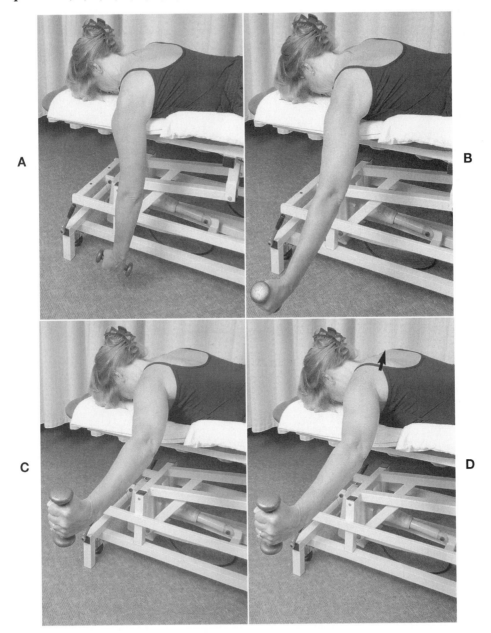

Exercise 4—Prone Lying Forward Humeral Elevation

Beginning Position: Lie in a comfortable prone position with a light weight in hand. The table height permits complete scapular protraction without weight touching the floor. Forward elevate and externally rotate the humerus with final scapular upward rotation and retraction.

Focus: Complete scapular upward rotation.

Sequence: A, B, C, B, A.

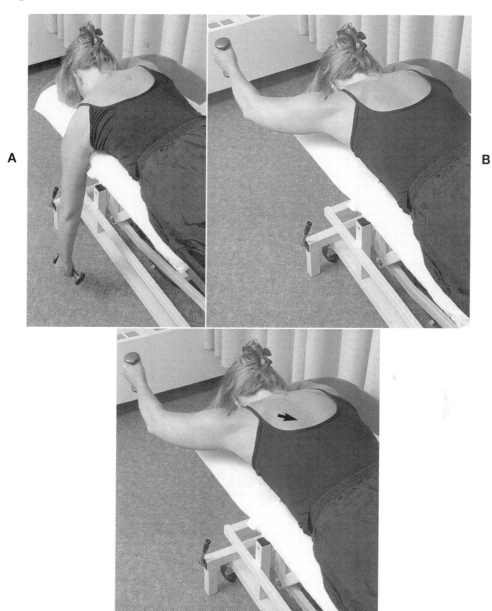

A

B

C

Exercise 5—Prone Lying Resisted Scaption

Beginning Position: Lie in a fully supported position on a table high enough that the arms can hang down freely. Flex, abduct, and externally rotate the humerus to the horizontal position. Hold arm position isometrically, pause, and then perform a few complete repetitions of scapular retraction and humeral external rotation. Pause and reverse.

Focus: Externally rotating the humerus and the quality of scapular motion.

Sequence: A, B, C, D, C, D, B, A.

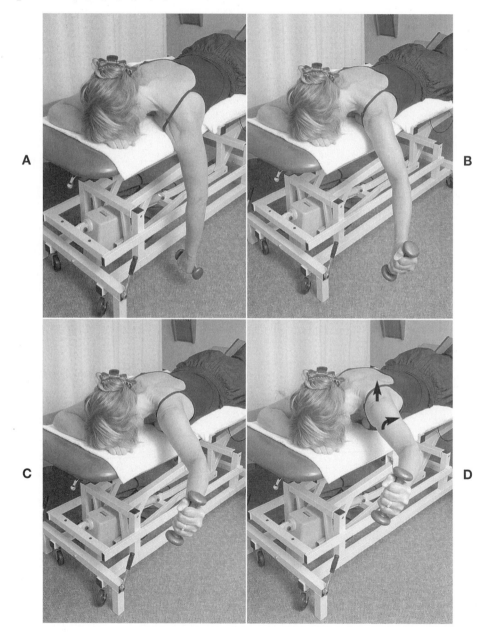

Exercise 6—Prone Lying Humeral Extension With Internal Rotation

Beginning Position: Lie in a comfortable prone position with a light weight in hand. The table height permits complete scapular protraction without weight touching the floor. Extend and slightly internally rotate humerus to the horizontal position, and then retract the scapula. Perform one or more scapular retractions before returning to the starting position.

Focus: Complete scapular retraction.

Sequence: A, B, C, D, C, D, C, B, A.

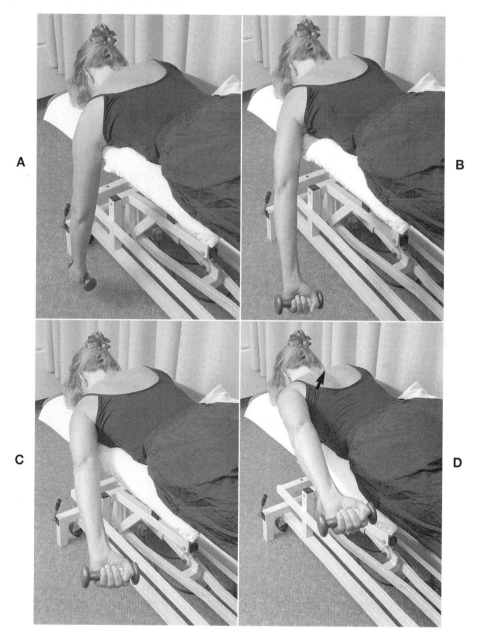

Exercise 7—Prone Lying Humeral Extension With External Rotation

Beginning Position: Lie in a comfortable prone position with a light weight in hand. The table height permits complete scapular protraction without weight touching the floor. Extend while externally rotating the humerus. Pause and retract the scapula. Perform one or more scapular retractions before returning to the starting position.

Focus: Complete scapular retraction.

Sequence: A, B, C, D, C, D, B, A.

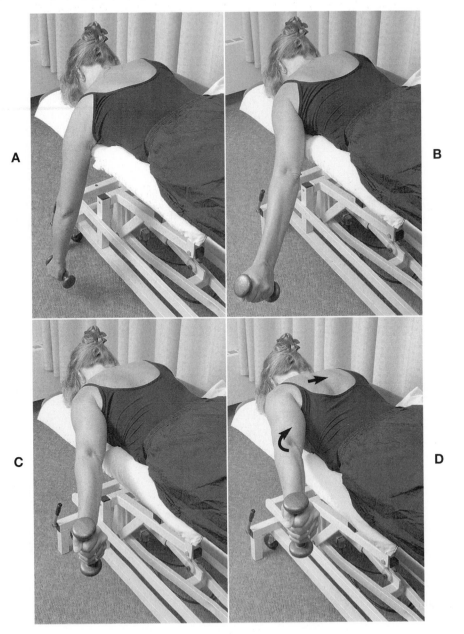

Exercise 8—Seated Scapular Elevation and Retraction With Dumbbells

Beginning Position: Sit up straight with a dumbbell in each hand; scapulae are fully depressed. Elevate and retract scapulae, keeping arms straight. Pause and reverse.

Focus: Isolating the motion to the scapulae, and the last portion of scapular elevation and retraction (up and back, squeeze).

Sequence: A, B, A.

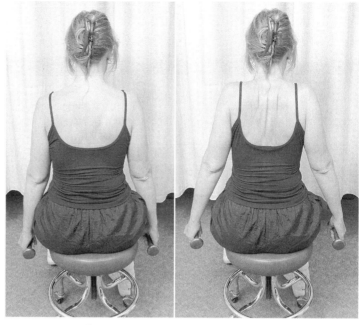

A   B

Exercise 9—Seated Humeral Forward Elevation

Beginning Position: Sit up straight with a dumbbell in each hand. Forward elevate and externally rotate the humerus in the scapular plane until weights are overhead. Vary planes of motion from straight abduction to humeral flexion.

Focus: External rotation of humerus during humeral forward elevation.

Sequence: A, B, C, B, A.

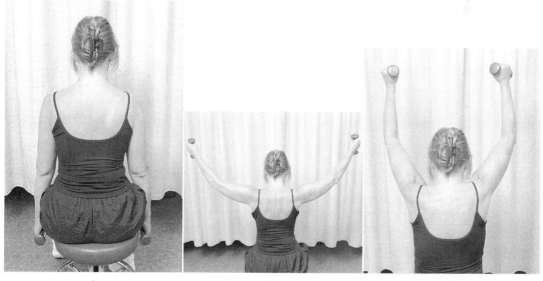

A   B   C

Exercise 10—Seated Forward Elevation and Upward Rotation of the Scapula

A
B

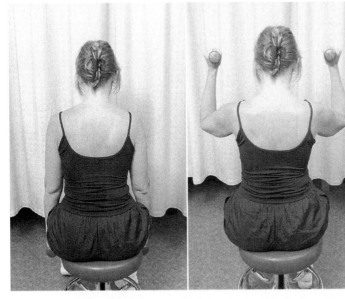

C

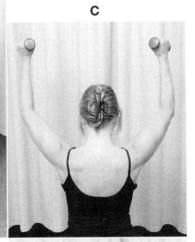

Beginning Position: Sit up straight with a dumbbell in each hand. Flex elbows and abduct humerus in scapular plane; push dumbbells overhead. Keep forearms in a neutral position. Push the front of the dumbbell up in a curvilinear motion, rotating the scapulae upward as high as possible (squeeze). Pause and retract scapulae, keeping arms straight. Repeat a number of times, then return arms to the starting position.

Focus: Isolating the movement to the scapulae and completing the range in forward elevation. The focal point is the interior angle of the scapulae.

Sequence: A, B, C, D, C, D, C, B, A.

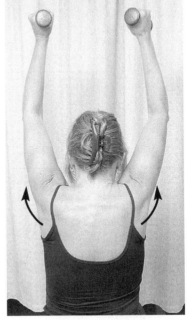

D

Exercise 11—Seated Scapular Elevation and Retraction With Humeral Abduction and External Rotation Using Dumbbells

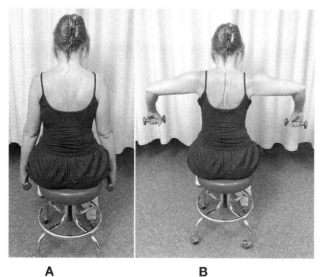

A   **B**

Beginning Position: Sit up straight with a dumbbell in each hand; scapulae are fully depressed. Elevate and retract scapulae; abduct and slightly externally rotate the humerus. Squeeze, pause, and reverse.

Focus: Slight external rotation of the humerus after full scapular elevation (up and back, squeeze, pause, reverse).

Sequence: A, B, A.

Exercise 12—Single-Armed Dumbbell Row

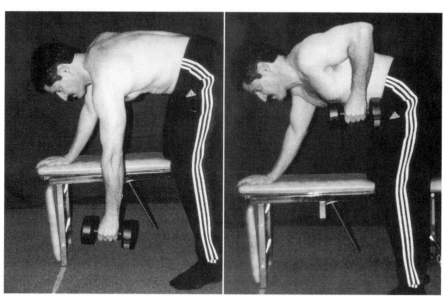

A   **B**

Beginning Position: Place one knee and ipsilateral arm on bench with other foot on the floor, and place dumbbell in the other hand with the left scapula fully protracted. Flex elbow, extend humerus, retract the scapula, and slightly rotate trunk. Make sure to maintain the midrange position of the contralateral scapula and lumbar spine.

Focus: Full scapular retraction.

Sequence: A, B, A.

Exercise 13—Seated Row, High Range With No Spinal Motion

Beginning Position: Sit up straight with scapulae fully protracted. Extend the humerus and retract the scapulae (do not extend lumbar spine past the neutral position). Pull cable to eye level. Pause and reverse.

Focus: The last portion of scapular retraction.

Sequence: A, B, C, B, A.

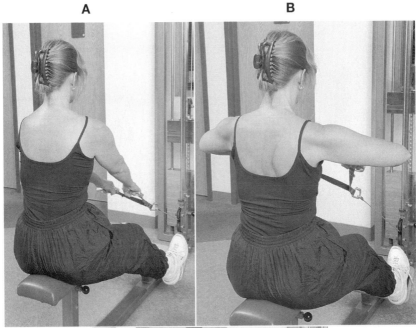

A   **B**

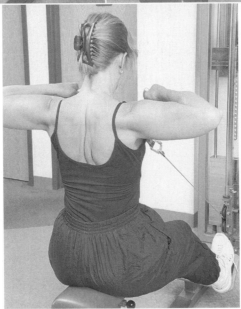

C

Exercise 14—Seated Row, Midrange With Trunk Flexed

Beginning Position: Sit and bend forward with spine flexed and scapulae fully protracted. Slightly extend the head, pull the humerus and scapulae back, sit up straight (do not extend the lumbar spine past the neutral position), and retract (squeeze) both scapulae. Pull cable to lower rib cage. Pause and reverse.

Focus: The last portion of scapular retraction.

Sequence: A, B, C, D, C, B, A or E, F, E.

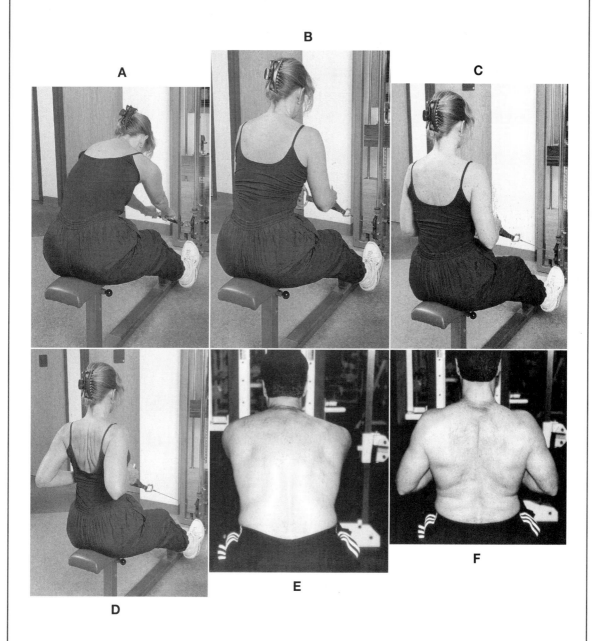

Exercise 15—Seated Row, High Range With Trunk Flexed

Beginning Position: Sit and bend forward with spine flexed and scapulae fully protracted. Slightly extend the head and neck, extend the humerus, retract the scapulae, and extend the spine to the neutral position (do not extend the lumbar spine past the neutral position). Pull cable high to eye level. Pause and reverse.

Focus: The last portion of scapular retraction (squeeze).

Sequence: A, B, C, B, A.

A   B

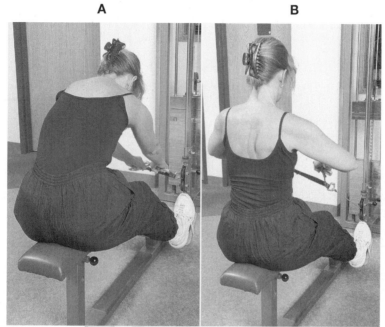

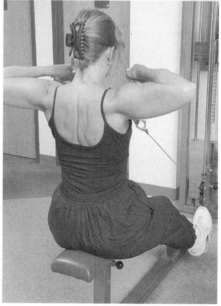

C

Exercise 16—Latissimus Dorsi Pull-Down, Wide Grip

Beginning Position: Sit up straight and use wide grip; stabilize thighs under pad. Lean back and pull cable down to mid-chest. Pause and reverse.

Focus: Pulling bar down in front, and scapular depression and retraction.

Sequence: A, B, C, B, A or D, E, D.

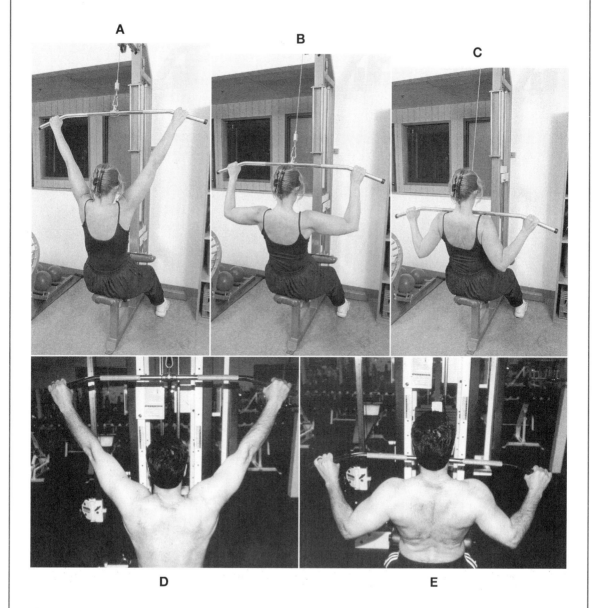

Exercise 17—Latissimus Dorsi Pull-Down, Narrow Grip

Beginning Position: Sit up straight and use narrow grip; stabilize thighs under pad. Lean back and pull cable down to mid-chest. Pause and reverse. NOTE: Compared with the wide grip lat pull-down, this position and movement can produce more force and may need more resistance.

Focus: Pulling handle down in front, and scapular depression and retraction.

Sequence: A, B, C, D, C, B, A.

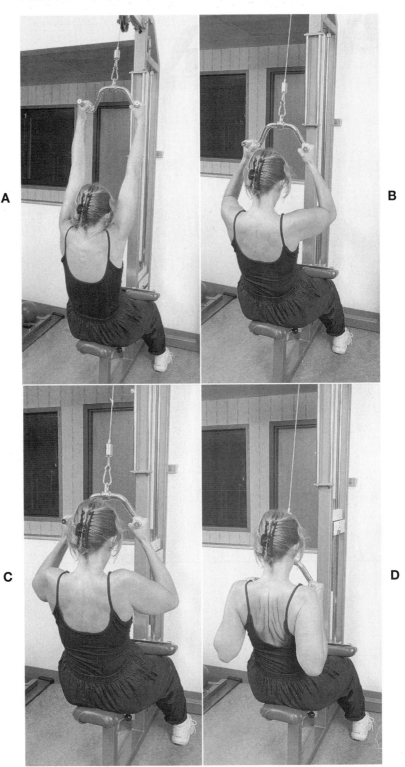

Exercise 18—Pull-Up, Gravity Assisted

Beginning Position: Stand on platform. Flex, abduct, and externally rotate humerus, and grasp bar. Extend and adduct humerus, and downwardly rotate the scapulae. NOTE: This exercise requires specialized equipment that permits adjustment to counterbalance (minimize) body weight.

Focus: Complete coordinated, smooth motion.

Sequence: A, B, C, B, A.

A   B

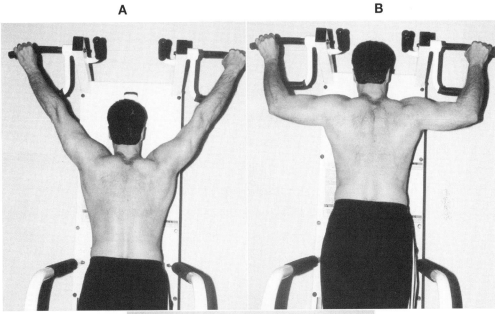

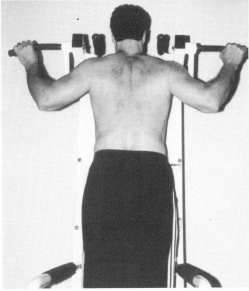

C

Exercise 19—Standing High Row, Midrange

Beginning Position: Stand with one foot forward and both scapulae fully protracted and elevated. Slightly flex trunk. Pull cable down to the zyphoid process of the sternum while transferring weight to back foot and retract the scapulae. Pause and slowly reverse. Do not extend the lumbar spine.

Focus: Retraction and downward rotation of the scapulae.

Sequence: A, B, C, D, C, B, A.

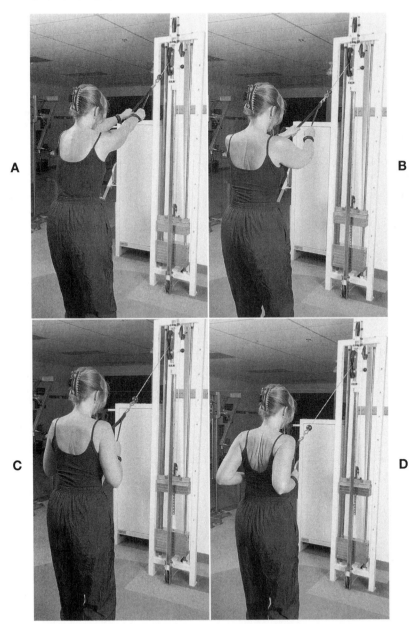

Exercise 20—Standing High Row, Low Range

Beginning Position: Stand with foot forward and scapulae fully protracted and elevated. Pull cable down to mid-thighs while transferring weight to back foot, pull rib cage slightly down toward the top of the pelvis (crunch), and extend humerus and retract scapulae.

Focus: Slight trunk flexion (crunch) and scapular retraction at the end.

Sequence: A, B, C, D, C, B, A.

OR

Focus: Emphasize scapular depression and trunk flexion.

Sequence: A, B, C, E, F, C, B, A.

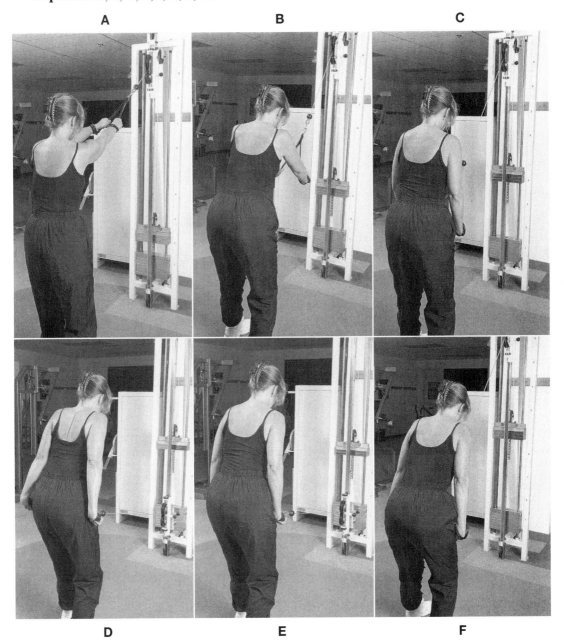

A   B   C

D   E   F

Exercise 21—Standing Two-Handed Diagonal High Row

Beginning Position: Stand facing pulley, then turn left to a 90-degree angle from the pulley. Reach up across with both hands (note hand placement) and pull cable down and across. NOTE: The motion is an 80% push with the top (right) hand and a 20% pull with the bottom (left) hand. Use varying degrees of motion. Slow down and even stop a few times during the eccentrics to enhance the training effect.

Focus: Smooth and controlled weight transfer passing from the closest foot to the pulley to the back foot while flexing and slightly rotating the trunk with full scapular protraction.

Sequence: A, B, C, D, C, B, A.

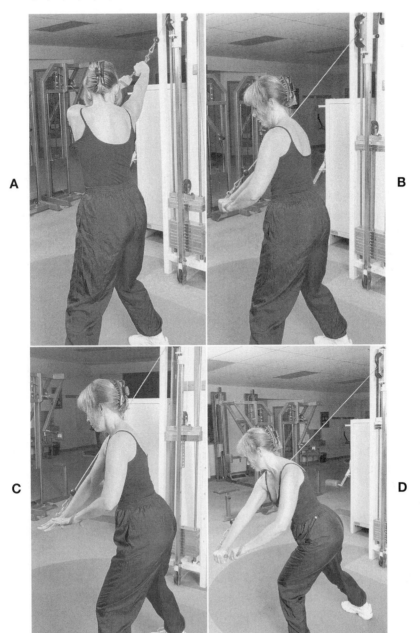

Exercise 22—Standing One-Armed Diagonal High Row
With External Rotation

Beginning Position: Stand facing pulley, then turn left to a 90-degree angle from the pulley. Reach up across with scapula fully protracted and upwardly rotated. Pull cable down, high to low, extending and externally rotating the humerus while retracting and depressing the scapula and rotating the trunk. Use varying degrees of motion.

Focus: Smooth and controlled weight transfer, and scapular retraction and trunk rotation at the end.

Sequence: A, B, C, B, A.

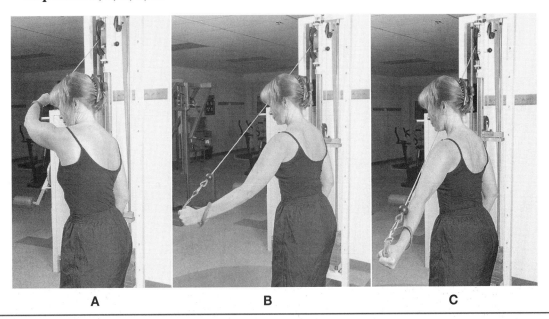

A   B   C

Exercise 23—Standing Mid-Row, Midrange

Beginning Position: Stand with one foot forward and both scapulae fully protracted. Pull the cable straight back to belt line while transferring weight to back foot. Pause and reverse.

Focus: Full scapular retraction (squeeze).

Sequence: A, B, C, B, A.

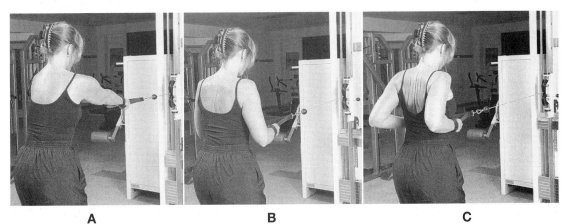

A   B   C

Exercise 24—Standing Mid-Row, High Range

Beginning Position: Stand with one foot forward and both scapulae fully protracted. Pull the cable back and up to chin level, and squeeze the scapulae together. Pause and reverse.
Focus: The smoothness of scapular motion and the tight squeeze at the end of the motion.
Sequence: A, B, C, D, C, B, A.

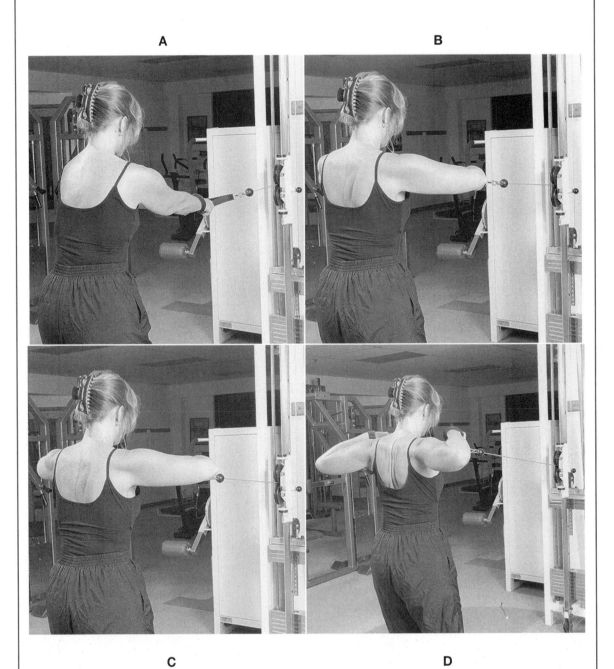

A

B

C

D

Exercise 25—Standing Mid-Row, Low Range

Beginning Position: Stand with one foot slightly forward and scapulae fully protracted. Arms are straight. While transferring weight from the front foot to the back foot, pull the cable to mid-thighs by extending and depressing the humerus and flexing the trunk (crunch) at the end.
Focus: Humeral depression and crunch at the end.
Sequence: A, B, C, D, C, B, A.

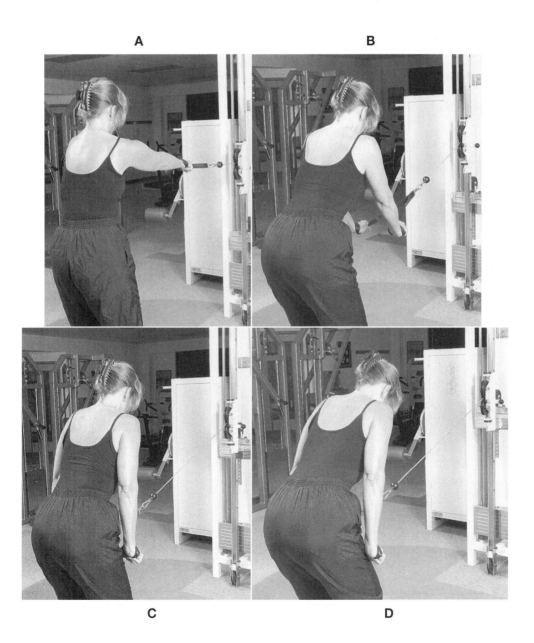

A

B

C

D

Exercise 26—Standing One-Armed Mid-Row, Midrange With External Rotation

Beginning Position: Stand facing pulley, then turn left to a 90-degree angle from the pulley. Reach across body with scapula fully protracted. Pull cable straight across, extending and externally rotating the humerus, retracting the scapula, and slightly rotating the trunk. Use varying degrees of humeral motion and trunk flexion.

Focus: Smooth and controlled weight transfer, and humeral external rotation and scapular retraction.

Sequence: A, B, C, B, A.

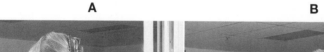

A   B

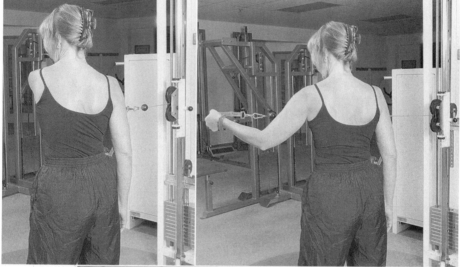

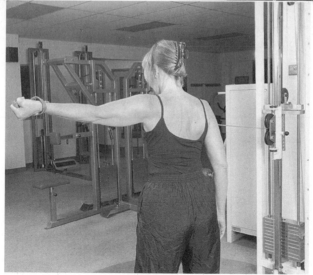

C

Exercise 27—Standing One-Armed Diagonal Mid-Row With Increased Trunk Motion

Beginning Position: Stand facing pulley, then turn to a 90-degree angle from the pulley. Bend forward, side bend to the right, slightly rotate trunk to the right, and transfer weight to the right foot with scapula fully protracted. Pull up and out, transferring weight from the right foot to the left foot and extending, abducting, and externally rotating the humerus while at the same time retracting the scapula. Pause and protract the scapula forward (lunge). Use varying degrees of motion.

Focus: Smooth and controlled weight transfer, and scapular retraction, stabilization, and protraction at the end.

Sequence: A, B, C, B, A.

A

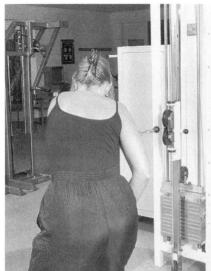

B

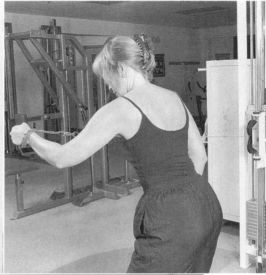

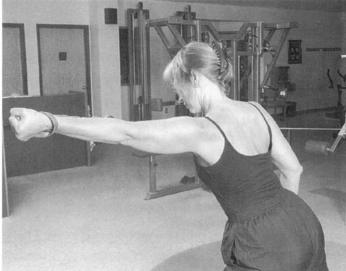

C

Exercise 28—Standing One-Armed Punch

Beginning Position: Stand facing away from pulley with one foot (left) forward, humerus extended, elbow fully flexed, scapula fully retracted, and trunk rotated to the right. Transfer weight forward onto the front foot while performing a horizontal punch. Pause, then perform a few repetitions of scapular protraction before returning to the starting position.
Focus: Smooth and controlled weight transfer and complete scapular protraction at endrange.
Sequence: A, B, C, D, C, B, A.

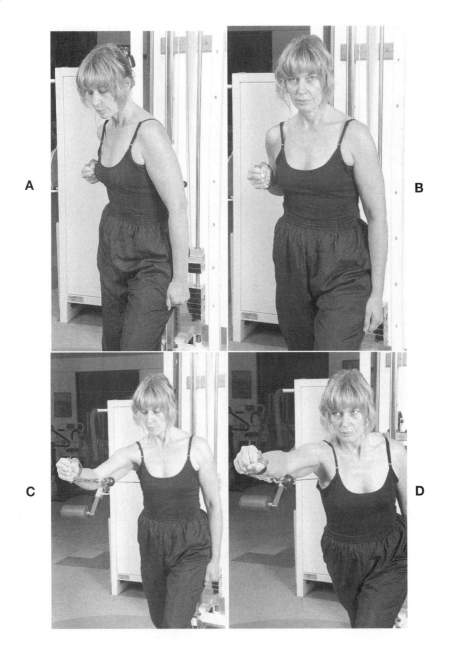

Exercise 29—Standing Low Row, High Range

Beginning Position: Stand with one foot forward and flex knee, hip, and lumbar and cervical spine. Slightly extend the head, extend and abduct the humerus, retract and elevate the scapula, and pull cable to the middle of the eyes. Pause and reverse; return to starting position with smooth and controlled motion.

Focus: Spinal extension and smooth weight transfer.

Sequence: A, B, C, D, E, D, C, B, A.

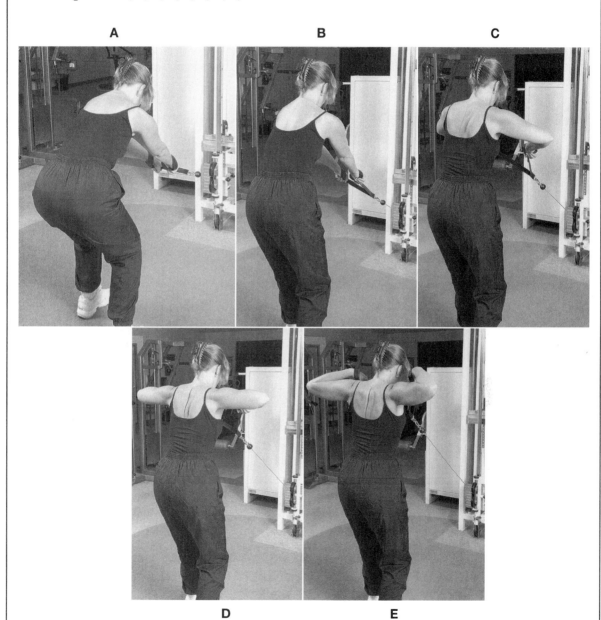

A   B   C

D   E

Exercise 30—Standing Low Row, Midrange

Beginning Position: Stand with one foot forward, slightly flex spine, and fully protract scapula. Slightly extend the spine, transfer weight to back foot, and retract the scapula while pulling cable to the belt line.

Focus: Transfer weight to back foot without extending the lumbar spine past the neutral position and complete scapular retraction.

Sequence: A, B, C, D, C, B, A.

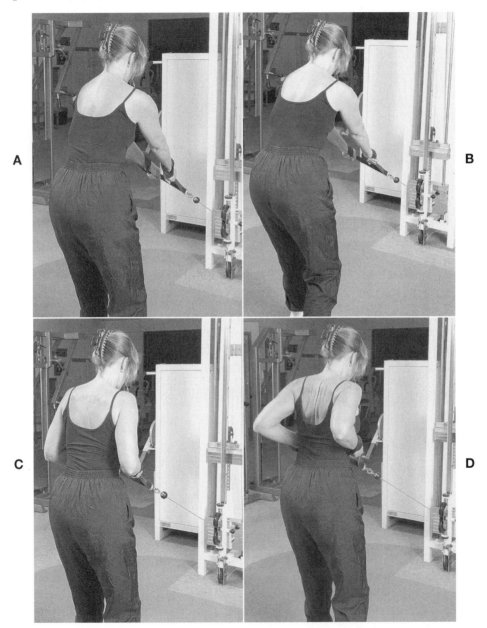

Exercise 31—Standing Low Row, Scapular Elevation

Beginning Position: Stand with neck and thoracic spine slightly flexed and scapulae fully protracted, depressed, and downwardly rotated. Pull scapulae straight up and back. Pause and reverse. Permit elbows to flex only slightly.

Focus: Elevating and retracting the scapulae.

Sequence: A, B, A.

OR

Beginning Position: Stand with neck and thoracic spine slightly flexed and scapula fully depressed and downwardly rotated. Pull scapulae up, flex elbows, and bring hands to the chin. Pause and reverse. Abduct while extending the humerus.

Focus: Elevating and retracting the scapulae by emphasizing the final scapular "pinch."

Sequence: A, B, C, D, C, B, A.

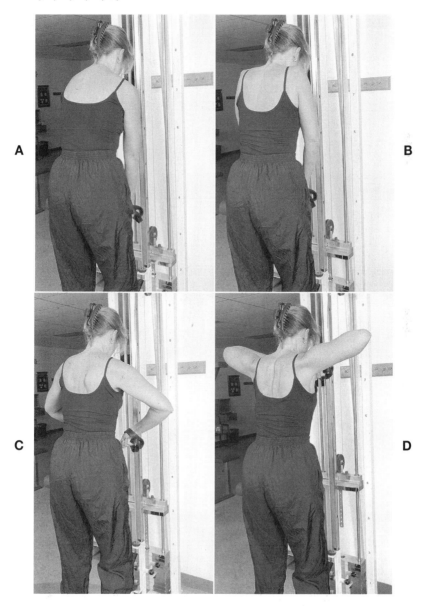

Exercise 32—Standing One-Armed Diagonal Low Row

Beginning Position: Stand facing pulley, then turn left to a 90-degree angle from the pulley. Flex and slightly rotate trunk to the right with scapula fully protracted. Pull cable up, low to high, extending and externally rotating the humerus, retracting and elevating the scapula, and rotating the trunk. Use varying degrees of motion.

Focus: Smooth and controlled weight transfer, trunk rotation, and scapular elevation and retraction at the end.

Sequence: A, B, C, B, A.

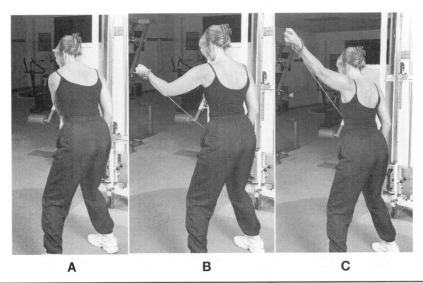

A   B   C

Exercise 33—Standing Humeral Abduction, External Rotation

A   B

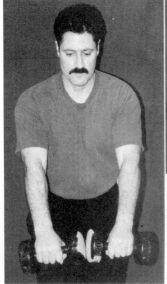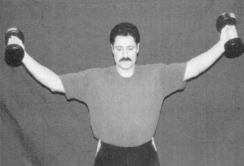

Beginning Position: Stand with one foot in front and dumbbell in each hand, stabilize the trunk, and rotate humerus internally. Forward elevate and externally rotate the humerus and retract the scapulae. Begin moving in the scaption plane. Pause and return to the starting position, making sure to internally rotate the humerus and touch the ends of the dumbbell. Vary the plane of motion.

Focus: Scapular elevation and retraction and humeral rotation.

Sequence: A, B, A.

Exercise 34—Standing Diagonal Low Row, Bilateral

Beginning Position: Stand in the middle and slightly back between two low pulleys. Slightly flex trunk, cross arms, and grasp opposite handles. Slightly extend trunk and abduct and externally rotate the humerus. Retract and elevate the scapulae. Be careful not to extend lumbar spine beyond the neutral position.

Focus: Coordinated, smooth movement and complete scapular elevation and retraction.

Sequence: A, B, C, B, A.

A   B

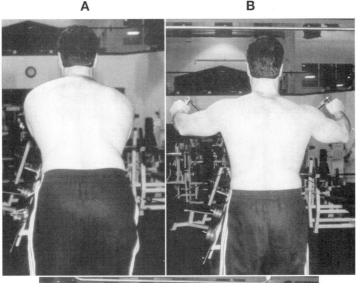

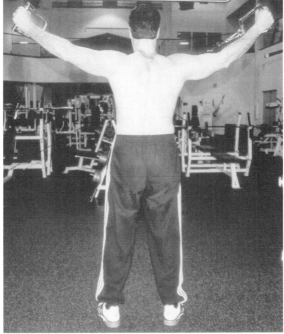

C

Exercise 35—Seated Diagonal Low Row, Bilateral

Beginning Position: Sit on a chair or inflated ball between two low pulleys. Stabilize trunk and equalize weight between the pelvis and feet. Cross arms and grasp opposite handles. Abduct and externally rotate the humerus and retract and elevate the scapulae. Pause. Be careful not to extend lumbar spine beyond the neutral position.
Focus: Coordinated, smooth movement and complete scapular elevation and retraction.
Sequence: A, B, A.

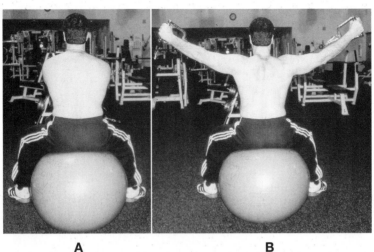

A   B

Exercise 36—Seated Dumbbell Curls

Beginning Position: Sit on the edge of the bench or chair, one foot forward and the other back. Shift weight forward over feet, dumbbell in each hand and elbows straight with wrists pronated. Supinate and flex one elbow. As you lower arm, begin to flex the other arm. Learn to develop a smooth (no pause) movement.
Focus: Sustain trunk and scapular position.
Sequence: A, B, A, B.

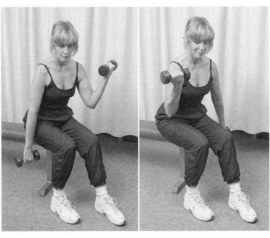

A   B

Exercise 37—Supine Flys

Beginning Position: Lie on a narrow bench with feet comfortably placed either on the floor or up on the bench. With a dumbbell in each hand, slowly lower the weight as the elbows flex and the humerus abducts to horizontal position. Push up while externally rotating the humerus and supinating the forearm slowly until the bottoms of the dumbbells touch. Pause and slowly return to the horizontal position.

Focus: Rotary motion required to touch the bottoms of the dumbbells. Do not go down beyond the horizontal position.

Sequence: A, B, C, B, C, B, A.

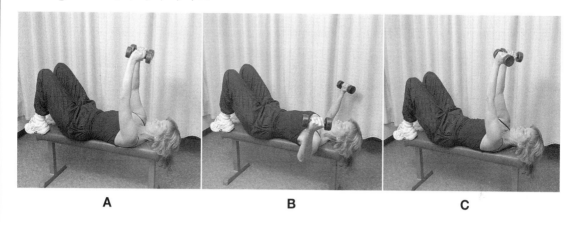

A   B   C

Exercise 38—Inclined Bench Press

Beginning Position: Lie on an inclined bench, holding a barbell across the chest. Push straight up and forward, making sure that the humerus tracks in midrange and the scapulae are completely protracted. Pause and return to the horizontal position. Be cautious when extending the humerus below the horizontal position.

Focus: Complete scapular motion and full but safe range of humeral motion.

Sequence: A, B, A.

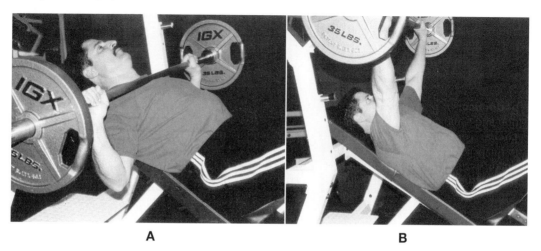

A   B

Exercise 39—Diagonal Push-Ups

Beginning Position: Stand and lean on a high countertop or the wall. Start with scapulae fully protracted. Keep arms straight and fully retract and protract scapulae. Pause at the endrange.
Focus: Complete protraction.
Sequence: A, B, C, B, A.

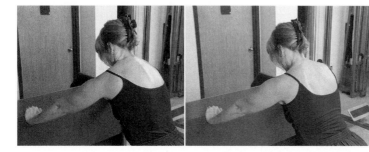
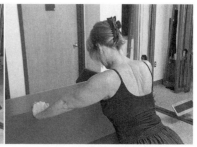

A   **B**   **C**

Exercise 40—Push-Ups

Beginning Position: Use a medicine ball and assume a push-up position. Accomplish three movements: **A,** with arms straight, protract and retract scapulae, **B,** slowly flex the elbows, lowering the chest toward the ball, and **C,** push up, making sure to fully protract the scapulae.
Focus: Movement of the scapulae around the rib cage.
Sequence: A, B, C

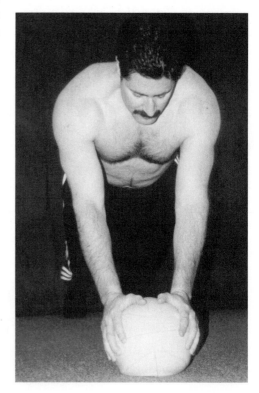

Exercise 41—Supine Lying Resisted Humeral Extension

Beginning Position: Lie on a narrow bench with feet comfortably placed either on the floor or up on the bench with arms extended and holding a weight. Slowly permit the weight to fall back overhead. Take the weight to the desired endrange of motion. Permit the rib cage to rise. Pause and return by first pulling the rib cage, and then the arms, up to the starting position. Bending the elbows lessens the resistance.

Focus: Abdominal activity at the rib cage, either isometric or dynamic.

Sequence: A, B, A.

A

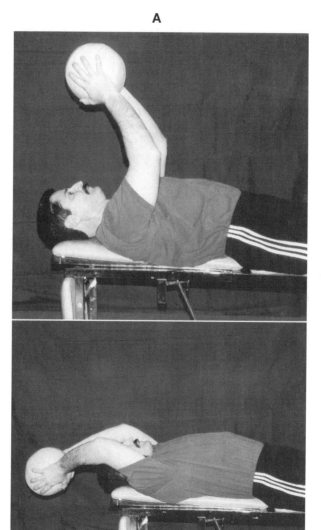

B

Exercise 42—Supine Lying Resisted Humeral Extension, Combined

Beginning Position: Lie on a narrow bench with feet comfortably placed either on the floor or up on the bench and arms straight and holding a weight (dumbbell). Slowly permit the weight to fall back overhead. Take it to the desired endrange of motion. Permit the rib cage to rise. Pause and return by first pulling the rib cage, and then the arms, up to the starting position. Continue the movement by pushing the front of the dumbbell up in a curvilinear motion, rotating the scapula forward and upward. Tuck chin, slightly flex trunk, and complete the scapular motion (squeeze). Pause and retract scapulae, extend the humerus (keeping arms straight), and permit the weight to move overhead.

Focus: Coordinated, smooth, complete motion. Focal point is the abdominal contraction (isometric or dynamic) at the rib cage and movement of the inferior angle of the scapulae.

Sequence: A, B, A, C, D, C, A.

A   B

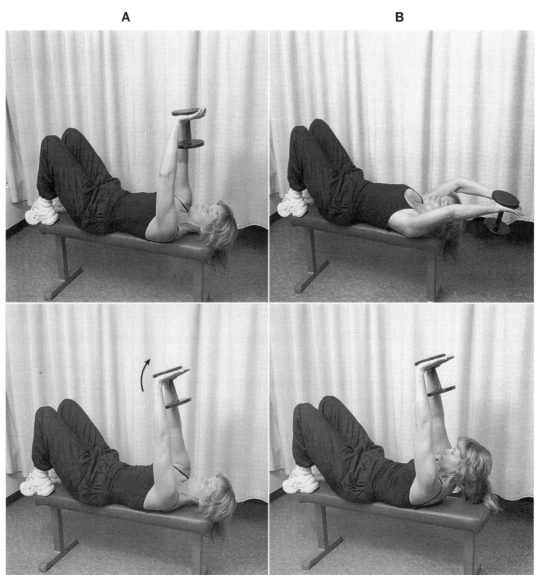

C   D

Exercise 43—Supine Lying Scapular Protraction, Isolated

Beginning Position: Lie on a narrow bench with feet comfortably placed either on the floor or up on the bench. Hold dumbbells with arms straight. Push the front of the dumbbells up in a curvilinear motion, rotating the scapulae forward and upward. Tuck chin, slightly flex trunk, and complete the scapular motion (squeeze). Pause and retract scapulae, keeping arms straight.
Focus: Isolating movement to and complete forward elevation of the scapulae. Focal point is movement of the inferior angle of the scapulae.
Sequence: A, B, A, B, A.

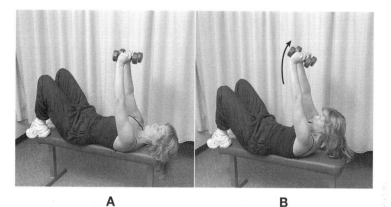

A   B

Exercise 44—Upward Rotation of the Scapula

Beginning Position: Sit with dumbbell or on special equipment. Elevate humerus forward to approximately 140 degrees. Push weight up and forward. Pause and return to straight arm position.
Focus: Curvilinear motion isolated to the scapula. Focal point is the inferior angle of the scapula.
Sequence: A, B, A, B, A.

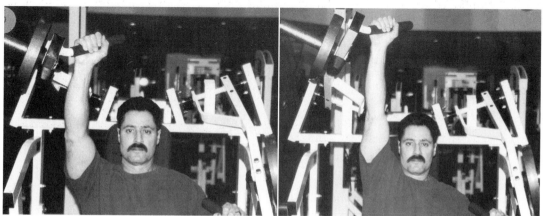

A   B

Exercise 45—Supine Lying Resisted Push

Beginning Position: Lie on a narrow bench with feet comfortably placed either on the floor or up on the bench. Flex elbows and hold dumbbell close to chest. Extend elbows and protract the scapulae. Slightly tuck chin, push weight in a curvilinear motion up, and pull rib cage down toward the pelvis (crunch). Complete range of motion and return to the starting position, permitting weight to just barely touch chest.

Focus: Coordinated, smooth, complete motion.

Sequence: A, B, C, D, C, B, A.

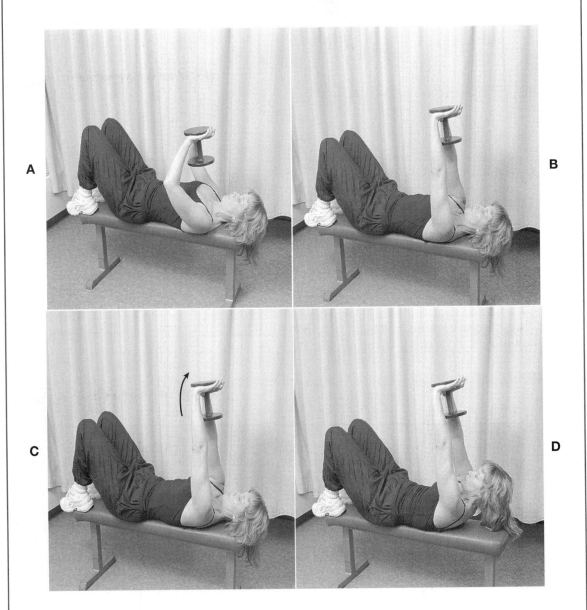

A B

C D

Exercise 46—Resisted Functional Training (Tramp), Two-Handed Straight On

Beginning Position: Stand facing the inclined trampoline, one foot forward. With both hands, throw and retrieve a weighted ball into the trampoline. Vary the range of motion (high, low, side-to-side).
Focus: Loads imparted to the shoulder and the smooth transfer of weight through the spine.
Sequence: A, B, A, C, D, C, A.

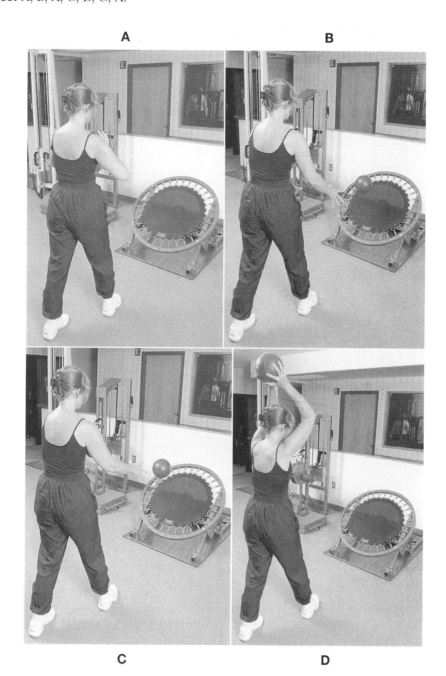

A

B

C

D

Exercise 47—Resisted Functional Training (Tramp), One-Handed Diagonal With Isolated Movement

Beginning Position: Stand facing the inclined trampoline, then turn left to a 90-degree angle from the trampoline. Throw and retrieve a weighted ball into the trampoline. Vary the range of motion (high, low) and gradually use as much of the spine and lower body as possible.

Focus: Loads imparted to the shoulder and the smooth transfer of weight through the spine.

Sequence: A, B, C, D, B, C, A.

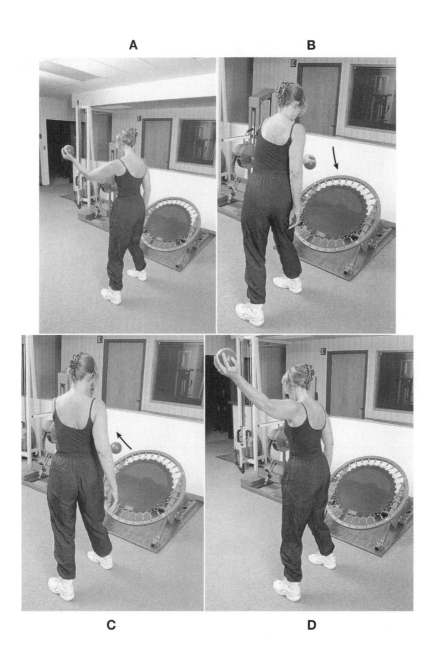

Exercise 48—Resisted Functional Training (Tramp), One-Handed Diagonal With Full Movement

Beginning Position: Stand facing the inclined trampoline, then turn left to a 90-degree angle from the trampoline. Throw and retrieve a weighted ball into the trampoline. Vary the range of motion (high, low) and gradually use as much of the spine and lower body as possible.

Focus: Loads imparted to the shoulder and the smooth transfer of weight through the spine.

Sequence: A, B, A, B, C, A, B, A.

A   **B**

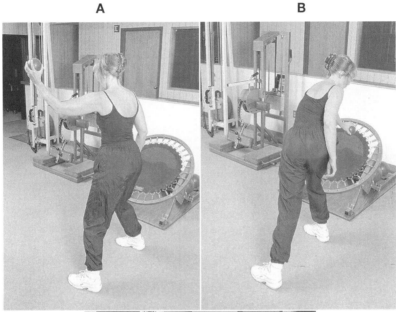

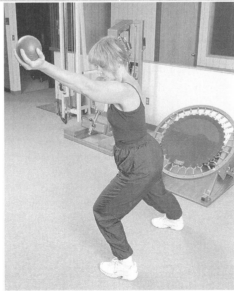

C

CLINICAL EXAMPLES: PATHWAYS OF CARE FOR SHOULDER DISORDERS CORRELATED WITH THE OBJECTIVES OF TREATMENT

Impingement Syndromes and Disorders Related to Soft Tissues of the Coracoacromial Arch: Nonsurgical Management

We discussed the pathomechanics contributing to impingement syndromes in previous chapters because many interventions focus on altering those mechanical factors that might contribute to compromise of tissues in the subacromial space. The problem arc is typically forward rather than lateral, with impingement occurring against the anterior third of the acromion and inferior aspect of the acromioclavicular joint. The structures most commonly involved are the supraspinatus tendon, the anterior aspect of the infraspinatus tendon, the bursal covering associated with these two tendons, and the long head of the biceps tendon. Several biomechanical considerations guide the clinician in the development of a comprehensive treatment plan:

- Scapulothoracic muscle weakness contributes to increased stress of the soft tissues in the subacromial space through failure to provide scapular stability; muscle weakness results in a relatively downwardly rotated position and protracted position during shoulder motions, leading to subacromial impingement.
- Glenohumeral joint capsular restrictions result in the inability of the humerus to remain centered on the glenoid during humeral movements and the loss of the ability of the glenohumeral joint to reach the degree of external rotation required to allow the greater tuberosity to be positioned behind the acromion process during overhead activities (see Chapter 4).
- Rotator cuff weakness or early fatigue of the cuff musculature results in the inability of the musculature to center and maintain the head of humerus within the glenoid fossa during glenohumeral motion (see Chapter 3).
- Excessive tensile loading that may occur with deceleration activities results in significant stress placed on the posterior rotator cuff muscles during the deceleration phase of throwing, especially the

supraspinatus, infraspinatus, and teres minor; tendon attrition begins, and tearing can be a sequelae.

The objective of treatment that is the primary focus during the initial patient treatment session is effective *modulation of pain*. Pain and swelling must be controlled first before addressing the mechanics associated with impingement. There are several ways to control pain and the associated inflammatory response:

- Nonsteroidal antiinflammatory drugs (NSAIDs)
- Ice, which is particularly effective following the application of cross friction techniques
- Phonophoresis or iontophoresis: these modalities can be effective because the subacromial region of the shoulder is relatively subcutaneous; when applying these modalities, the following patient positioning should be considered in order to optimize exposure of the medicinal ions:

1. Subacromial exposure—the best exposure is with hand in small of back, but care must be taken that excessive adduction of humerus does not occur.
2. Biceps long head—the best exposure is with the humerus in slight external rotation and hyperextension.

- Injection of inflammation reducing agents into the subacromial space
- Grade I and II accessory mobilizations to provide mechanoreceptor input into the joint, potentially modulating pain

The next objective of treatment to implement is the clinician's application of *passive and active stresses to promote and encourage pain-free, active movements* by the patient. This is an extremely important objective because often it directly deals with the shoulder pathomechanics considered to be contributing factors to the syndrome. The following list summarizes some of the most strategic interventions to consider:

- *Stretching of the glenohumeral joint capsule in order to increase all physiological motions, especially external rotation.* External rotation of the glenohumeral joint is essential to clear the greater tuberosity from under the head of the humerus during overhead motion; to be most effective with this passive stretching technique, use varying degrees of flexion and abduction with the stretches into external rotation.
- *Accessory motion joint mobilization techniques of the glenohumeral joint both in the neutral position and in varying*

degrees of glenohumeral elevation. The accessory mobilization maneuvers need to be translations of the head of the humerus on the glenoid in the anterior, posterior, and inferior directions. If the intent of joint mobilization maneuvers is to modulate pain, the techniques should be applied with the glenohumeral joint in the loose packed position. If the intent is to increase the mobility of the glenohumeral joint capsule, then the techniques should be applied with the glenohumeral joint in varying degrees and planes of glenohumeral elevation.

- *Stretching of pectoralis major muscle.* This is indicated if the examiner notes adaptive changes of the soft tissues of the anterior shoulder girdle that are contributing to the forward head, rounded shoulder posture; an internally rotated humerus, such as might occur with tightness of the pectoralis major muscle, will increase compression under the coracoacromial arch during any forward elevation movements.
- *Stretching of pectoralis minor.* This might also be necessary as a result of the adaptive changes that occur with a rounded shoulder posture; a protracted scapula would require an even greater range of glenohumeral external rotation in order to provide clearance of the greater tuberosity from under the acromion during overhead movements.
- *Mobilization of the scapulothoracic articulation for a hypomobile scapulothoracic articulation in superior-inferior, protraction-retraction, and upward rotation–downward rotation motions.* Scapulothoracic hypomobility leads to increased glenohumeral compression stresses associated with repetitive overhead efforts.

There are several effective ways to stretch these tissues, from the prolonged passive stretch and oscillations for connective tissue structures to a contract-relax and hold-relax technique that affects the neuromuscular elements.

With the inflammatory process under reasonable control, the clinician can initiate treatment to *enhance neuromuscular performance.* Strengthening the rotator cuff musculature is often the primary focus, although it is essential to prescribe strengthening exercises for the muscles of the scapulothoracic articulation, especially the scapula retractors, elevators, and upward rotators, and the extrinsic muscles of the shoulder girdle. The rationale for emphasizing the rotator cuff muscles is to optimize their ability to maintain the central position of the head of the humerus in the glenoid fossa during motions that bring the arm overhead. We often

prefer to begin with rotator cuff strengthening before initiating strengthening of the extrinsic muscles because a weak rotator cuff in the presence of stronger extrinsic shoulder muscles results in superior migration of the humerus.

While isolated rotator cuff exercises can be a point from which to begin a resistance exercise program for the rotator cuff muscles, broad patterns of movement incorporating the intrinsic cuff muscles, extrinsic shoulder muscles, scapulothoracic muscles, abdominal mechanism, and spinal extensors are the most functional and practical way to progress the training effect for the muscles. The general principles of strengthening the rotator cuff muscles in the patient with impingement syndrome are to emphasize correct form and positioning, to stay within the pain-free range, to carefully observe the weight and repetitions to avoid muscle substitution, and to progressively incorporate eccentric activities in a carefully monitored manner. If tears of the rotator cuff muscles have already developed as a result of chronic deceleration stresses or impingement, the clinician must cautiously overload the muscles because a consequence of excessive overload may be an even greater tear of the rotator cuff.

Exercises mentioned in Chapter 3 and earlier in this chapter have an important training effect on the rotator cuff muscles. The specific muscles and related exercises considered to have an excellent training effect on them when monitored closely and performed with exacting shoulder girdle and trunk mechanics include:

- *Supraspinatus.* Military press activities and scaption exercises, both performed with the humerus in external rotation, are excellent functional exercises for training this muscle (we do not use an internally rotated glenohumeral joint position for any resisted shoulder elevation exercise).
- *Subscapularis.* Scaption exercises take advantage of the subscapularis function of centering the humeral head; additional exercises include internal rotation against the resistance of free weights or pulleys, military press exercise with the humerus maintained in external rotation, and shoulder flexion exercises. We prefer to avoid any positions of overhead motion against resistance without the humerus being maintained in external rotation. When the muscle fiber orientation of the subscapularis is closely examined, it is clear that pulling the arm down and across the body against resistance incorporates the trunk, extrinsic shoulder muscles, and intrinsic subscapularis muscle.

- *Infraspinatus and teres minor.* Horizontal abduction with external rotation, external rotation against resistance, scaption with external rotation, and shoulder deceleration exercises are all excellent ways to introduce a specific training stimulus to these key posterior cuff muscles.

Often the clinician prescribes exercises using resistance tubing or other elastic resistance. Use such exercise equipment cautiously with suspected rotator cuff injuries in impingement conditions because the resistance the tubing offers increases throughout range of motion. Thus the resistance force of the elastic increases as the muscle begins to lose its efficiency in the motion. This may place excessive stress on injured tissues.

Strengthening of scapular muscles is an essential but often overlooked aspect of exercise in the management of impingement disorders. The rationale for emphasizing strong upward rotators of the scapula is to ensure that the coracoacromial arch of the scapula moves up and away from the humeral head during shoulder motion. The primary upward rotators of the scapulothoracic articulation are the serratus anterior and the force couple provided by the upper and lower trapezius muscles.

Several exercises can be incorporated to maximize the training effect to specific muscles of the scapulothoracic articulation:

- *Serratus anterior.* "Bench press," or pushing motions against resistance with a strong protraction at end of motion; a push-up "plus," which is a standard push-up incorporating a strong protraction at the end of the motion; pullover exercises from the supine position; and complete shoulder arcs of motion through full range using light weights in order to emphasize upward rotation of the scapula are excellent exercises for the serratus anterior. The patient must be closely monitored with any exercises that require the humerus to elevate above the horizontal plane in order to avoid exacerbation of an impingement problem.
- *Trapezius, rhomboids, and levator scapula muscles.* Shoulder shrugs, scapula retraction pulling exercises such as one-arm rowing, emphasize the scapular retraction component of bilateral rows and pull downs; proprioceptive neuromuscular facilitation (PNF) patterns, which focus on scapular motion and setting of the scapula, are also effective manual resistance exercises for these muscles as well.

The remaining objective of treatment refers to *patient education in the form of biomechanical counseling.* By this, we mean teaching the patient those motions, positions, and activities that potentially compromise the soft tissues involved with the impingement syndrome. Very often the instructions given to the patient for this condition must be sport or occupation specific. For example, advise swimmers to decrease internal rotation of the arm as it enters the water (thumb should not enter water first), decrease their body roll during the freestyle and backstroke, and increase their body lift during the butterfly stroke. In addition, advise them to avoid using hand paddles because of the potential increased stress as a result of increased lever arm length acting over the shoulder.

In athletes involved in throwing sports, closely monitor the number of throws, pitches, the velocity of the throw, and the distance thrown. It is often wise to progress a thrower from gentle "lobs" to throws of incrementally increasing distance.

Teach overhead workers in the industrial setting to pay close attention to scapular strength, how much overhead work is being done, and how much repetitive stress occurs in their workstation. Small adjustments in the workstation can significantly change the stresses to the tissues of the shoulder, especially if the work requires prolonged overhead positioning or repetitive overhead motions.

Postsurgical Rehabilitation Considerations Related to Impingement Disorders: Rotator Cuff Tears and Subacromial Debridement

Surgery for shoulder impingement disorders is generally reserved for conditions classified as stages II and III in the Neer classification scheme for shoulder impingement (see Table 5-2). Decisions to operate on Stage II disorders are often reserved for the patient over 40 years of age. Types of surgery performed to decompress the suprahumeral space include excision of anterior third of acromion, release of coracoacromial ligament, rotator cuff tendon debridement, and bursectomy. The variability of the surgical approach, coupled with the varying degrees of cuff and subacromial debridement or reconstruction performed, makes a general discussion of rehabilitation difficult.

For ease of discussion, we will describe the rehabilitation concepts behind three surgical approaches of increasingly greater tissue disruption:

1. Arthroscopic debridement of the subacromial space
2. Arthroscopic debridement of the subacromial space and open cuff repair through separation of the fibers of the deltoid
3. Open repair via detachment of the deltoid from its clavicular and anterior acromial attachments

We have summarized the surgical approaches in this manner to emphasize that the rehabilitation for each of these varies not only in terms of time lines but also in the aggressiveness with which the patient can pursue active exercise and resistive exercise and return to sport or activities of daily living. Postsurgery rehabilitation for each of these patients begins with communication with the surgeon in order to gain an understanding of the specific tissues and the health of those tissues involved in the surgery. In all three conditions, the patient must understand that continuing his exercise program is essential for his condition, even after completing his course of rehabilitation.

In the postsurgical management following *arthroscopic debridement,* a more rapid recovery is expected because the deltoid attachment has not been compromised. We begin passive and active assistive motion immediately following surgery with a particular emphasis on external rotation. When performing passive glenohumeral elevations in any plane, we apply a very small inferior glide simultaneous with the elevation movements. Rotation exercises are relatively safe within the first 30 degrees of glenohumeral elevation, but above that level the clinician must carefully monitor rotations because they can simply "grind" the cuff tendons within the subacromial space.

Isometric exercises for the extrinsic and intrinsic shoulder muscles are also initiated immediately after surgery. When range of motion is full and relatively pain free, we then commence the use of free weights and pulleys to progressively strengthen the intrinsic, extrinsic, scapulothoracic, and trunk muscles. Depending on the degree of tissue surgically debrided or repaired, patients can typically return to full activity at 3 to 5 months if range of motion is full and pain free and optimal muscular strength and endurance are present.

If open repair of the rotator cuff is performed concurrent with an arthroscopic debridement, the surgical approach typically splits the deltoid along the lines of its fibers rather than detaching it from its origin. Consequently, there is more tissue disruption than with arthroscopy alone but less than in open procedures that take down the deltoid.

The rehabilitation time line is also determined by the viability and size of the tendon defect repaired. Older tendon tears do not present the surgeon with an optimal amount of tendon tissue to reattach to the humerus, and the size of the tendon tear is one of the determining factors of healing time. Consequently the tendon repair of a large defect is not as strong and cannot be stressed as early or as vigorously as a repair of a smaller, acute tear in a younger individual.

Immediately after surgery the patient uses a shoulder sling for the first few weeks to counter the gravitational stress of the humerus on the glenoid and to minimize motion. We typically begin mild isometric exercises and careful passive and active assistive range of motion exercises within a pain-free range during this healing period. Range-of-motion exercises remain the essential aspect of treatment during the first 2 to 3 months, and depending on the strength and size of the repair, strengthening exercises can be progressed using light resistance through controlled motions at the 3- to 4-month mark. Typically a more advanced exercise program for all of the shoulder muscle groups is not initiated until the fourth or fifth month, but during this time, the clinician is closely monitoring the gains in range of motion and working to ensure that a full range of pain-free motion is present before any aggressive strengthening regimen is initiated. Again, the size of the repair and viability of the tissue, coupled with the activity or sport the patient is returning to, determine the time frame at which he can return to activity. Patients with a smaller, acute repair may be able to return to activity following gain of full motion and neuromuscular performance in 5 to 6 months, whereas patients with repairs at the opposite end of the spectrum may not be able to return to activity for 9 to 12 months.

The *open repair* of the cuff tendon in which the deltoid is detached to present a larger subdeltoid field features the greatest tissue disruption discussed. As such, the shoulder joint must be protected to a greater extent early on, and stresses to the repaired tissues must be introduced in a very controlled manner.

The early aspects of rehabilitation primarily consist of passive and very guarded active assistive range of motion for the first 2 to 3 months, depending on the size of the repair. Depending on the degree of tissue disruption, we do not typically begin resistance exercises until the third or fourth month, again based on the surgeon's opinion of the strength of the repair. Return to activity often takes 1 year or more because of the length of time needed for optimal tissue fixation and the return of fully functional shoulder motion and neuromuscular control.

Nonsurgical Management for Shoulder Instability

Several factors determine the aggressiveness of treatment for individuals who have instability of the glenohumeral joint. Combinations of the factors noted below warrant caution in the early stages of management:

- Can the examiner detect excessive translation with passive translational stresses?
- Is the anterior glenoid rim palpably tender?
- Is there a suspicion of anterior rim of labrum involvement (palpable tenderness; clicks and pops anteriorly)?
- What has been the frequency of dislocations and resultant reductions, and how many have occurred?
- Does arm transiently "go dead," and is there sudden pain with subluxation?
- Is there an associated impingement phenomenon?

The body type and onset of instability also guide the clinician in selecting the most appropriate treatment regimen. Shoulder instability problems can be characterized as:

- Atraumatic: the patient with general hypermobility, lax connective tissue framework, often female, with generalized weakness and poor posture
- Microtraumatic: the 15- to 35-year-old athlete or worker whose activities require much overhead movement that results in gradual stretching of connective tissue restraints (usually this patient has associated pathology such as impingement or overuse syndromes)
- Traumatic: the patient with a single, identifiable, initial episode of dislocation of the glenohumeral joint that may now have resulted in recurrent episodes of dislocation

The use of a nonsurgical rehabilitation program for shoulder instability depends on such factors as the severity of the glenohumeral joint injury, the frequency of dislocations and subluxations, the age and activity level of the patient, and the status of the surrounding tissues, particularly the rotator cuff musculature. If connective tissue structures such as the glenohumeral joint capsule and the glenohumeral ligaments are excessively lax or the glenoid labrum is torn or partially avulsed from the glenoid, there is little chance that exercises can result in complete stability of the glenohumeral joint. Perhaps more than in any of the other shoulder syndromes, the patient must clearly understand the importance of his participation throughout the rehabilitation process and be willing to avoid or decrease those activities that render the shoulder vulnerable to subluxation or dislocation.

As with the impingement syndrome, it is useful to plan the interventions along the four objectives of treatment. If pain is a primary complaint, then the first objective is to address *modulation of pain*. Modalities to desensitize the region include ice or electrical stimulation and the use of NSAIDs. The concept of "active rest" also becomes important with instability problems. Motion within very controlled ranges while the pain settles is important in this pain modulation phase.

The clinician's application of *passive and active stresses to promote and encourage pain-free, active movements* by the patient must be applied in a very judicious manner. Aggressive stretching and joint mobilization have very few indications with an instability problem because this problem is primarily one of decreased stability between the humerus and the glenoid. If a forward head, rounded shoulder kyphotic posture is present, it may be necessary to inspect the length of anterior chest muscles but avoid specific stretches to the glenohumeral joint structures. Likewise, mobility exercises and stretches for the lower cervical and thoracic spine, especially thoracic extension, may be necessary because limitations of motion in the spine increase the motion requirements for the glenohumeral joint during overhead activities.

Following an acute injury of the glenohumeral joint that has resulted in instability, it is important to initiate isometric exercises to the rotator cuff and extrinsic muscles of the shoulder early in the rehabilitation process. Isometric exercises should not exacerbate the pain and are well tolerated by the patient. Instruct the patient to perform them in ranges of motion that do not compromise the weakened connective tissues. The purpose of such isometric exercises is to prevent atrophy of the cuff muscles and to place very controlled forces through the joint capsule through the actions of the rotator cuff.

Enhancing neuromuscular performance is one of the more important objectives in management of the patient with shoulder instability. The primary focus of treatment with instability disorders of the glenohumeral joint is enhancing the strength, power, and endurance of the intrinsic and extrinsic musculature of the shoulder girdle complex. In addition to the important rotator cuff muscles, exercises for the powerful extrinsic muscles of the shoulder, such as the latissimus dorsi, deltoid, pectoralis major, coracobrachialis, and biceps brachii, and for the muscles of the scapulothoracic articulation, such as the trapezius, levator scapula, rhomboids, and the serratus anterior, must be included (see Chapter 3 and previously in this chapter).

As noted in Chapter 3, it is also essential for the clinician to incorporate exercises that increase strength of the trunk and lower extremities because of the linkages between the muscles and through the key fascial systems. Although many different exercises have been suggested for strengthening the shoulder girdle, we prefer to use diagonal patterns against resistance through the invulnerable ranges of motion because these exercises incorporate trunk muscle activation (abdominal mechanism and spinal extensors), scapula muscles, extrinsic shoulder muscles, and the rotator cuff. While there has been a tendency in the past to focus on the anterior shoulder muscles with the more common anterior subluxations and dislocations, strengthening of the external rotators, particularly the infraspinatus and teres minor complex, is the more logical focus for managing anterior instability (see Chapter 3). Ultimately, a global approach incorporating total shoulder girdle and trunk strengthening is the most comprehensive treatment strategy.

The use of rhythmic stabilization exercises in varying ranges of motion is very effective in the nonsurgical management of instability.[1] In the later stages of rehabilitation, exercises against resistance and co-contraction exercises can be performed from the apprehension position with the intent being to develop kinesthetic and proprioceptive awareness of vulnerable shoulder positions and the appropriate neuromotor responses to such positions. Plyometric exercises using varying sizes and weights of medicine balls are also effective ways to train the neuromuscular complex about the shoulder and are especially effective in dealing with athletes.[27]

During the physical examination (see Chapter 5) the clinician gains information regarding the vulnerable and invulnerable positions of the shoulder and the ease with which the humerus translates over the glenoid. This allows for the careful planning of the motions and positions relative to the glenohumeral joint for safe and effective strengthening programs. This is the essential aspect of enhancing neuromuscular performance with shoulder instability: overloading and challenging the neuromuscular system but not overwhelming the already compromised specialized connective tissues. We recommend beginning the development of the exercise prescription using the invulnerable ranges of motion and carefully progressing to more functional ranges during the course of rehabilitation. The patient must understand that no matter how strong or how hypertrophied the musculature becomes, most likely there will be portions of the range that have the potential for subluxation or dislocation.

Biomechanical counseling in the nonsurgical management of instability disorders requires that clinician and patient carefully assess activities of daily living, work postures and requirements, and sport activities in order to determine the limits of motion and loading patterns to the shoulder. The patient also is counseled to avoid the slumping postures and the glenohumeral apprehension position (abduction and external rotation) with sleeping.

Part of the educational process for a patient with instability is that he realize the strengthening program for his shoulder is not just a temporary phenomenon. Because of the high incidence of rotator cuff tendonitis and impingement related disorders associated with glenohumeral joint instability, an exercise program must be maintained even after pain has subsided.[9,12] Shoulder and trunk exercises need to be continued on a regular and habitual basis.

Surgical Management for Shoulder Instability and Postsurgical Considerations

Numerous procedures have been described to surgically stabilize the glenohumeral joint. The clinician needs to understand the extent and type of surgical procedure performed, because each has its own set of unique precautions and protocols that influence the rehabilitation process.

The general principle behind surgical procedures designed to enhance the stability of the glenohumeral joint is to directly restore the anatomy, particularly the glenohumeral joint capsule, glenohumeral ligaments, and glenoid labrum, to as normal an anatomical relationship as possible or to use the surrounding tissues to support the glenohumeral joint and minimize aberrational movement between the humerus and the glenoid fossa. The challenge is to bolster the stability of the joint but still maintain functional range of motion and strength throughout the range of motion.

Anatomical reconstruction of the compromised tissues, specifically the glenohumeral ligament complex and glenoid labral tears, can be accomplished using open or arthroscopic procedures. The size and extent of these lesions have become better recognized with the increasing use of diagnostic arthroscopy. The greater the extent of repair needed to the glenohumeral ligament and labral complex, however, the smaller the potential to effectively reach all of the necessary tissue via the arthroscope, increasing the necessity for an open repair. In addition to labral reattachment, capsular shift procedures are designed to tighten the joint capsule, thereby removing the slack and redundancy from the capsule-ligament complex.

The rehabilitation process uses each of the four objectives of treatment, and the timing of the introduction of each objective depends on many factors such as the presurgical status of the tissue, viability of tissues involved with the surgical procedure, and the time frames associated with surgical healing. Pain and swelling are controlled immediately after surgery through the use of a sling and scaption support, which places the glenohumeral joint at approximately 30 degrees of scaption plane motion and 30 degrees of external rotation. This helps protect the surgically repaired capsulolabral complex.

During the first 2 months of rehabilitation the primary focus is on passive and active assistive range of motion (application of controlled stresses). The clinician must have a keen tactile sense of end feel during any passive motions and be able to clearly discern muscle guarding from connective tissue tension. The connective tissues are gently "coaxed" out toward full motion. While all patients present as unique cases, we typically strive to have full range of motion reached by 2 to 3 months.

Strengthening (enhancing neuromuscular performance) is begun with light isometric exercises at approximately the second or third week. As the patient makes gains in the range of motion, we encourage isometric muscle strengthening in these newly gained ranges. Usually by the end of the first month the patient can also perform light resistance exercises through varying arcs of acquired motion. The clinician must monitor

the patient to avoid placing excessive stress on the anterior capsule, so we typically do not position the patient in any way that might result in the arm being pulled into uncontrolled external rotation by any free weight, pulley, or medicine ball. It is important at this time also to monitor the contribution of the scapulothoracic and trunk muscles to the motion carefully because these are integral components of the strengthening program.

Finally, patient education (biomechanical counseling) is important. The patient must understand the importance of a long-term commitment to his exercise program. He must also understand the activities and positions that can compromise the repair. Throwing especially increases loading to the repaired tissues, and while gentle lob throws can be started at approximately the eighth or ninth month, full speed throwing must often be delayed for about a year after surgery.

Another surgical approach that attempts to deal directly with the lax capsular tissue is thermal capsular shrinkage. The postsurgery rehabilitation plan for this procedure includes passive range of motion of glenohumeral joint to tolerance, including external rotation with the glenohumeral joint placed at 45 degrees abduction during the first month. Passive techniques are followed by the initiation of antigravity motion as tolerated. Posterior-to-anterior accessory joint mobilization techniques are carefully avoided in order to minimize any forces against the anterior wall of the joint capsule. Submaximal resistance exercises are used with a particular emphasis on rhythmic stabilization.

After the first month we include active and passive range-of-motion exercises to tolerance, including accessory mobilizations. Posterior capsule stretches are incorporated using across-the-body horizontal adduction, but care must be taken to stabilize the scapula in order to properly and completely apply such a stretch. Resistance exercises using light weights and pulleys are initiated with scaption plane elevations and external rotation in varying positions of glenohumeral abduction and flexion. Along with the strengthening programs noted, exercises that ultimately incorporate the combined actions of the trunk, scapulothoracic articulation, and glenohumeral joint are the eventual goal. The key is to monitor symptoms and recognize the healing constraints of the surgically managed tissues.

Several other surgical procedures do not deal with the involved connective tissues directly but instead seek to offer increased joint stability by using surrounding bone or muscle tissue to provide a physical restraint to excessive glenohumeral translation. These techniques are used less often today because of recent advances in arthroscopic and open techniques to the capsule and labrum but are presented here for the sake of completeness.

The Bristow procedure, in which the tip of the coracoid process, with the attached short head of the biceps brachii and coracobrachialis, is removed and then reattached to the anterior aspect of the glenoid, is one such surgical approach.[24] The bone (coracoid) and muscular sling (biceps and coracobrachialis) create a barrier to anterior subluxation of the humerus. Limitations in external rotation typically occur with this surgery, and the clinician must be cognizant of exercises, especially resistance exercises, that may place increased loads through the biceps or coracobrachialis muscles.

The Putti-Platt procedure uses the subscapularis muscle to reinforce the anterior aspect of the glenohumeral joint. The subscapularis tendon is divided medial to its insertion, allowing a medial and lateral flap of subscapularis muscle to then be overlapped and attached to the anterior aspect of the joint to provide an additional restraint to anterior subluxation. Like the Bristow, the Putti-Platt often results in limited range of motion, especially external shoulder rotation, and a loss of strength.[21] In addition, excessive tightening of the subscapularis has been attributed to promoting early degenerative joint changes in the glenohumeral joint.[11]

SUMMARY

We have provided treatment techniques, as well as a thought process to organize a treatment approach along the four objectives. Although there are many different treatment techniques, the similarity in techniques lies in their purported effects. Thus, as reviewed early in this chapter, it is the intended effect or *intent of treatment* that is most important in the development of a treatment program. When treating a patient with shoulder problems, it is important to recognize the following as essential aspects: range of motion of the glenohumeral joint, strengthening of the rotator cuff musculature, strengthening of the extrinsic musculature of the shoulder, strengthening of the scapulothoracic muscles, and strengthening of the trunk musculature. Regardless of the clinical problem

that is seen, these five aspects remain the mainstays of successful shoulder rehabilitation.

REFERENCES

1. Adler SS, Bekers D, Buck M: *PNF in practice*, London, 2000, Springer Verlag.
2. Bigliani LU, Pollock RG, Soslowsky LJ, et al: Tensile properties of the inferior glenohumeral ligament, *J Orthop Res* 10:187, 1992.
3. Biundo J, Mipro BC, Djuric V: Peripheral nerve entrapment, occupation related syndromes, sports injuries, bursitis and soft tissue problems of the shoulder, *Curr Opin Rheumatol* 7:151, 1995.
4. Blenman PR, Carter DR, Bequpre GS: Role of mechanical loading in the progressive ossification of a fracture callus, *J Orthop Res* 7:398, 1989.
5. Buckwalter JA: Musculoskeletal tissues and the musculoskeletal system. In Weinstein SL, Buckwalter JA, editors: *Turek's orthopaedics: principles and their application*, Philadelphia, 1991, Lippincott.
6. Buckwalter JA, Mow VC, Ratcliffe A: Restoration of injured or degenerated articular cartilage, *J Am Acad Orthop Surg* 2:192, 1994.
7. Flowers KR, LaStayo PC: Effect of total end range time on improving passive range of motion, *J Hand Ther* 7(3):150, 1994.
8. Frank C, Amiel D, Woo SL, et al: Normal ligament properties and ligament healing, *Clin Orthop* 196:15, 1985.
9. Fu FH, Harner CD, Klein AH: Shoulder impingement syndrome: a critical review, *Clin Orthop* 269:162, 1991.
10. Hardy MA: The biology of scar formation, *Phys Ther* 69(12):1014, 1989.
11. Hawkins RJ, Angelo RL: Glenohumeral osteoarthritis: a late complication of the Putti-Platt repair, *J Bone Joint Surg Am* 72(8):193, 1990.
12. Hawkins RJ, Kennedy JC: Impingement syndrome in athletes, *Am J Sports Med* 8:151, 1980.
13. Komi PV: Training of muscle strength and power: interaction of neuromotoric, hypertrophic, and mechanical factors, *Int J Sports Med* 7(Suppl):10, 1986.
14. Larsson SE, Bengston A, Bodegard L, et al: Muscle changes in work related chronic myalgia, *Acta Orthop Scand* 59:552, 1988.
15. LaStayo PC, Jaffe R: Assessment and management of shoulder stiffness: a biomechanical approach, *J Hand Ther* 7(2):122, 1994.
16. MacKinnon SE, Novak CB: Clinical commentary: pathogenesis of cumulative trauma disorder, *J Hand Surg* 19(5):873, 1994.
17. Mankin HJ: The response of articular cartilage to mechanical injury, *J Bone Joint Surg Am* 64(3):460, 1982.
18. Misamore GW, Ziegler DW, Rushton JC: Repair of the rotator cuff: a comparison of results of two populations of patients, *J Bone Joint Surg* 77(9):1335, 1995.
19. Modl JM, Sether LA, Haughton VM, et al: Articular cartilage: correlation of histological zones with signal intensity at MR imaging, *Radiology* 181(3):853, 1991.
20. Pelmear PL, Taylor W: Hand-arm vibration syndrome: clinical evaluation and prevention, *J Occup Environ Med* 33:1144, 1991.

21. Regan WD Jr, Webster-Bogaert S, Hawkins RJ, et al: Comparative functional analysis of the Bristow, Magnusson-Stack, and Putti-Platt procedures for recurrent dislocation of the shoulder, *Am J Sports Med* 17(1):42, 1989.

22. Sapaega AA, Quedenfeld TC, Moyer RA, et al: Biophysical factors in range of motion exercise, *Physician Sports Med* 9:12, 1981.

23. Stone MH: Implications for connective tissue and bone alterations resulting from resistance exercise training, *Med Sci Sports Exerc* 20(Suppl):S162, 1988.

24. Torg JS, Balduini FC, Bonci C, et al: A modified Bristow-Helfet-May procedure for recurrent dislocations and subluxations of the shoulder: a report of 212 cases, *J Bone Joint Surg Am* 69(6):904, 1987.

25. Tyson LL, Crues J: Pathogenesis of rotator cuff disorders: magnetic resonance imaging characteristics, *Magn Reson Imaging Clin N Am* 1(1):37, 1993.

26. van der Muelen JCH: Present state of knowledge on processes of healing in collagen structures, *Int J Sports Med* 3:4, 1982.

27. Wilk KE, Arrigo CA: Current concepts in the rehabilitation of the athletic shoulder, *J Orthop Sports Phys Ther* 18:365, 1993.

28. Wolffe CJ: Generation of acute pain: central mechanisms, *British Med Bulletin* 47:523, 1991.

29. Zarin B: Soft tissue injury and repair: biomechanical aspects, *Int J Sports Med.* 3:9, 1982.

INDEX

Page numbers followed by f indicate figures;
t, tables.